Qualitative Research Methodologies for Occupational Science and Occupational Therapy

This comprehensive text provides a practical introduction to the range of qualitative methodologies and methods being used by occupational science and occupational therapy researchers today, enabling readers to produce and critique high-quality qualitative research themselves.

Showcasing a diverse range of qualitative research from both academic scholarship and the wider community of health professionals, each chapter combines both foundational knowledge and therapeutic applications. Importantly, the book lucidly explains the synergy between research problem, choice of methodology, and methods. It also fosters a best-practice approach, ensuring that qualitative research is epistemologically sound while reflecting the values and beliefs of the diverse communities within which research is conducted.

This new edition, featuring an international range of authors, also addresses new and cutting-edge research methodologies, including Indigenous methodologies, netnography, the visual arts, and Big data. It is the ideal textbook for any student, practitioner, or researcher of occupational science and occupational therapy.

Shoba Nayar is a New Zealand trained and registered occupational therapist. Since completing her PhD in occupational science, she has held various roles in academic institutions in New Zealand, the United Kingdom, and India. Shoba currently works as an independent academic, offering consultation services to academic institutions and postgraduate students in the area of qualitative research.

Mandy Stanley is a Professor in the School of Medical and Health Sciences at Edith Cowan University, Perth, Australia. Mandy is a senior academic with an established program of funded research who has taught qualitative research to both undergraduate and postgraduate students, and successfully supervised higher degree students writing qualitative theses and more than 30 Honors students.

Qualitative Research Methodologies for Occupational Science and Occupational Therapy

Second Edition

Edited by Shoba Nayar and Mandy Stanley

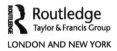
Routledge
Taylor & Francis Group

LONDON AND NEW YORK

Designed cover image: © Getty Images

Second edition published 2024
by Routledge
4 Park Square, Milton Park, Abingdon, Oxon, OX14 4RN

and by Routledge
605 Third Avenue, New York, NY 10158

Routledge is an imprint of the Taylor & Francis Group, an informa business

First edition published by Routledge 2015

British Library Cataloguing-in-Publication Data
A catalogue record for this book is available from the British Library

Library of Congress Cataloging-in-Publication Data
Names: Nayar, Shoba, editor. | Stanley, Mandy, editor.
Title: Qualitative research methodologies for occupational science and occupational therapy / edited by Shoba Nayar and Mandy Stanley.
Description: Second edition. | Milton Park, Abingdon, Oxon ; New York, NY : Routledge, 2024. | Includes bibliographical references and index.
Identifiers: LCCN 2023025263 | ISBN 9781032597799 (hardback) | ISBN 9781032312637 (paperback) | ISBN 9781003456216 (ebook)
Subjects: LCSH: Medicine, Industrial. | Occupational therapy. | Qualitative research--Methodology.
Classification: LCC RC963 .Q38 2024 | DDC 615.8/515--dc23/eng/20230817
LC record available at https://lccn.loc.gov/2023025263

ISBN: 978-1-032-59779-9 (hbk)
ISBN: 978-1-032-31263-7 (pbk)
ISBN: 978-1-003-45621-6 (ebk)

DOI: 10.4324/9781003456216

Typeset in Galliard
by SPi Technologies India Pvt Ltd (Straive)

With love and thanks to
Krish and Val Nayar
Jeremy, Erin, Wit, Annette, Gilmour and Suea Noi

Contents

List of Figures   ix
List of Tables   x
Acknowledgments   xi
Foreword   xii
Editors   xiv
List of Contributors   xv

1 Introduction to the Second Edition   1
   SHOBA NAYAR AND MANDY STANLEY

2 Tenets of Qualitative Research: Deepening Understandings   12
   MANDY STANLEY AND SHOBA NAYAR

3 Connections, Disruptions, and Transformations: Decolonizing
   Qualitative Research   30
   ISLA EMERY-WHITTINGTON, LANA DRAPER AND CHONTEL GIBSON

4 Qualitative Descriptive: A Very Good Place to Start   52
   MANDY STANLEY

5 Grounded Theory   68
   KATE D'CRUZ AND SHOBA NAYAR

6 Phenomenology   88
   KIRK REED

7 Case Study Methodology   105
   SIMON LEADLEY, MARGARET JONES AND CLARE HOCKING

8 Narrative Inquiry   127
   JENS SCHNEIDER, LAETITIA ZEEMAN, NATALIE EDELMAN AND LEE PRICE

9 Ethnography   149
   SUZANNE HUOT AND ANNE-CÉCILE DELAISSE

10 Critical Discourse Analysis   169
   DEBBIE LALIBERTE RUDMAN AND SILKE DENNHARDT

11 Participatory Action Research   187
   TANYA ELIZABETH BENJAMIN-THOMAS AND DEBBIE LALIBERTE RUDMAN

12 Visual Arts-Based Methodologies   208
   LAURA R. BOWMAN AND KATIE MAH

13 Visual Methodologies: Photovoice in Focus   230
   ERIC ASABA, MELISSA PARK, MARGARITA MONDACA AND DEBBIE LALIBERTE RUDMAN

14 Community-Based Research   252
   ROSHAN GALVAAN AND PAM GRETSCHEL

15 Qualitative Evidence Synthesis   272
   CAROLYN MURRAY, KATIE ROBINSON AND MANDY STANLEY

16 Netnography   289
   AMY WALLIS

17 Big Qualitative Data   304
   MANDY STANLEY

18 Best (or Better?) Practices   318
   SHOBA NAYAR

   Index   *332*

Figures

3.1   A continuum of Indigenous control in occupational science and occupational
      therapy research   42
7.1   Case study methodology   106
7.2   Continuum of case study designs   109
7.3   Analysis of Coco's occupations: active and passive   117
12.1 (a and b) Sample of visual data generated by Katie's participants 219
12.2 (a and b) Body map storytelling data generation process from Laura's study 220
12.3 Researcher analyses individual body maps as products in Laura's study 222
13.1 Overview of the photovoice process   237
16.1 Visual presentation of themes and sub-themes   295

Tables

3.1	Questions from the CREATE tool	45
3.2	Roles and responsibilities of researchers in Indigenous research	47
4.1	Examples of research questions studied with a qualitative descriptive methodology	54
4.2	Sampling frame for 'Driverless car' study	55
4.3	Example of open coding of the transcript	60
4.4	Contrasting descriptive themes from early analysis with conceptual dimensions	62
6.1	Key phenomenologists over time	89
7.1	Data table relating to key assumption/issue statement #4	115
7.2	Example of data analysis table showing data, source, and emerging themes	116
8.1	Assigning elements of a Deweyan inquiry to parts of narratives	135
9.1	Data collection methods across the two critical ethnographies	155
9.2	Observation table	159
11.1	Research purposes identified within exemplar occupation-based participatory action research projects	191
11.2	Guiding questions to guide critical analysis of participatory action research and best practice recommendations	198
12.1	Common reasons for considering a visual arts-based methodology	210
12.2	Considerations when undertaking visual arts-based methodological inquiry	212
12.3	Examples of process and product data	217
13.1	Authors' photovoice projects drawn upon for this chapter	233
13.2	Potential risks and strategies for working with risks	243
14.1	Characteristics of community-based research	253
14.2	Example of grouping codes into themes	262
14.3	Questions for critiquing literature	268
15.1	Examples of qualitative evidence synthesis questions framed using the SPIDER, SPICE, and PerSPecTiF frameworks	275

Acknowledgments

We would like to thank the community of occupational science academics and occupational therapy practitioners who have offered their support for a second edition of this book. We are always humbled to hear how well used and received the first edition has been for many of our colleagues and students.

With regards to this, the second edition, we thank Professor Davina Porock, School of Nursing and Midwifery, Edith Cowan University, Australia, for her critical read and feedback of Chapter 2.

Priya Nayar and Samantha Jorgensen—we are so appreciative of your willingness to host our writing retreat, which enabled us to meet face to face for the first time in three and a half years, and provided a space to write, talk, and laugh. And a special thanks Priya for the amazing catering!

Foreword

My late friend Gary Kielhofner was fond of noting that the idea of occupation as a therapeutic medium is so powerful that if occupational therapy failed to realize its potential by fully embracing it (as it almost did); it would surely be taken up by another profession with the wisdom and resolve to nurture it to greatness. That nurturing would necessarily require theory and research.

Dr. Kielhofner was among the earliest occupational therapy scholars to employ qualitative research (Kielhofner & Miyake, 1981). He recognized that fully comprehending the meaning and significance of agency in the lives of individuals required a deeper understanding of the lived experiences of people—particularly those whose situations might interfere with their opportunities to live optimally fulfilling lives.

It is notable that Kielhofner gained recognition in the 1980s, arguably the most transformative decade for research in occupational therapy. The importance of theory-based practice and the need for a deeper understanding of the 'occupational being' were emphasized. Five new occupational therapy scholarly journals were launched (Reed, 1988); and the discipline of occupational science was established (Yerxa et al., 1989). Perhaps serendipitously, it was also the decade in which qualitative research began, described then as an emerging paradigm for naturalistic inquiry in the social sciences (Lincoln & Guba, 1985).

Possibly no occupational therapy scholar at that time was more convinced of the value of qualitative methods than Elizabeth Yerxa. In 1991, she organized the first special issue of the *American Journal of Occupational Therapy* devoted exclusively to qualitative inquiry. In that issue, she suggested that research on occupation should rely exclusively on qualitative methodologies (Yerxa, 1991), largely arguing that understanding the subjective experiences of doing was far more important than knowing objective facts about occupational pursuits. Yerxa later moderated her views, advocating for an integrative approach to research that includes qualitative and other methodologies (Yerxa, 2009).

Although my early research training was based on quantitative methods, my feet are now planted firmly in both qualitative and other approaches. I'm certain my development as an investigator would have advanced more quickly if a complete and accessible book like this one had been available two or three decades ago. Nayar and Stanley therefore deserve our gratitude for their enduring commitment to advancing qualitative inquiry in the occupational sciences.

Charles Christiansen
Professor Emeritus, The University of Texas Medical Branch at Galveston
Rochester, Minnesota, USA

References

Kielhofner, G., & Miyake, S. (1981). The therapeutic use of games with mentally retarded adults. *American Journal of Occupational Therapy*, *35*(6), 375–382. https://doi.org/10.5014/ajot.35.6.375

Lincoln, Y. S., & Guba, E. G. (1985). *Naturalistic inquiry*. SAGE.

Reed, K. L. (1988). Occupational therapy articles in serial publications: An analysis of sources. *Bulletin of the Medical Library Association*, *76*(2), 125.

Yerxa, E. J. (1991). Seeking a relevant, ethical, and realistic way of knowing for occupational therapy. *American Journal of Occupational Therapy*, *45*(3), 199–204. https://doi.org/10.5014/ajot.45.3.199

Yerxa, E. J. (2009). Infinite distance between the I and the it. *American Journal of Occupational Therapy*, *63*(4), 490–497. https://doi.org/10.5014/ajot.63.4.490

Yerxa, E. J., Clark, F., Jackson, J., Parham, D., Stein, C., & Zemke, R. (1989). An introduction to occupational science: A foundation for occupational therapy in the 21st century. *Occupational Therapy in Health Care*, 6(4), 1–17. https://doi.org/10.1080/J003v06n04_04

Editors

Shoba Nayar is a New Zealand trained and registered occupational therapist. Since completing her PhD in occupational science, she has held various roles in academic institutions in New Zealand, the United Kingdom, and India. Shoba currently works as an independent academic, offering consultation services to academic institutions and postgraduate students in the area of qualitative research. Shoba has authored numerous scholarly journal articles, reports, and book chapters; as well as being an active reviewer of qualitative manuscripts for international journals including *Journal of International Migration and Integration, Journal of Advanced Nursing, International Journal of Therapy and Rehabilitation*, and the *Canadian Journal of Occupational Therapy*. She has served on the Editorial board and Executive of the *Journal of Occupational Science*.

Mandy Stanley is Professor in the School of Medical and Health Sciences at Edith Cowan University, Perth, Australia. She lives and works on Whadjuk Noongar country. Mandy is a highly experienced academic who has taught qualitative research to both undergraduate and postgraduate students over her long academic career, and successfully supervised higher degree students writing qualitative theses and more than 30 Honors students. Mandy is recognized internationally for her expertise in qualitative methodologies and received the award of Fellow of OTAustralia Research Academy in 2021 for her contributions to occupational science and occupational therapy research. Mandy is immediate Past President of the Australasian Society of Occupational Scientists, and has served on the Editorial board and Executive of the *Journal of Occupational Science*.

Contributors

Eric Asaba is an Associate Professor with joint appointment at the Division of Occupational Therapy, Department of Neurobiology, Care Sciences and Society, Karolinska Institutet, Huddinge, Sweden and Unit for Research, Education, Development, and Innovation, Stockholms Sjukhem, Stockholm, Sweden. His special research interests include occupation intersected with illness prevention/health promotion, working life, disability, migration, and identity; participatory and collaborative research, narrative and visual methods.

Tanya Elizabeth Benjamin-Thomas is an Assistant Professor in the School of Occupational Therapy at Texas Woman's University. Tanya's teaching areas include evidence-based practice, qualitative research methods and methodologies, and innovations in occupational therapy practice. Her research interests include working alongside children experiencing marginalization within local to global contexts through participatory action research and creative methodologies.

Laura R. Bowman is a Project Manager of Research and Evaluation for the Employment Pathways team at Holland Bloorview Kids Rehabilitation Hospital, Ontario, Canada. Her research interests include transitions through the pediatric system and into adult life for children living with disabilities and their families.

Kate D'Cruz is a Senior Research Fellow at the Summer Foundation and Adjunct at La Trobe University, Melbourne. With a background in occupational therapy, Kate is a qualitative researcher with a particular interest in partnering with people with disability in co-designing research that is relevant to the lives of people living with disability.

Anne-Cécile Delaisse is a PhD candidate at the University of British Columbia. Her research examines occupations in the context of immigration, using qualitative methods and a critical approach. Her dissertation is a critical ethnography about recent Vietnamese migrants transnational occupations and belongings in Vancouver, Canada, and Paris, France.

Silke Dennhardt is a Professor in the interdisciplinary Physiotherapy/Occupational Therapy Program at the Alice Salomon Hochschule, University of Applied Sciences, in Berlin and chair of the German occupational science association (dOS). Her research interests lie in qualitative methodologies, the mental health care field and the social construction of occupation and its consequences, especially for people in so-called vulnerable circumstances.

Lana Draper is a Ngiyampaa woman and works as an occupational therapist in the LINKS Trauma Healing Service (DCJ) which delivers trauma focused, evidence-based support to children in out-of-home-care. Her research focuses on generating knowledge about the ways that culture can be integrated into the child protection system for better outcomes for Aboriginal and Torres Strait Islander children, young people, and families.

Natalie Edelman is a Principal Research Fellow at the School of Sport and Health Sciences, University of Brighton in the United Kingdom, and a member of the British Association of Sexual Health and HIV. Her research interests include psychosocial and sexual health, reproductive health, public health, and research ethics.

Isla Emery-Whittington has affiliations to Rereahu, Ngāti Kauwhata, and Ngāti Kahungunu ki Wairarapa. She works at SHORE Whariki Research Institution, Massey University, Aotearoa New Zealand. Her research interests lie in the area of decolonizing occupation praxis.

Roshan Galvaan is a Professor of Occupational Therapy and the Head of the Department of Health and Rehabilitation Sciences, Faculty of Health Sciences, University of Cape Town. She is also an adjunct professor at Dalhousie University. Her research interests include critical occupational science and occupational therapy, community development practice, decoloniality, and social transformation. She focuses on experiences and situations of marginality, exploring individual and collective possibilities for transformation in everyday life.

Chontel Gibson is a Kamilaroi woman, who trained as an occupational therapist, holds a Master's in Public Health, and completed a PhD in relation to Aboriginal health and well-being. She is a Research Fellow in the School of Indigenous Studies, Poche Centre for Indigenous Health, University of Western Australia.

Pam Gretschel is a Senior Lecturer in the Occupational Therapy Division, Department of Health and Rehabilitation Sciences in the Faculty of Health Sciences at the University of Cape Town. Her teaching and research interests are focused on collaborative practice with parents and caregivers, and participatory research methods.

Clare Hocking is a registered kaiwhakaora ngangahau/occupational therapist in Aotearoa New Zealand. She is a Professor of Occupational Science and Therapy at the Auckland University of Technology and Executive Editor of the *Journal of Occupational Science*. Clare's scholarship centers on occupational justice and health equity.

Suzanne Huot is an Assistant Professor in the Department of Occupational Science and Occupational Therapy at the University of British Columbia. Her research program centers on the axes of occupation, immigration, and Francophone minority communities. Her studies primarily address the occupational implications of international migration to Canada through focused, critical examination of governmental legislation, policies, and discourses; of service providers and their roles; and of the experiences of individual immigrants, refugees, and asylum seekers.

Margaret Jones is a registered kaiwhakaora ngangahau/occupational therapist in Aotearoa New Zealand. She is a Senior Lecturer at the Department of Occupational Therapy at the Auckland University of Technology. Margaret's research activities focus on children's participation in occupations within their communities, and the ways that their participation promotes health and development. Her expertise is in qualitative research methods, particularly in the use of case study research as a means of exploring people's participation experiences.

Debbie Laliberte Rudman is a Distinguished University Professor in the School of Occupational Therapy at the University of Western Ontario, as well as field leader of the Occupational Science field in the Health and Rehabilitation Sciences program at the same Canadian university. Within her research, she employs diverse critical qualitative methodologies to deepen understanding of the socio-political production of occupational inequities and collaborate with marginalized collectives and community organizations to address occupational inequities.

Simon Leadley (he/him) is a kaiwhakaora ngangahau/occupational therapist, currently working as a Senior Lecturer at the School of Occupational therapy/Te Ohu Ora, Otago Polytechnic/Te Kura Matatini ki Otago, Te Pukenga. He is completing a PhD exploring the influences of poverty on tamariki/children's patterns of and participation in occupation, development, health and well-being. He has a broad interest in primary and public health, and health equity.

Katie Mah is a postdoctoral associate at Western University. She is a critical qualitative health researcher who focuses her research on challenging the pervasive covert and overt societal ways of considering and engaging young people in clinical and research practices that primarily concern them.

Margarita Mondaca is an Assistant Professor in the Division of Occupational Therapy, Department of Neurobiology, Care Sciences and Society, Karolinska Institutet, Huddinge, Sweden. Margarita's special research interests include everyday life among groups in situations of vulnerability, migration, aging, health inequalities and advances in use of collaborative research.

Carolyn Murray is a Senior Lecturer in Occupational Therapy at the University of South Australia. Carolyn has extensive experience in working with qualitative data with research focusing on living with brain injury (including stroke), spinal cord injury ageing, dementia, and processes of workforce development. Carolyn supervises higher degree by research students and teaches occupational therapy students at both graduate entry masters and undergraduate levels.

Shoba Nayar is a New Zealand trained and registered occupational therapist. Since completing her PhD in occupational science, she has held various roles in academic institutions in New Zealand, the United Kingdom, and India. Shoba currently works as an independent academic, offering consultation services to academic institutions and postgraduate students in the area of qualitative research.

Melissa Park is an Associate Professor in the School of Physical & Occupational Therapy, Faculty of Medicine and Health Sciences, McGill University; Professional Affiliations: Lady Davis Institute, Jewish General Hospital; Centre for Interdisciplinary Research in Rehabilitation; and the Culture & Mental Health Research Unit, Division of Social and Transcultural Psychiatry, McGill University. Her special research interests include aesthetics, transformative processes; narrative and critical phenomenology; participatory; community-engagement.

Lee Price is a retired occupational therapist and principal lecturer in occupational therapy from the United Kingdom. His research interests include the lived experiences of LGBTQ+ people: issues of human occupation, inclusion, exclusion, isolation, and health and social care.

Kirk Reed is an experienced occupational therapy academic having worked in both Aotearoa New Zealand and Australia. He is currently Associate Professor, Occupational Therapy at Deakin University. Predominantly a qualitative researcher with expertise in phenomenology, Kirk's research focus is related to the lived experience of mental health issues and occupational therapy practice in mental health.

Katie Robinson is a Senior Lecturer in Occupational Therapy at the University of Limerick, Ireland. Katie's research focuses on ageing and rehabilitation and she has published several syntheses of qualitative research in these thematic areas.

Jens Schneider is a Professor for Applied Therapeutic Sciences with a focus on Occupational Therapy at the Trier University of Applied Sciences in Germany. His research interests include LGBTQIA+ people especially transgender and gender diverse people, gender and sexuality, theories and concepts of occupation, pragmatism according to John Dewey, and transactional perspectives.

Mandy Stanley is a Professor in the School of Medical and Health Sciences at Edith Cowan University, Perth, Australia. Mandy is an established academic who has taught qualitative research to both undergraduate and postgraduate students for more than ten years, and successfully supervised higher degree students writing qualitative theses and more than 30 Honors students.

Amy Wallis is an occupational therapist with over 20 years of experience as a clinician in the corporate and private health sectors and academia, where she currently teaches at Edith Cowan University in the areas of physical rehabilitation, physiology of health conditions, and self-management of chronic conditions. Amy is particularly interested in qualitative research in the areas of cancer supportive care, cancer survivorship, and palliative care.

Laetitia Zeeman works at the Centre for Transforming Sexuality and Gender, University of Brighton (UK) and specializes in the field of gender, sexualities, and health.

1 Introduction to the Second Edition

Shoba Nayar and Mandy Stanley

In 1991, Hasselkus wrote:

> At this time in the history of research in occupational therapy, a rather amazing shift in the balance of paradigms is occurring. Qualitative research is in. Or, at the very least, it is standing in the doorway rather than down the hall and around the corner.
>
> (p. 3)

Over three decades later, we argue that qualitative research has now left the doorway, crossed the threshold, and made itself at home in the lives (or at least the offices) of many occupational science and occupational therapy researchers. Yet, if that is indeed the case, why do we need another textbook on qualitative research; and that too, one that is targeted at a specific audience—researchers situated within occupational science and occupational therapy? We suggest that it is because human engagement in occupation is a complex, multifaceted experience that cannot be understood from one perspective. Why is it complex? Well, simply because people are complex; and without people, there would be no research. People are needed to design, conduct, participate in, and write—without which research would not happen. Without the research, there would be a lack of much needed knowledge to drive forward change at individual, community, societal, and global levels—change that truly makes a difference for all our lives and well-being.

Historically, quantitative research has been given priority for research funding and being able to generate data that bring about change. More recently, researchers are acknowledging that mixed methods research—the combination of qualitative and quantitative approaches—has increasing benefits for society. While we agree that mixed methods research is useful for answering an array of questions and expanding our understandings of the world, we argue that the diversity of qualitative methodologies now available for use may not be well understood. Further, without a solid understanding of qualitative methodologies, there is first, the risk that they are poorly implemented in the conduct of mixed methods studies; and second, that any outcomes from such studies will not translate to practice.

At this point, it is important to acknowledge that while the focus of this text is very clearly on qualitative research it is not to say that we do not value quantitative research. In our view, approaches to research form a continuum with quantitative and qualitative at opposite ends and mixed methodology claiming middle ground. We certainly do not want to perpetuate any debates of quantitative versus qualitative work as each has its own value and purpose. For us it is about choosing the right approach for the research question. Currently the questions in occupational science and occupational therapy that energize us and call to be answered are, by and large, best served by a qualitative methodology.

DOI: 10.4324/9781003456216-1

In the occupational therapy practice arena there is a strong push from funders and clients to have practice that is evidence based. Evidence-based practice, developed out of evidence based medicine, is defined as practice that is informed by a combination of client preference, practitioner expertise and the research evidence (Sackett et al., 2000). In our experience that definition, which emphasizes the combination of the three areas, is played out with the research evidence trumping practitioner experience and expertise. Further, the research evidence is then classified into a hierarchy by eminent governing bodies of research such as the National Institute of Health (United States) and National Health and Medical Research Council (Australia). In those evidence hierarchies qualitative research ranks quite low on the hierarchy.

When it comes to single studies examining questions about effectiveness of interventions randomized controlled trials, often considered to be the gold standard, will provide the best research evidence. There has been a concerted push for robust trials and systematic reviews; however, in many areas of occupational therapy, evidence from randomized controlled trials just do not exist. Much of what occupational therapists do in practice is difficult to reduce to discrete variables that can be measured and controlled; in large part due to the complexity of occupational engagement, the diversity of individuals and environments, and the nature of the relationship between the occupational therapist and the client. Other authors have critiqued the philosophical fit between occupational therapy and evidence-based practice (Gustafson et al., 2014), but it would be remiss of us not to address the issue in this text.

The need for evidence for practice is not being questioned; what we are questioning is the place of qualitative research within that evidence. For questions related to the client's view of a particular intervention then use of a qualitative methodology will provide the best research evidence. Qualitative research methodologies can account for the complexity of occupational engagement situated in context. As such Tomlin and Borgetto (2011) proposed an alternative hierarchy of evidence which is a three-dimensional pyramid with three sides and a base. One of the sides is a hierarchy of qualitative evidence with qualitative studies utilizing one source of data at the lowest rank on the hierarchy and meta-syntheses which combine a number of related qualitative studies at the top. The authors acknowledge that there are some limitations to their proposed model; however, it is worthy of consideration. Given the historical placement of qualitative research as 'inferior' to that of quantitative studies, our focus in this book is on promoting the use of qualitative research that is done well, robust, and showcases a depth of understanding on the part of the researcher.

We began our journey into the complex field that is qualitative research in 2014 with the publication of the first edition of *Qualitative Research Methodologies for Occupational Science and Therapy*. The motivation for the book came from a number of informal conversations that we had whenever we would meet regarding the development of qualitative research and the robustness of qualitative research within occupational science and occupational therapy. Underpinning these conversations were our experiences of working with the *Journal of Occupational Science* and supervising postgraduate students, writing an article in which we explored what quality meant in qualitative research from conceptualization to publication (Stanley & Nayar, 2014), and particularly during a workshop at the New Zealand Association Occupational Therapy 2012 national conference where we presented the initial idea for such a book. Some years later, the landscape of qualitative research more generally, and within occupational science and occupational therapy specifically, has witnessed substantial change.

Situating Qualitative Research in Occupational Science and Occupational Therapy

The discipline of occupational science seeks to better understand the role of engaging in occupations in everyday life, and qualitative approaches provide an array of ways for accessing that kind of information (Carlson & Clark, 1991); information that cannot be enumerated or captured by measurement without losing some of the richness and depth of meaning. Further, there is resonance between the aim of occupational therapy in working with people to engage in meaningful occupations, and qualitative research in the ability to explore meaning or how people make sense of the world. Given these alignments it is not surprising that the vast majority of research conducted within occupational science and occupational therapy has historically, and still is to date, been of a qualitative nature.

That said, tracking the history of when occupational therapy researchers started to use qualitative approaches proved more difficult than we imagined! Online searching and indexing tools that are extensively used today do not reach back to the early beginnings of occupational therapy journals. Hence, unless someone performs the laborious and enormous task of hand searching journals from across the globe, we are unable to say definitively when the first qualitative studies appeared in the professional literature. Frank and Polkinghorne (2010) contended that qualitative approaches had been adopted by occupational therapy researchers since the 1970s, and it appears that some of the early work came out of the University of Chicago Illinois, in the United States, a university department well known for its strength in scholarship and theory development, as well as qualitative research practices.

Although Gary Kielhofner (1982) championed the "special harmony between the concerns of occupational therapy and the paradigm and methods of qualitative research" (p. 162), his review of qualitative methodologies indicated that the use of qualitative research in health care fields was not wide spread. Nearly a decade later, Cheryl Mattingly (1991), another of the early pioneers, published her seminal work on clinical reasoning making comparisons with the phenomenological tradition. Both Kielhofner and Mattingly, as with Carlson and Clark (1991), noted, however, that the qualitative research tradition emerged largely from the disciplines of sociology and anthropology. Within the field of health, much pioneering work in terms of the development of qualitative research methodologies was carried out by nurse researchers and was, subsequently, used to inform occupational therapy research.

It appears that Gary Kielhofner was one of the early pioneers of qualitative research in the occupational therapy profession (Hasselkus, 1991), publishing studies undertaken with children (Kielhofner et al., 1983) and 'mentally retarded persons' (Kielhofner & Takata, 1980) in the early 1980s in the *American Journal of Occupational Therapy*. The next flurry of qualitative studies to be published in occupational therapy journals happened in the early 1990s, including Suto and Frank's (1994) ethnographic study on daily occupations of persons with chronic schizophrenia; Hasselkus' (1992) research into activities in day care for persons with Alzheimer disease; and studies exploring occupational therapy students' perspectives of fieldwork (Herzberg, 1994; Swinehart & Meyers, 1993). Around this time, qualitative research in occupational science was also emerging.

Tracing the development of qualitative research within occupational science is somewhat easier. In 1990, Yerxa and colleagues named a variety of research approaches they believed were suited for the study of occupation. Although no rationale was offered for their selection, that list included commonly employed qualitative research methodologies such as ethnography, life history, naturalistic inquiry, and case method. In the early days of using qualitative approaches within occupational therapy, ethnographic studies were the most common. Over time, that research broadened to include the use of phenomenology – mirroring movements in nursing research. Latterly, we have seen the growth of methodologies such as grounded theory and action research. In 1993, the *Journal of Occupational Science* was launched (known as *Journal of Occupational Science: Australia* in the beginning). Many of the earlier publications were theoretical in nature and early time use studies were quantitative (e.g., Pentland et al., 1998; Stanley, 1995); however, predominantly the studies published within the *Journal of Occupational Science* are qualitative. Today, the qualitative studies being produced in occupational science span a range of topics and methodologies.

In the early days, qualitative research within occupational science and occupational therapy was primarily either of a qualitative descriptive nature or aligned with one of the three main qualitative methodologies—ethnography, phenomenology, and grounded theory (Frank & Polkinghorne, 2010). That said, much of the early work did not differentiate the research design and was simply labeled a qualitative study. From these early studies, there has been substantial growth in the variety of qualitative methodologies used by occupational science and occupational therapy researchers. For instance, when we compiled the first edition of this book, we included methodologies such as critical discourse analysis, narrative, and visual methodologies. Nearly a decade later, we are now encountering newer methodologies such as Big data and embracing Indigenous ways of knowing as a means of both advancing Indigenous research as well as supporting a decolonial approach to more traditional qualitative methodologies. Hence, more than ever, it is imperative that researchers keep abreast of qualitative methodologies in order to make informed decisions when designing studies to further the discipline of occupational science and profession of occupational therapy.

Engaging with Qualitative Research

In the first edition, we argued that occupational science and occupational therapy qualitative research and publications needed to be of a high quality for three main reasons. First, ensuring a high standard is maintained throughout the research process goes towards demonstrating a level of respect and justice for participants who volunteer time and allow researchers to enter aspects of their personal lives. Considering the notion of respect, we then contended that to be taken seriously by service users, funding bodies, and other professions, occupational science and occupational therapy researchers must show they can produce and disseminate quality studies. To not do so, leaves the profession's body of knowledge, and thus the profession itself, open to judgment by other researchers and practitioners.

Our third argument centered on the push for evidence-based practice which places a demand for quality occupational science and occupational therapy research from conceptualization of the study through to publication. Integral to the quality of evidence-based research is the fit between choice of topic, appropriate methodology, and associated methods. We believe that the alignment between topic, methodology, and method, is often not clearly articulated or is misrepresented in the publication of studies, thus diminishing the quality of the research which has implications for the implementation of evidence-based practice and professional reputation. If the occupational therapy profession wants practice to be based on research evidence, then it must be quality evidence to inform practice. Yet, if practitioners are drawing on published studies that are low quality then it will not be the best evidence for quality occupational therapy practice and, therefore, positive outcomes for clients.

While, to some degree, these concerns remain, we have been heartened to witness the growth in quality, rigor, debate, application, and readership of occupational science and occupational therapy qualitative research internationally. However, the world of research is ever evolving and researchers must keep on top of current and best practices. For instance, the COVID-19 pandemic has been a catalyst for qualitative researchers to rethink how they engage in the research process given the restrictions of social distancing and lockdowns.

Therefore, as qualitative researchers with experience as university academics, supervision of research students, and teaching qualitative methodologies, we believe it is timely for a second edition of this book. Additionally, as occupational scientists and occupational therapists who review for a number of occupational therapy and health-related journals, including working with the *Journal of Occupational Science*, we believe that our disciplines have reached a stage of maturity that warrants the publication of occupation focused research texts. Since the publication of the first edition, we have engaged in work wherein we have increasingly partnered with researchers from other fields such as psychology, social work, nursing, exercise science, and gerontology. Therefore, despite the explicit focus on occupational science and occupational therapy, researchers from other disciplines may well find something useful and relevant in this book.

Without making claims to know it all, we have set out to create a text that we believe will provide some guidance to students and novice researchers or to experienced researchers who want to extend their knowledge and skills into methodologies less familiar to them. We offer that guidance with humility and recognize our limitations, so it is not the definitive text; rather, we put it forward as a contribution to ongoing understandings within the field of qualitative research. Our intent right from the beginning was to have a strong international flavor. Thus, a key feature of this book is the inclusion of chapter contributions from leading occupational science and occupational therapy researchers from across the globe, bringing variety, depth, and breadth.

Diversity is not confined to the array of researchers and scholars contributing to this book. Although qualitative research has been used in both occupational science and occupational therapy research for some time, the diversity of approaches can make defining the term 'qualitative research' tricky. So what do we mean when we the use term qualitative research? Nkwi et al. (2001) stated that "Qualitative research involves any research that uses data that do not indicate ordinal values" (p. 1). This is deliberately a broad and all-encompassing definition. While still maintaining the breadth, Denzin and Lincoln (2005) offered a somewhat more refined definition, "Qualitative researchers study things in their natural settings, attempting to make sense of, or to interpret, phenomena in terms of the meanings people bring to them" (p. 3).

In this book, and in our practice, we conceptualize qualitative research as a process of engagement either with oneself and/or with others, be they individuals or groups, through conversations, texts, images, observations—any form of data that are not numbers. As the nature of engagement can vary, so too do different approaches within qualitative research. Some are descriptive, some are more in-depth, some are designed with a specific purpose to understand or get inside a topic … we could go on. Essentially, we believe, as with any good interaction, qualitative research is about authentic engagement with the context within which one is situated for the purpose of advancing understandings in the topic of interest. In order to fully develop those understandings, the interaction requires thought and planning, as well as a commitment to ensuring a rigorous process, which is not without its challenges. Thus, in choosing to undertake qualitative research, one should not underestimate the demand or the effort required to do it well. We do not say this to scare off anyone who is just at the point of commencing their journey into qualitative research! Undertaking qualitative research can (and we would argue should) be an exciting experience. Thus, we offer this book as a guide to perhaps instigate or help sustain the excitement.

The Second Edition

The purpose of this second edition is to offer a practical introduction to the range of qualitative methodologies and methods currently being used by occupational science and occupational therapy researchers, while exploring how each research methodology and the range of methods are shaping the future of these disciplines. To produce rigorous qualitative research that is credible both within academic scholarship and the wider community of health professionals, occupational scientists and occupational therapists need to have a solid understanding of the match between topic, question, methodology, and methods. As we have stated before, without these understandings translated into good research practice, there is a risk that the discipline and profession fail to produce quality evidence that can be taken seriously and used judiciously by those who hold and sit outside of an occupational perspective. This book takes a rigorous approach to ensuring the match between the research problem, methodology, and methods through offering examples of credible research both within academic scholarship and the wider community of health professionals. The emphasis is on developing the reader's ability to produce and critique high quality qualitative research that is epistemologically and ontologically sound and rigorous, as well as reflective of the values and beliefs of the diverse communities within which occupational scientists and occupational therapists currently work to enable people to live healthy and fulfilling lives.

As a contribution to building research capacity, to generate the research evidence for occupational therapy, we see this book as a first stop for occupational scientists or occupational therapists interested in undertaking qualitative research with an explicit occupational focus. That said, we do not believe that it is the only stop. Within the chapters, authors have directed readers to other quality resources for more in-depth consideration of the chosen methodology. Thus, we encourage readers to use this book as a springboard in their learning of qualitative research and explore the offered resources and further readings, while knowing they can always return to this text that it is 'grounded in occupation.'

The intended audience is primarily graduate students in the fields of occupational science and occupational therapy with a basic understanding of qualitative research approaches; however, graduate students and researchers from other health disciplines may also benefit. The aim of the first edition was to produce a book that addressed a range of qualitative methodologies identified, at that time, as being used by occupational scientists and occupational therapists in their research. As well as presenting the core features of the methodology, the book introduced readers to a range of different research areas being explored at that time, as well as key questions to ask when reviewing studies purporting to use a specific qualitative methodology. The second edition updates relevant elements and content of traditional qualitative methodologies; as well as introducing new and cutting-edge research methodologies within a qualitative paradigm that reflect current advances in qualitative research. Additionally, across all chapters, this second edition is an opportunity to expand discussions regarding how qualitative methodologies are responding to current social movements such as countering racism, decolonization, climate change, and marriage equality.

The Chapters

In keeping with the focus on delivering a book that provides examples of robust qualitative research grounded in occupational science or occupational therapy, the lead author of each chapter is an occupational scientist or occupational therapist who has experience in the particular methodological approach. Throughout the chapters, examples of research pertaining to occupation, in terms of both foundational knowledge (occupational science) and therapeutic applications (occupational therapy), are used to showcase the design and utilization of the methodological approach. The aim is to develop the reader's ability to produce high quality qualitative research that is philosophically sound and rigorous, and to be a skilled critical reader of qualitative research.

Having positioned ourselves as editors, shared the story of how we came to write this book, and declared our intent for the book, here in Chapter 1, we turn to Chapter 2 where we set forth some shared understandings that lay the foundation for robust qualitative research including a brief discussion of paradigms; consideration of epistemology, ontology, and axiology; differentiating between methodology and methods; making explicit researcher positioning and reflexivity; and appreciating the complexity of the interplay between researcher and context. These last two points, in particular, are brought to the fore in the next chapter.

In Chapter 3, Isla Emery-Whittington (Aotearoa New Zealand; Ngāti Unu, Ngāti Kahu), Chontel Gibson (Australia; Kamilaroi yinarr), and Lana Draper (Australia; Ngiyampaa winarr) offer their insights into decolonizing qualitative research in occupational science and occupational therapy. They challenge researchers to both think about and articulate their call to engaging in research with Indigenous communities, and how such engagement may perpetuate research as a function of coloniality as opposed to becoming a tool for equity and justice. We believe that the ideas these authors put forth have relevance not just for Indigenous research but are important principles for all researchers to be cognizant of, no matter what their choice of qualitative methodology.

The specific methodology chapters begin with contributions from Australasian researchers. In Chapter 4, Mandy Stanley (Australia) draws on her experience of conducting qualitative descriptive research with a team to explore older Australians' perspectives of driverless cars. While no less complex than the other methodologies presented in this book, we believe qualitative descriptive is a good starting point for anyone new to qualitative research and methods of analysis in particular. Next, in Chapter 5, Kate D'Cruz (Australia) and Shoba Nayar (India, Aotearoa New Zealand) discuss the process involved with undertaking a grounded theory study that sought to uncover the relational process of narrative storytelling in brain injury rehabilitation.

Continuing with authors from the Southern Hemisphere, in Chapter 6, Kirk Reed (Australia) delves into the world of hermeneutic phenomenology, a methodology he chose for exploring the meaning of occupation for adults from Aotearoa New Zealand who had experienced a disruption to their occupations. Next, Simon Leadley, Margaret Jones, and Clare Hocking (Aotearoa New Zealand) discuss the application of case study methodology in Chapter 7. Their chapter highlights the strength of qualitative research in studying the complexity of occupational engagement in context as they employ a unique multiple layered approach to analysis, both literally and figuratively, to better understand a young girl's occupational choices for individual and community participation.

From the Southern Hemisphere we travel north where, in Chapter 8, Jens Schneider (Germany) and colleagues Lee Price, Laetitia Zeeman, and Natalie Edelman (United

Kingdom) describe how narrative inquiry and occupation can be philosophically under-pinned with Deweyan pragmatism; and how narrative inquiry was applied to explore expe-riences of meaningful occupations of transgender men during their gender transition process.

Still within the Northern Hemisphere, Chapters 9 and 10 have a Canadian influence. Suzanne Huot and Anne-Cécile Delaisse (Canada) consider a well-established qualitative school of inquiry—critical ethnography—and draw on two studies undertaken with the Francophone community in Canada to illustrate some of the key features of this method-ology. In Chapter 10, Debbie Laliberte Rudman (Canada) and colleague Silke Denhardt (Germany) introduce readers to critical discourse as a qualitative methodology for advanc-ing understanding of occupation and occupational therapy as contextually situated and inherently political. They draw on two examples of Foucauldian-informed critical discourse analysis studies addressing occupational possibilities to showcase this methodology in action. Issues of power and participation continue to be highlighted in the next group of chapters which draw on researchers from around the globe. In Chapter 11, Tanya Benjamin-Thomas (United States) and Debbie Laliberte Rudman draw on Tanya's experience using participatory action research methodology to demonstrate its transformative power for studying phenomena in context and embedding occupational science concepts into occu-pational therapy practice. In Chapter 12 Laura Bowman and Katie Mah (Canada) bring in illustrative examples of their work with young people living with acquired brain injury to show how visual arts-based methodologies can be used by occupational scientists or occu-pational therapists, as researchers and co-producers of knowledge, to facilitate the mean-ingful inclusion of people in research processes that can impact their future occupational engagement.

Keeping with visual methodologies, in Chapter 13, Eric Asaba and Margarita Mondaca (Sweden) and colleagues Debbie Laliberte Rudman and Melissa Park (Canada) give more focused consideration to photovoice. Using illustrations and reflections from photovoice projects spanning three countries, these authors argue that photovoice is inherently occu-pational in the sense that engagement in the project means that people will plan things, do things, reflect on their plans and engagements, share in other people's experiences, as well as communicate their realities and reflections visually, textually, and/or verbally. In round-ing out this group of chapters with a focus on community participation, in Chapter 14 Roshan Galvaan and Pam Gretschel (South Africa) describe their use of community-based research to address social injustices and how, through its alignment with decolonial per-spectives, this methodology enriches occupational science to re-orient knowledge produc-tion away from dominating paradigms, opening opportunities for exploring the plurality and diversity of human occupation.

Chapters 15 to 17 explore newer qualitative methodologies that have developed in response to a growing body of available, occupation focused research, technology, social media, and large data sets. In Chapter 15, Carolyn Murray (Australia), Katie Robinson (Ireland), and Mandy Stanley tackle some of the issues of undertaking metasynthesis methodology in a field where there is sometimes very limited literature, and provide a useful framework for undertaking this form of research. Next, in Chapter 16, Amy Wallis (Australia) delves into the world of netnography, a form of qualitative, social media research drawn from ethnography, and uses a study on the experience of occupational participation for bloggers living with leukemia to highlight the process of conducting netnography research and demonstrate its usefulness for occupation-focused research. In rounding out the methodology specific chapters, in Chapter 17, Mandy Stanley introduces us to Big data within a qualitative context. As the world in which we research becomes more multi-faceted, Big qualitative data offers researchers a pathway for dealing with larger, more complex data sets.

To close the book, in Chapter 18, Shoba Nayar draws readers' attention to areas of best (or we would argue better) practice when undertaking qualitative research, regardless of the specific methodology. In the words of Hasselkus (1991), "flexibility and freedom within guidelines, not orthodoxy, support this experiential research process" (p. 7); thus, this chapter is written as a way of stimulating further researcher reflexivity as opposed to being a mandated set of rules for undertaking robust qualitative research.

How to Navigate the Book

The order the chapters are presented in has been deliberate. We began with setting the scene regarding some of the key tenets we believe need to be embedded in qualitative research. Subsequently, authors of the specific methodology chapters have continued the discussion of these tenets as they have presented their work such as reflexivity and author positioning. Readers will also find themes related to culture, decoloniality, and power as introduced by Isla and colleagues in Chapter 3 have also been picked up in subsequent chapters.

We have chosen to start the section on specific methodologies with what might be considered the more traditional pillars of qualitative research methodologies (e.g., qualitative descriptive, grounded theory, phenomenology, case study, and narrative). As the chapters progress we move towards methodologies that reflect more directly engagement with the issues of culture, power, and injustice seen in society. These chapters start off with more traditional methodologies (e.g., ethnography, critical discourse, participatory action research) and move towards methodologies that are gaining in popularity (e.g., visual arts, photovoice, community-based research). Finally, we introduce some newer qualitative methodologies that are starting to be seen and utilized in occupational science and occupational therapy research (e.g., metasynthesis, netnography, Big data). As is noted within each chapter, there is not one right way to go about applying the research methodology. In reality, it is much more nuanced and researchers can choose from variations within a methodology and from a range of methods. Each author offers one particular slant on a methodology in which there are multiple variations. In a text such as this, we believe it is not possible nor is it helpful, to cover every variation. Thus, we make it explicit that our intention has not been to write another *SAGE Handbook of Qualitative Research* (Denzin & Lincoln, 2005)!

We received overwhelmingly positive feedback from readers regarding the accessibility to content enabled by the structure of the chapters. Therefore, we have endeavored to retain this format beginning with an introduction to the methodology and philosophy. Consideration is given to what the methodology aims to do and suitable topics/questions that might be asked. This leads to the selection of the particular research methods including recruitment and sampling, data collection, and analysis. Throughout, authors draw on their own work to provide examples of the different methods in play. Following the methods, there is a section on ensuring rigor within a study and issues of ethics particular to the chosen methodology. Next, authors offer a set of questions to ask when critiquing studies using the methodology, before providing examples of how the given form of qualitative research contributes to expanding knowledge within occupational science and occupational therapy. The chapter concludes with authors' personal reflections on their fit/choice of the methodology. At the end of each chapter further resources in the form of additional readings and websites to quality sources are offered to readers to further extend their knowledge and skills. Thus, while each chapter has a similar structure, variations are inevitable and these reflect the style and methodological approach of the contributing author(s). Readers have the choice of beginning with Chapter 1 and reading through to the final chapter or dipping in and out of chapters as needed. The consistent framework in each chapter enables the reader to readily locate the material of interest. That said, we would strongly recommend that readers start with Chapters 2 and 3 before going into the specific methodology chapters.

Having described our intent behind the book and what readers can expect, we turn to Chapter 2 to continue our discussion. In particular, our conversations here include a closer examination of key issues to consider related to qualitative research; including, reflexivity; researcher knowledge, including epistemology, axiology, and ontology; differentiating between methodology and methods; and a consideration of the research context. This chapter provides a foundation for understanding some of the principles which contribute to robust qualitative research; principles which are then expanded upon or tailored according to the specific methodology.

We hope you will enjoy and benefit from the ideas contained within this book, and we wish you well in your research journey.

References

Carlson, M. E., & Clark, F. A. (1991). The search for useful methodologies in occupational science. *American Journal of Occupational Therapy*, 45(3), 235–241. https://doi.org/10.5014/ajot.45.3.235-

Denzin, N., & Lincoln, Y. (Eds.). (2005). *Handbook of qualitative research* (3rd ed.). SAGE.

Frank, G., & Polkinghorne, D. (2010). Qualitative research in occupational therapy: From the first to the second generation. *OTJR: Occupation, Participation and Health*, 30(2), 51–57. https://doi.org/10.3928/15394492-20100325-02

Gustafson, L., Molineux, M., & Bennet, S. (2014). Contemporary occupational therapy practice: The challenges of being evidence based and philosophically congruent. *Australian Occupational Therapy Journal*, 61(2), 121–123. https://doi.org/10.1111/1441-1630.12110

Hasselkus, B. R. (1991). Qualitative research: Not another orthodoxy. *The Occupational Therapy Journal of Research*, 11(1), 3–7. https://doi.org/10.1177/153944929101100101

Hasselkus, B. R. (1992). The meaning of activity: Day care for persons with Alzheimer disease. *American Journal of Occupational Therapy*, 46(3), 199–206. https://doi.org/10.5014/ajot.46.3.199

Herzberg, G. L. (1994). The successful fieldwork student: supervisor perceptions. *American Journal of Occupational Therapy*, 48(9), 817–823. https://doi.org/10.5014/ajot.48.9.817

Kielhofner, G. (1982). Qualitative research: Part two. Methodological approaches and relevance to occupational therapy. *Occupational Therapy Journal of Research*, 2(3), 150–170. https://doi.org/10.1177/153944928200200303

Kielhofner, G., Barris, R., Bauer, D., Shoestock, B., & Walker, L. (1983). A comparison of play behavior in nonhospitalized and hospitalized children. *American Journal of Occupational Therapy*, 37(5), 305–314. https://doi.org/10.5014/ajot.37.5.305

Kielhofner, G., & Takata, N. (1980). A study of mentally retarded persons: Applied research in occupational therapy. *American Journal of Occupational Therapy*, 34(4), 252–258. https://doi.org/10.5014/ajot.34.4.252

Mattingly, C. (1991). What is clinical reasoning? *American Journal of Occupational Therapy*, 45(11), 979–986. https://doi.org/10.5014/ajot.45.11.979

Nkwi, P., Nyamongo, I., & Ryan, G. (2001). *Field research into socio-cultural issues: Methodological guidelines.* International Center for Applied Social Sciences Research and Training/UNFPA.

Pentland, W., Harvey, A., & Walker, J. (1998). The relationship between time use and health and well-being in men with spinal cord injury. *Journal of Occupational Science, 5*(1), 14–25. https://doi.org/10.1080/14427591.1998.9686431

Sackett, D. L., Strauss, S. E., Richardson, W. S., Rosenberg, W., & Haynes, R. B. (2000). *Evidence-based medicine: How to practice and teach EBM* (2nd ed.). Churchill Livingstone.

Stanley, M. (1995). An investigation into the relationship between engagement in valued occupations and life satisfaction for elderly South Australians. *Journal of Occupational Science: Australia, 2*(3), 100–114. https://doi.org/10.1080/14427591.1995.9686400

Stanley, M., & Nayar, S. (2014). From conceptualisation to publication: Ensuring quality in occupational therapy qualitative research. *New Zealand Journal of Occupational Therapy, 61*(1), 6–12.

Suto, M., & Frank, G. (1994). Future time perspective and daily occupations of persons with chronic schizophrenia in a board and care home. *American Journal of Occupational Therapy, 48*(1), 7–18. https://doi.org/10.5014/ajot.48.1.7

Swinehart, S., & Meyers, S. K. (1993). Level I fieldwork: Creating a positive experience. *American Journal of Occupational Therapy, 47*(1), 68–73. https://doi.org/10.5014/ajot.47.1.68

Tomlin, G., & Borgetto, B. (2011). Research pyramid: A new evidence-based practice model for occupational therapy. *American Journal of Occupational Therapy, 65,* 189–196. https://doi.org/10.5014/ajot.2011.000828

Yerxa, E. J., Clark, F., Frank, G., Jackson, J., Parham, D., Pierce, D., et al. (1990). An introduction to occupational science: A foundation for occupational therapy in the 21st century. *Occupational Therapy in Health Care, 6*(4), 1–17.

Additional Resources

Finlay, L., & Ballinger, C. (Eds.). (2006). *Qualitative research for allied health professionals: Challenging choices.* John Wiley & Sons.

Liamputtong, P. (Ed.). (2019). *Qualitative research methods in health* (5th ed.). Oxford University Press.

Taylor, R. R. (2017). *Kielhofner's research in occupational therapy: Methods of inquiry for enhancing practice.* F. A. Davis.

2 Tenets of Qualitative Research
Deepening Understandings

Mandy Stanley and Shoba Nayar

In Chapter 1 we recounted a brief history of qualitative research in occupational science and occupational therapy, our rationale for the second edition, and introduced the forthcoming chapters. As part of navigating this book, we suggested that readers start with Chapter 2 before they begin exploring the individual methodologies in each chapter. Our reason for this was our continued drive for and belief in the need for robust, rigorous, qualitative research. To that end, the purpose of this chapter is to take a number of tenets of qualitative research and consider these in greater depth. These tenets include (1) articulating epistemology, ontology, and axiology; (2) differentiating between methodology and methods; (3) making explicit researcher positioning and reflexivity; and (4) appreciating the complexity of the interplay between researcher and context.

We have chosen the first three key points based upon our experiences in researching, teaching, reviewing, and editing qualitative studies. Often students and novice researchers grapple with the new concepts and the nuances of language used in qualitative research; in particular the terms epistemology, ontology and axiology. Indeed, we frequently notice that the latter two—ontology and axiology—are completely absent in published studies. Then there lies the confusion between methodology and methods. The confusion of terms is compounded when the choices are not made explicit, or the use of language is conflicting within the published literature. A second area for debate, which often flows on from epistemology, is the critique of qualitative research in terms of subjectivity. Thus, we want to discuss the issue of researcher positioning and reflexivity, and the importance of making the researcher's position evident within the research.

Lastly, we turn to the fourth key point of appreciating the complexity of the interplay between researcher and context. As with the previous points, our experiences of engaging in qualitative research from multiple perspectives has brought this tenet to our attention. However, it is also our philosophical values and ethics as researchers and as occupational scientists that really fuels our desire for a considered approach to qualitative research. In reading through Chapters 3 to 17, it is evident that there are many ways of undertaking a qualitative study. In this increasingly changing digital world, fast forwarded by the global COVID pandemic beginning in 2019, researchers may choose to undertake studies on their own, with a team, across countries, or to connect more globally through the use of online platforms. Hence, in rounding out this chapter we pay attention to some of the issues that researchers need to consider when undertaking qualitative research in different contexts, including those hard to grapple notions of privilege, power, and colonization. We weave these notions beginning with thinking very close to 'home,' then expanding the discussion to researching in 'unfamiliar territory' and utilizing emerging technologies.

DOI: 10.4324/9781003456216-2

Before we turn to exploring each of the four tenets raised above, and in line with tenets 3 and 4 regarding research positionality and context, we would like to use this space to position ourselves in relation to how and why we have come to editing this book. We met back in early 2006 through our involvement with the *Journal of Occupational Science*. Discovering we were both grounded theorists who shared a love for process quickly led to conversations, musings, and writings regarding qualitative research. These discussions eventually became more focused around the quality of the qualitative studies that were being produced within occupational science and occupational therapy literature. We were frustrated that several of the studies we read lacked the detail needed to determine the quality of the study or else the detail provided did not showcase the robustness and rigor required. Eventually our discussions led to the first edition of this book being published in 2014.

While some of our initial frustrations remain, we acknowledge that there is a far better understanding and appreciation for how to conduct and report robust qualitative research for the benefits of the communities we serve. Indeed, our own thinking has shifted significantly over the years as the field of qualitative research has grown and expanded. That said, by no means do we claim to be 'experts' when it comes to qualitative research. We are passionate. We have expertise. We have a depth of understanding across a range of methodologies; but this book would in no way be possible without a group of international contributing authors who have contributed their knowledge. We are constantly learning.

I (Mandy) am a Professor in Occupational Therapy working in Australia on Noongar Whadjak country (Perth). I have over 35 years' experience as an academic. I supervise higher degree students, have a large program of funded research including nationally competitive funding, and have had sustained involvement (29 years) with the *Journal of Occupational Science*, including a role as Associate Editor. My program of research focuses on understanding the ways in which older people and those living with a disability adapt their occupations for health and well-being. I use a range of methodologies, predominantly qualitative, including descriptive qualitative, grounded theory, and some discourse analysis; and have worked with colleagues from different parts of the globe including Ireland, Sweden, and Thailand. Qualitative research approaches provide me with the tools to satisfy my curiosity about humans as occupational beings and to foreground the perspective of those with lived experience. That speaks to both the occupational scientist and occupational therapist within me.

I (Shoba) have had a somewhat less traditional path when it comes to academia. As an immigrant, I have lived, worked, and researched in multiple countries and contexts. I have worked with the *Journal of Occupational Science*, in various roles, including Senior Associate Editor, for a number of years; and have had the privilege of walking alongside postgraduate students during their research, supporting them with interviewing styles, reviewing, and editing their studies. Over the years I have also been fortunate to be invited on to research writing teams and have assisted colleagues in publishing in an array of different disciplines and journals. More recently I have been working with colleagues in India, providing training in qualitative research and building capacity with analysis and publication of qualitative studies. While I have always considered myself to be a grounded theorist, the scope of my work has offered me the opportunity to learn about and engage with different methodologies such as qualitative descriptive, narrative, photovoice, and Indigenous ways of researching.

Having positioned ourselves, we turn to a brief discussion on paradigms. It is not our intention to go into a detailed discussion of paradigms as there are other texts (cf. Guba & Lincoln, 1994; Willis, 2007) available that provide this information. However, we recognize that to write a book on qualitative methodologies it would be remiss not to include a discussion of paradigms; particularly as the paradigms overarch the four key tenets that we espouse here as being foundational to qualitative research.

Paradigms

The number and names of paradigms in research vary depending upon the research field and the author (c.f., Denzin & Lincoln, 2018). A paradigm helps to define the philosophical standpoint taken toward building scientific knowledge. In general terms a researcher's philosophical standpoint will determine three inter-related things: First, how the researcher sees reality—is there just one reality that can be known through observation and empirical measurement, or multiple realities seen from multiple perspectives? (ontology). Second, how the researchers understand what can be known and how to know it—is it known objectively or subjectively? (epistemology). And finally, what the researcher values about knowledge and how it is obtained and constructed into theory or evidence—is the information assumed by experts or agreed by co-creators? (axiology). In health research, there are broadly three key paradigms that are referred to: positivist, interpretivist, and critical. Each of these paradigms have an expected stance on epistemology, ontology, and axiology.

Work within a positivist paradigm is based on the assumption that there is a single, agreed reality and that it can be measured in some objective way. The positivist paradigm in health and medicine sees research as the means to generate and test theory developed from empirical observation that is measurable. It is predominantly presented in the form of numbers (quantified) and statistical analyses to make inferences (hypotheses) about pre-determined relationships between or among variables. Generally, the researcher is seen as the expert in the field, building on existing knowledge which favors the maintenance of the status quo in terms of what is considered and valued as scientific knowledge.

Work within an interpretivist paradigm is predominantly qualitative and acknowledges subjectivity in the naturalistic setting indicating multiple views of reality can and do exist, thus requiring data analysis to involve interpretation. Interpretivist research generates theory by bringing together multiple observations or perspectives of a phenomenon usually from firsthand experience. The researcher in the interpretivist tradition is not the expert; rather the instrument through which 'experts by experience' are given a voice. Knowledge revealed and built in the interpretivist paradigm shapes different perspectives on what is valued as science and how scientific knowledge is generated. When interpretivist research first became recognized in the 20th century, mainly in sociology (Schwartz-Shea & Yanow, 2020), it was seen as an enormous challenge to the notion of science. Over the last 100 years it has become mainstream, and a very useful and popular approach in health sciences generally, and occupational science specifically, enabling the full extent of occupational practice to be included as scientific knowledge.

A critical paradigm takes the stance of addressing disadvantage and issues of social justice or, in occupational science and occupational therapy, occupational justice. The aim of research within this paradigm is to draw attention to issues of power and control and the outcome is transformative. In a postmodern critical paradigm, the researcher analyzes data or discourse through the lens of a critical theory to bring to light the 'taken for granted.' Shining a light on social structures that perpetuate disadvantage provide an avenue for change.

In addition to the three paradigms noted above—positivist, interpretivist, and critical—we also recognize two more paradigms. The first of these is a pragmatist paradigm which provides a bridge to the opposing positions of positivism and interpretivism. Within a pragmatic paradigm the researcher chooses the approach that is the best fit for the research question. The emphasis is on finding the best fit for the situation. Use of a mixed-methodology approach comes within this pragmatist paradigm.

We contend that a second, and further paradigm needs to also be considered—Indigenous knowledges. In this post-colonial paradigm, the aim is to decolonize and address existing structural disadvantage that is a result of colonization (refer to Denzin et al., 2008). In a post-colonial paradigm, researchers bring Indigenous ways of knowing to the research endeavor which respects and foregrounds culture, community, and relationships (Emery-Whittington, 2021). The aim is to repair harms that have been created through white colonizing research and to work towards healing. While we have articulated five broad paradigms, within each paradigm there are different beliefs about ways of knowing (epistemology) and how knowledge is created (ontology), and it is to these concepts to which we now turn our attention.

Articulating Epistemology, Ontology, and Axiology

Engaging with any new body of knowledge or undertaking any new skill requires learning a new language particular to that area; and it is no different with qualitative research. While there are several terms to become familiar with—many of which will be introduced in the specific chapters that follow—there are three in particular that apply across the different approaches; these are epistemology, ontology, and axiology. Before we define these terms, we refer you to Textbox 2.1 and ask you to pause a moment to consider the reflection questions posed. The purpose of this reflection exercise is to start you thinking, if you have not done so already, about how you make sense of the terms. Consider writing your responses in a reflective journal as a way of crystallizing your thinking and to be able to revisit your thoughts from time to time in your development as a qualitative researcher or consumer. It is vital that you understand your perspectives on epistemology, ontology, and axiology as they determine the standpoint you take in approaching knowledge development. This in turn ultimately underpins your choice(s) for methodology and indeed the specific methods you will use.

Textbox 2.1   Reflection Exercise

1 What am I aiming to understand?
2 How do I make sense of the world?
3 What does reality mean to me?
4 How can I know reality?
5 What values do I bring to my role as the researcher in this study?

Having spent a few minutes thinking about and writing your answers to the questions above, read the definitions below and review your answers.

Epistemology is the study of knowledge and considers the ways of knowing and understanding the world. It also considers how knowledge is constructed, which is why it is an important ingredient for determining the methodological approach to be taken. When considering epistemology in a qualitative study, researchers need to address what they believe is possible to know and how that knowledge is obtained (Given, 2008). Within contemporary occupational science and occupational therapy research, new knowledge is often understood to be jointly constructed between researchers' and participants' shared experiences which mirrors the therapeutic encounter which upholds the principle of client/family centered practice. Further, new knowledge is understood to only ever be one perspective and it may change over time or in different contexts. Since the turn of the 21st century, there has been growing discussion regarding the need for culturally informed epistemologies (Iwama, 2003), as well as specific forms of epistemologies such as pragmatist (Morrison, 2016) and critical (Farias et al., 2016) for underpinning occupational science and occupational therapy practice and research. We would encourage those embarking upon research to take the time to read the literature and become informed of these ways of knowing.

Where epistemology encourages researchers to consider how knowledge is constructed, ontology deals with the fundamental nature of reality—what can be known (Ayyala et al., 2006; Willig, 2009). Ontology is "concerned with the existence of, and relationship between different aspects of society, such as social actors, cultural norms and social structures" (Barron, 2006, p. 301). From our perspective, ontology tends to span a continuum, with the idea of a single, objective reality at one end moving towards multiple, subjective, and constructed realities at the other. The positioning of most qualitative research, particularly within occupational science and occupational therapy literature, is towards that of multiple realities. However, depending what one's ontology is, will shape the subjective stance underpinning those multiple realities. For instance, researchers who come from an interpretivist paradigm (such as ourselves) argue that one's reality is changed and shaped by their interactions with others or the social world; whereas critical theorists might take a more political stance in seeking to expose dominant ways of thinking that shape the realities within which society operates (Cruickshank, 2012).

The epistemological and ontological stance taken by the researcher will influence the entire process of the study and the outcome; hence, it is important to be clear about one's epistemology and ontology before embarking on a research project. It is not something that can be determined at the end, in retrospect, or even halfway through. In time we have come to understand that our epistemology and ontology are interwoven and shape our stance as qualitative researchers and our preference towards utilizing grounded theory methodology for our research.

For instance, as we have come to know ourselves, and each other, we have recognized and deepened a shared personal preference for an understanding of processes. For example, we both like to engage in a consultative process of decision making rather than being given a predetermined outcome. Such a worldview plays out in our everyday work, and in our writing and our thinking, as illustrated by a writing project where we combined our grounded theory studies to produce a journal manuscript on occupational adaptation as a social process in everyday life (Nayar & Stanley, 2014). Although these studies were conducted separately for our doctorates, our preferred ways of knowing the world and our views of how knowledge and reality are constructed meant that we could bridge the two studies to highlight a bigger process at play.

Having considered our epistemological and ontological positions, we turn now to axiology. This term is probably the least discussed by researchers; yet, for us, is what holds us accountable to ensuring we conduct and publish high quality research. Broadly, axiology is the philosophical study of values (Given, 2008); and, in research, comes to the fore when thinking about ethics which encompasses moral values and code of conduct. More specifically, it is about the shared values and beliefs we—Mandy and Shoba—hold about the importance of occupation and its relation to health and well-being. Knowing what our values are, and being firm in our belief of these values, has meant that we always seek to bring an occupational perspective to the fore in our research, while recognizing that we are not the experts and that we need the engagement of participants in order to generate knowledge and recommendations for practice and future research. Indeed, our experience is that stakeholders advise engagement of participants at a minimum, and there is ever growing emphasis on the active involvement of participants all the way through the research process including co-design, co-researching, and co-creating.

At this point we would like to acknowledge that it is not easy to come to grips with the terminology and concepts that begin to appear when one enters the field of qualitative research. It has taken us many years of readings and discussions to understand these concepts, and even now we will turn back to the texts for a refresher. So, we encourage you not to be disheartened. This is a process of learning. It is something you need to keep working at and over time you will come to a deeper understanding—it will not happen overnight or in one reading, but it will happen … as we noted in Chapter 1, humans, occupation, and qualitative research are all filled with complexity! Take a moment now to think about a research project you are intending to undertake or are currently engaged in. Revisit Textbox 2.1 and consider if your answers have changed in the context of your chosen area of research.

Ensuring there is alignment between your epistemological, ontological, and axiological positioning is critical for developing a credible qualitative study. Similarly, understanding the difference and alignment between the terms 'methodology' and 'methods' is also important. We turn now to the second key tenet.

Differentiating Between Methodology and Methods

There is a tendency to conflate the terms methodology and methods or to use them interchangeably when in fact they mean different things (Nicholls, 2009a). This is something that we have seen done by both novice and experienced researchers. Alternatively, we have seen authors simply avoid defining or using these terms altogether. Although they are intricately linked, it is important to know the difference between the terms; thus, throughout the following chapters, a key aim is to ensure congruence in how they are used. This particular aim speaks back to the call from Frank and Polkinghorne (2010) for a better understanding of the difference between methods and theory and the place of theory in guiding the approach.

Methodology is the theoretical or philosophical orientation "of how research should, or ought, to proceed given the nature of the issue it seeks to address" (Hammell, 2006, p. 167). A change in orientation will change the process and outcome of the study. For example, the outcome of a phenomenological study is to obtain a rich description and/or the meaning of the lived experience compared to, for example, a grounded theory study where the outcome is to derive an explanatory theory about a social process. Within each of these approaches the theoretical orientation might be drawn from a range of theorists, for example phenomenology may draw on the works of Husserl, Heidegger, or Gadamer; the grounded theory study from symbolic interactionism from Glaser and Strauss, or social constructivism from Charmaz. Again, it is important that researchers clearly articulate their theoretical or philosophical orientation as this will help the reader understand how the data were interpreted and the findings are presented, as well as be able to judge the rigor of the study.

Methods, then, are the actual tools for implementing the research (Mills & Birks, 2014). It is the detail of the steps taken by the researcher in conducting the study; for example, the steps of recruitment, participant selection, ethical protocols, data collection approach, phases in analysis, and the strategies to implement rigor. The choice of methods will be influenced by the epistemology and methodology (Lune & Berg, 2017).

It is possible, at times, for epistemologies and methods to overlap around different methodologies. For example, a theoretical orientation in symbolic interactionism could inform both grounded theory and ethnography; and interviews are a common data collection technique used across qualitative methodologies. Interviews are a way of engaging with participants to elicit their stories and perspectives regarding particular phenomenon. However, variations exist within interviews, just as there are variations within qualitative research. Therefore, the questions that are asked in an interview, and how they are asked, need to be congruent with the chosen epistemology and methodology (Nicholls, 2009b); for example, a semi-structured phenomenological interview is not the same as a narrative interview. Thus as, Frank and Polkinghorne (2010) noted, it is critical "that the relationship must be re-established between methods and theories" (p. 56) if the aim is to have occupational science and occupational therapy qualitative research be taken seriously.

Having acknowledged the possibility for an overlap in epistemologies and methods, one source of frustration for us is when we hear researchers engage in what has been termed 'method slurring' (Baker et al., 1992)—a blending of approaches to research without consideration of the alignment between epistemology, ontology, and methodology. Our advice to researchers—new and experienced—is that if you choose to use a mix of approaches in your study, clearly articulate your rationale for doing so and acknowledge any conflicts that may exist with regards to philosophical positioning.

By now, we trust that you, the reader, are coming to appreciate the complexity that is qualitative research. As researchers, it is imperative that we take ownership of our chosen approach and what it has to offer, along with the appropriate amount of humility, rigor, and robustness! Equally, it is important for readers of qualitative research to be astute critical consumers in order to judge the quality of the research and its usefulness for practice. To that end we have included questions for critiquing studies in each chapter. These questions will be useful to readers of qualitative research and to researchers who can critique the robustness of their own application of the methodology; which leads us into our next key tenet—researcher positioning and reflexivity.

Making Explicit Researcher Positioning and Reflexivity

One of the critiques of qualitative research is that it is 'subjective' in nature. We believe that one cannot really do qualitative research without engaging as a person; all researchers come to a study with their experience and knowledge (epistemology), shaped by their culture (axiology), and their own views of reality (ontology). Therefore, at the outset, we position ourselves by explicitly stating our assumption that qualitative research is a subjective endeavor and that one way in which subjectivity is managed is through explicating the "lens through which every researcher sees her or his research" (Hasselkus, 1997, p. 81). While there are different ways to position oneself according to different methodologies— as will be discussed in upcoming chapters—here we set the scene for our understanding.

It is important to bear in mind, that keeping in line with the complexity of qualitative research noted thus far, positioning and reflexivity cannot be considered in isolation; they influence each other and the progression and outcome of the study.

Positionality

Positioning is the process of making explicit one's personal and epistemological beliefs as a researcher within a given study (Manohar et al., 2017). Given the subjective nature of qualitative research, the analysis of data is always going to be filtered through the researcher's particular lens. If the researcher positions themselves, then readers view the research findings knowing the researcher's lens and can make their own judgments about the data presented. Positioning oneself is important throughout the study—not just in the final reporting, but at all stages of the research process from study design through to data collection and analysis—as a way of staying open to data that may not have been anticipated. One way of making positioning explicit is in the reporting, and researchers stating how they came to do the study and how it relates to them personally. For instance, as an Indian woman and an immigrant, Shoba has often identified closely with participants in studies and the stories they were sharing (Nayar, 2011; Nayar et al., 2012; Nayar & Wright-St. Clair, 2018; Wright St. Clair & Nayar, 2018).

However, one of the challenges for novice qualitative researchers is that positioning is not always evident in publications. Journal requirements such as word limits, may stymie the opportunity to report one's positioning. Yet it is possible to position oneself in a sentence or two, as Shoba did in reporting her study:

> The focus of this research stemmed from the first author's experiences as an occupational therapist working with immigrants in a mental health service, and self-identification as an Indian immigrant woman who has witnessed and experienced the challenges of settling in a new environment.
>
> (Nayar et al., 2012, p. 65)

Ensuring the participants and readers of her research knew Shoba was an Indian immigrant woman herself, was important both in terms of enabling the women to talk openly and assisting the readers to understand what it was the women were sharing in their stories.

Reflexivity

Being conscious of, and explicitly positioning oneself as a researcher, requires an ability to engage in thinking and writing reflexively. Reflexivity can be defined as "the capacity of any system of signification to turn back upon itself, to make itself its own object by referring to itself" (Myerhoff & Ruby, 1982/1992, p. 307). It is the notion that a person's thoughts and ideas tend to be inherently biased; in other words, the values and thoughts of a researcher will be represented in their work. Thus, reflexivity is "consciousness about being conscious, thinking about thinking" (Frank, 1997, p. 87). It is a process that goes beyond reflecting on what worked or did not work to questioning and challenging oneself, particularly around assumptions. The aim is to gain a deeper level of insight than previously existed. Employing reflexivity will enable a researcher to get to new and richer insights. The challenge is not to remove the subjective nature of qualitative research and be free of bias, rather to use it as the focus for more intense and complete insight into the phenomenon of interest.

Reflexivity may be personal or epistemological in nature. Personal reflexivity encompasses a researcher's values, beliefs, interests, and relationships and how these influence the study. Depending on the topic there is the potential for reflexivity to take a more psychodynamic lens with a view to transference and counter transference. If it is a topic that is very close to one's personal experience, such as Shoba's description above, then there could be greater risk for issues of transference to occur. At the outset of a study, a researcher may be more focused on personal reflexivity; whereas epistemological reflexivity may come later in the process. Epistemological reflexivity is the attempt to identify the foundations of knowledge and the implications of any findings; situating the findings within the existing body of knowledge. This level of reflexivity adds a further layer of robustness to the study.

We recommend that before engaging in a study, the researcher undertakes a pre-understandings interview with an experienced qualitative researcher to uncover potential assumptions or understandings related to the field of study. Alternatively, the researcher may wish to journal, reflecting on the questions raised in Textbox 2.2.

Textbox 2.2   Questions to Ask for Reflexive Purposes

1 What do I think I might find in this study?
2 What is my interest in undertaking this study?
3 What current knowledge do I have about this topic?
4 What do I want the outcome of this study to be?
5 Why is it necessary to undertake this study?
6 How am I influencing the gathering and analysis of data?
7 What are the power differentials between me as the researcher and those I am researching?
8 Am I being true to the epistemology, ontology, and methodology of the study?

Whatever strategy one chooses to use, it is important to remember that reflexivity is not just thinking about assumptions—it is an active process of writing, talking, asking, questioning; until the researcher counters the 'aha moment' through examining the origins of their assumptions.

A further issue to consider, under the heading of researcher positioning and reflexivity, is that of ethics and power in the partnership between researcher and participant or participant groups. We believe it is not ethical to approach a qualitative study with the 'drive by' or 'hit and run' idea of engaging briefly with participants, doing the research, and then exiting to write up the thesis or publication with no intentions of making contact again. On the one hand, taking that approach reduces the likelihood of accessing participants who are willing to share their experiences. On the other hand, some people may volunteer to participate in the study, but given the lack of acknowledgement of the contribution and reciprocity, the next researcher who comes along is not going to be received so well. The approach taken to the relationship between the researcher and the researched relates back to axiology and the values that underpin the knowledge creation which emphasizes the importance of the researcher's axiological position. Ethics and ethical positioning is discussed further in Chapter 18 on best practice.

As researchers, it is important for the discipline and the profession to make a positive contribution in participants' lives and an equally useful contribution to knowledge; however, this requires that researchers are aware of sensitivities in negotiations with prospective participants and dissemination of findings. Thus, in the spirit of doing justice to both participants and methodological rigor, it is important to consider the research context and potential issues of power that may influence the study. Suggestions for reflexive questions to stimulate thinking about relationships with participants include: 'where is the power located?'; 'how can power differentials be addressed?'; and 'who is being advantaged or disadvantaged?'

Throughout Chapters 1 and 2 we have made statements regarding our position as qualitative researchers, academics, occupational therapists, and editors, and how we came to this text. Each of the authors have explicated their positioning in relation to the methodology, which you will see as a common feature of all chapters in this book. The purpose is to provide the reader with examples of how to frame one's positioning, as well as ensuring that we are being rigorous and true to what we are recommending as good practice.

Appreciating the Complexity of the Interplay Between Researcher and Context

Having considered issues of language and terminology, philosophical positioning and reflexivity, this section explores the fourth key tenet we believe is necessary for qualitative researchers to give consideration before embarking on their study—appreciating the complexity of the interplay between researcher and the varied contexts within which qualitative studies are conducted. The word context is derived from the Latin 'con-' meaning 'together,' and 'texere' meaning 'to weave.' In this final tenet, we weave together issues of privilege, power, and colonization; issues that cannot be avoided when engaging in studies that connect intimately with people, as occurs in qualitative research. In unpacking the interplay between researcher and context, we discuss three broad areas: (1) geographical location; (2) cultural considerations; and (3) researcher experience.

Geographical Location

The first aspect of interplay between research and context is that of geographical location, or where the research is conducted. Given that research questions often come from practice or experience, it may well be that the research study is located within one's own workplace or community. While on the surface this may seem to have immediate benefits, such as ease of access to participants, consideration must be given to how such proximity might influence people's roles and contributions. For instance, it might be that researching in one's own 'backyard' will impact on who will volunteer and what participants will be prepared to reveal. Potential participants may be wary about confidentiality of information shared and being easily identified and perceive that the research has a degree of power to either protect or expose them. Communicating openly about how participants' rights to retain confidentiality will be preserved and being sensitive to the potential for coercion and a sense of obligation to volunteer is vital. As a solo researcher, alleviating the issues raised here include being open about one's positionality in relation to the topic being research and the community in which the research is being undertaken. Further strategies may be to engage in research as part of a team or use online methods.

The advent of COVID-19 fueled a rapid growth in the use of online tools for conducting research and for generating research data, and social media sites as exciting opportunities for research, both in terms of people engaging in occupations online as well as the place of online or social media in the lives of clients of occupational therapy practice. When we wrote the first edition, online research was in its infancy but, thanks to COVID-19, that is no longer the reality. The worldwide pandemic forced many into finding new ways to conduct their daily work or research from within the confines of their homes.

In this short section we do not propose to provide extensive coverage of all the different types of tools or applications, nor do we have anything to gain from mentioning some products and not others; rather our intention is to talk more broadly about the ways that media might be used. Advances in technology—computers, tablets, mobile devices, and internet connections—have enabled researchers to continue their studies while adopting new research methods. There has been an upsurge in free or inexpensive applications with tools such as Skype®, Zoom®, or Microsoft Teams enabling research teams to connect in and across different geographical locations. The webcam has made it possible to see each other as well which is important for the non-verbal aspects of communication. Other tools furnished by the internet for storage and exchange of files (e.g., Dropbox, iCloud) and sharing bibliographic databases (e.g., Refworks, Endnote web) all provide ways to make the work of multi-site research easier. The tools just mentioned are available 24 hours, which is useful when working across diverse time zones.

The use of online forums, blogs, and social media provides researchers with a ready source of data, much of which is freely available in the public domain. While the emergence of online research presents increasing options for accessing data, such exciting opportunities raise a need for caution, the need to pause and consider the ethics associated with undertaking research where participants may not be willingly or knowingly consenting to having their ideas used for research when they write a blog or send a tweet. Ethical issues are around informed consent, or the lack of it, the inability to gain informed consent from the writer of the information and the inability to return to, the originator of the material and check the researcher's interpretations. Given the upsurge in online research, it should come as no surprise that this second edition of *Qualitative Research Methodologies for Occupational Science and Occupational Therapy* contains new chapters that will further explicate the practical and ethical issues touched upon here.

While there is an upsurge in internet based qualitative research, the literature in occupational science or occupational therapy on internet based qualitative research is still in its infancy. Within qualitative health research, Wilkerson et al. (2014) have provided researchers with two checklists: one for deciding between the use of online or offline data collection; and the second to guide decision making about when to begin online data collection. Drawing on their experience with several qualitative projects with hard-to-reach groups on sensitive topics, they offer a useful discussion on the use of online forums for recruiting and data collection. However, methodological literature from the perspective of occupational science or occupational therapy research, particularly with regards to use of other social media, is still needed.

Use of digital media and online methods are also being used to facilitate multi-site research activities. Increasingly, multi-site studies are the way forward for many researchers as funders look towards studies that incorporate multiple perspectives. Multi-site studies are still relatively uncommon within the fields of occupational science and occupational therapy. Within occupational science there are few examples of multi-site or multicultural studies; the most well-known being the food-centered occupations study conducted in New Zealand, Thailand, and the United States. Findings from the site-specific studies have been published separately (Shoredike & Pierce, 2005; Wright St. Clair et al., 2004) and in combination (Wright-St Clair et al., 2013), along with a methodology paper (Shoredike et al., 2010). Thus, while there is recognition, as part of the maturation of the discipline and profession, of the benefits in bringing together research teams to add further layers of complexity to the research process, there does, however, remain a paucity of literature within occupational science and occupational therapy regarding methodologies and processes that promote successful multi-site research.

Multi-site studies entail both richness and challenges. For example, having multiple perspectives or 'lenses' through which to view the data may result in deeper insights, with relevance of research findings beyond that of one profession. Further, online platforms can provide tools to assist the way researchers work and enable better communication. Alternatively, researcher positioning and reflexivity may pose a challenge if researchers' personal and epistemological perspectives do not align among members of the team. Therefore, key to engaging in a multi-site study is the researcher's ability to be a good communicator and willingness and commitment to engage in robust frank conversations, in a collaborative process, in order for the desired outcomes to be achieved, cultural values respected, and relationships preserved. Working effectively in teams is facilitated by clear documentation of team decisions, particularly in relation to ownership of data and what it can be used for, as well as agreements about allocation of tasks, timelines, intellectual property, publication, and authorship.

Multi-site studies within a country might be undertaken as a very strategic approach to increasing the chances of recruiting participants from different regions, as well as achieving sufficient participant numbers. Additionally, the findings from multi-site studies in the same country will hold broader application of the outcome and transferability. The researchers will make a commitment to answering the same research question and following the grant proposal or agreed protocols. The added complexity for researchers then is quite pragmatic about methods of communication across geographical locations, and possibly accounting for time zone differences both across countries and within countries like Canada, Australia, and the United States. When it comes to multi-country research, complexities are amplified. Working across more distant geographies brings additional challenges through different language and culture, time zones, institutional requirements for governance and ethics, governments, legislative requirements, and politics. With both of these configurations of multi-site research, additional time needs to be spent prior to writing the research proposal to engage in shared discussions about ways of working and epistemological positioning (Shordike et al., 2010).

Cultural Considerations

Epistemological, ontological, and axiological positioning are imperative when considering a second aspect of the interplay between research and context—that of culture. While we recognize that 'culture' is broader than ethnicity alone, for the purpose of our discussion here we have chosen to consider culture under two broad headings of ethnicity and insider/outsider perspectives. In part our rationale for doing so is due to a recent upsurge in recognition of the need for, and implementation of, Indigenous research methodologies.

When we published the first edition of this book, decolonizing methodologies for undertaking research involving Indigenous communities were only just beginning to emerge within the occupational science and occupational therapy research (Hammell, 2011; Yalmambirra, 2000). Similar to the lead taken by feminist researchers in the 1970s, the use of decolonizing methodologies places the disadvantaged group into a 'privileged' position epistemologically and ethically to protect the groups' interests and prevent further oppression or marginalization (Denzin et al., 2008; Tuhiwai Smith, 2012). More recently, occupational scientists and occupational therapy researchers are undertaking explorations using Indigenous ways of researching and knowing to shed light on occupations beyond a Western focus such as Ryan et al.'s (2020) "exploration of how Aboriginal and Torres Strait Islander people experience and express advocacy as an occupation, via an on-line platform" (p. 405) and Gibson et al.'s (2020) study revealing the importance of Aboriginal and Torres Strait Islander Elders and older people in "maintaining the cultural well-being of family, community, and country" (p. 193). Such studies are imperative both for diversifying understandings of occupations engaged in by various ethnic and Indigenous communities, as well as providing critical commentary on the historical reliance of methodologies stemming from the West.

However, just as multi-site studies are lacking in occupational science and occupational therapy research, so too are cross-cultural studies wherein the occupations of more than one ethnic group within the same country are explored in the one study. One example of such a study is that undertaken by Shoba and colleague Valerie Wright-St. Clair. Their cross-cultural study included older Korean, Chinese, and Indian immigrants' who resided in Auckland, New Zealand, for the purpose of better understanding how these different ethnic groups contribute to society through their everyday occupations (Wright St. Clair & Nayar, 2018). While they also published a methodology paper addressing how they dealt with cross cultural challenges in the processes of data collection and analysis (Nayar & Wright St. Clair, 2020) there is a need for more such studies.

In undertaking cross cultural studies or using Indigenous methodologies, questions are often raised regarding who is best suited for doing such research. The insider/outsider debate has been given much attention in the literature and it is not our intention to try to summarize the arguments or even offer solutions. Rather, we highlight some points here for researchers to consider at the outside of their study, many of which will be addressed again and in greater depth in the forthcoming methodology chapters.

More often than not, people come to research with a question (or multiple questions) either from practice or from their lived experience. If it is a question from practice, the researcher already has a body of knowledge from their education, reading, and practice experiences with clients or colleagues. Thus, as indicated above, it is impossible to enter the research field free of assumptions. Equally, if a person comes to a question from personal experience, the drive to pursue that question is because it has personal meaning, which, again, is accompanied by a set of assumptions based on that experience; thus, it is more of an embodied experience and comes with a different set of knowledges.

A balance is required in terms of having the drive and personal interest to pursue a question and, at the same time, recognizing the underlying assumptions and values, and how they might impact on the choice of methodology and methods used in the research. It is harder to reveal one's own assumptions and values if researching something closely related to personal experience. It is much harder to separate out the cognitive and emotive elements and the researcher will be naturally drawn to focus attention on data that speaks to their own experience. For instance, if the researcher's lived experience is of being a refugee who has resettled in a new country and is now involved in research with other refugees about their settlement experiences, it is particularly important to be vigilant in the analysis phase. Data that present alternative experiences to that experienced by the researcher need to be brought forward and the researcher must work hard to incorporate any 'outlier' data. It is much more difficult for the 'insider' to keep their own values and assumptions from influencing the analysis in certain ways; although there is much that a researcher with that experience brings to the analysis. For example, Wilson (2010), an occupational scientist and occupational therapist, drew on descriptive qualitative (Chapter 3) and auto-ethnographic (Chapter 7) methodologies, to write about her experience of weight loss surgery and the resultant change in occupational engagement and thus occupational identity.

Alternatively, there are times when one might come to a research field having very little personal experience of the topic area; for example, engaging in research with cultural groups of which one is not a part. In such an instance, strategies need to be employed by the researcher that demonstrate sensitivities in order to enter the field and to recruit participants and to leave the field in good standing. These strategies might include prolonged engagement and calling upon cultural advisors who can assist with the knowledge required to engage safely and respectfully. For example, in Thomas et al.'s (2012) study of use of time and links to well-being for people who were homeless, the first author "undertook more than 100 hours of fieldwork and observation in order to establish trust and rapport within the homeless community" (p. 784). Thus, it is possible to engage as a solitary researcher with a topic which one might have little knowledge of, through to a topic which one knows intimately. Either way, we strongly recommend having another researcher who can act as a critical friend and, using peer debriefing, assist the reflexive process throughout the study. The use of a critical 'friend,' mentor, or supervisor leads us to the last aspect of this fourth key tenet—interplay between researcher and context—that of researcher experience.

Researcher Experience

In our time with the *Journal of Occupational Science*, we both held roles as associate editors. This position afforded us the opportunity to read many manuscripts and work with authors to bring their work through to publication. What we noticed was that the quality of manuscripts varied greatly and one factor contributing to this quality was that of researcher experience; for instance, whether the author was a novice or experienced researcher, and whether they were an academic, practitioner, or student.

Occupational scientists and occupational therapists have clearly embraced qualitative research as a means of informing the discipline and profession. However, qualitative research is not a static 'thing,' as clearly indicated by the revised table of contents in this second edition. Methodologies and methods are constantly evolving and for novice researchers it can feel overwhelming. We believe that the profession has a responsibility to (a) develop capacity of those beginning their research journeys and (b) continue to take responsibility for continued learning and knowledge acquisition on the topic of qualitative research.

These days, research is no longer only the domain of the established academic. Increasingly therapists are also engaging in research activities; while students are encouraged to become researchers whether they are intending to graduate and pursue a career as a therapist or continue down the academic route. The area in which the researcher is situated may have a bearing on the motivation for pursuing their study. For instance, an academic may be expected to conduct research and secure research funding as part of their job description; therapists may pursue research with a desire to contribute to, and make changes in, the work setting; while students may undertake a small research study for the purpose of completing an assignment simply to graduate. Whatever the motivation, increasingly there is an expectation that the findings of the research will be disseminated, most commonly in the form of journal publications. While we uphold the belief that study outcomes need to be made accessible this should not be at the expense of quality.

One way in which more experienced researchers can assist with developing capacity of newer researchers is through mentoring and sponsorship. Mentoring is a direct relationship between two people wherein the mentor provides direct guidance, advice, feedback on skills to the mentee. In contrast, sponsorship entails support that goes beyond developing the internal capacity of the mentee (Ayyala et al., 2019). Sponsorship activities include advocacy, visibility, promotion, and connections. "Sponsors connect protégés with their network and by association, better position protégés to access people and resources they otherwise would not be able to access on their own" (DeWitty & McCamey, 2022). In this sense, where mentorship is a two-way relationship, sponsorship can be thought of as a three-way relationship between sponsor, recipient, and an external audience. While mentoring is evident, to a large degree, among occupational science and occupational therapy researchers, sponsorship is, perhaps, a lesser-known concept but one worth considering for the purpose of advancing occupation focused research and building capacity among researchers. Although it may seem that both mentorship and sponsorship are designed for the novice researcher, we see the benefits of more experienced researchers also engaging in these activities as the 'learner.' Morse (1994) put forth the notion of 'minus mentoring' wherein knowledge gained through the reading of texts gets passed from one student to another and in the process becomes diluted and the "description of how one does it (the method) has got to be elusive" (p. 216). Thus, taking the extra effort to build in time and space for mentoring and sponsorship within the research design can only result in greater knowledge and application of qualitative methodologies that produce robust knowledge to inform science and practice.

Summary

One of the key tenets we argue that underpins qualitative research is researcher positionality and reflexivity. Hence, it would have been remiss of us not to have introduced ourselves and what brought us to editing a book on qualitative research. Having situated ourselves in this context, we then chose to explore four key tenets that we believe underpin all qualitative research: (1) articulating epistemology, ontology, and axiology; (2) differentiating between methodology and methods; (3) making explicit researcher positioning and reflexivity; and (4) appreciating the complexity of the interplay between researcher and context. While we raise these as topics for conversation, it is not all that can be talked about. However, it is also not our intention to expand and replicate in this textbook what can be found elsewhere. We suggest that people seek out the abundant literature that is now readily accessible online, and refer to further readings and websites at the end of this and subsequent chapters in the book.

Qualitative research is not always what it appears to be; thus, it is important to emphasize the need to see beyond what one is told. Qualitative research is not formulaic. It is highly complex, evolving, and exciting. The following chapters further a number of the concepts that we have introduced here to reveal the creativity, complexity, and richness that is qualitative research.

References

Ayyala, M. S., Skarupski, K., Bodurtha, J. N., González-Fernández, M., Ishii, L. E., Fivush, B., & Levine, R. B. (2019). Mentorship is not enough: Exploring sponsorship and its role in career advancement in academic medicine. *Academic Medicine*, *94*(1), 94–100. https://doi.org/10.1097/ACM.0000000000002398

Ayyala, M. S., Skarupski, K., Bodurtha, J. N., González-Fernández, M., Ishii, L. E., Fivush, B., & Levine, R. B. (2006) Ontology. In V. Jupp (Ed.). *The SAGE dictionary of social research methods* (pp. 301–302). SAGE.

Baker, C., Wuest, J., & Stern, P. N. (1992). Method slurring: The grounded theory/phenomenology example. *Journal of Advanced Nursing*, *17*(11), 1355–1360. https://doi.org/10.1111/j.1365-2648.1992.tb01859.x

Barron, L. (2006). Ontology. In V. Jupp (Ed.). *The SAGE dictionary of social research methods*. SAGE. https://doi.org/10.4135/9780857020116

Cruickshank, J. (2012). Positioning positivism, critical realism and social constructionism in the health sciences: a philosophical orientation. *Nursing Inquiry*, *19*(1), 71–82. https://doi.org/10.1111/j.1440-1800.2011.00558.x

Denzin, N. K., & Lincoln, Y. S. (2018). *The SAGE handbook of qualitative research* (5th ed.). SAGE.

Denzin, N. K., Lincoln, Y. S., & Smith, L. T. (Eds.). (2008). *Handbook of critical and indigenous methodologies*. SAGE.

Emery-Whittington, I. (2021). Occupational justice: Colonial business as usual? Indigenous observations from Aotearoa New Zealand. *Canadian Journal of Occupational Therapy*, *88*(2), 153–162. https://doi.org/10.1177/00084174211005891

Farias, L., Laliberte Rudman, D., & Magalhães, L. (2016). Illustrating the importance of critical epistemology to realize the promise of occupational justice. *OTJR: Occupation, Participation and Health*, *36*(4), 234–243. https://doi.org/10.1177/1539449216665561

DeWitty, V. P., & McCamey, D. (2022). Mentorship and sponsorship: Viable strategies for increasing nursing school faculty. *Journal of Nursing Education*, *61*(9), 499–501. https://doi.org/10.3928/01484834-20220705-03

Frank, G. (1997). Is there life after categories? Reflexivity in qualitative research. *Occupational Therapy Journal of Research*, *17*(2), 84–98. https://doi.org/10.1177/153944929701700203

Frank, G., & Polkinghorne, D. (2010). Qualitative research in occupational therapy: From the first to the second generation. *OTJR Occupation, Participation and Health*, *30*(2), 51–57. https://doi.org/10.3928/15394492-20100325-02

Gibson, C., Dudgeon, P., & Crockett, J. (2020). Listen, look & learn: Exploring cultural obligations of Elders and older Aboriginal people. *Journal of Occupational Science*, *27*(2), 193–203. https://doi.org/10.1080/14427591.2020.1732228

Given, L. M. (Ed.). (2008). *The SAGE encyclopedia of qualitative research methods*. SAGE. https://dx.doi.org/10.4135/9781412963909

Guba, E. G., & Lincoln, Y. S. (1994). Competing paradigms in qualitative research. In N. K. Denzin & Y. S. Lincoln (Eds.), *Handbook of qualitative research* (pp. 105–117). SAGE.

Hammell, K. W. (2006). *Perspectives on disability and rehabilitation: Contesting assumptions, challenging practice*. Churchill Livingstone/Elsevier.

Hammell, K. W. (2011). Resisting theoretical imperialism in the disciplines of occupational science and occupational therapy. *British Journal of Occupational Therapy*, *74*(1), 27–33. https://doi.org/10.4276/030802211X129476860936

Hasselkus, B. R. (1997). In the eye of the beholder: The researcher in qualitative research. *Occupational Therapy Journal of Research*, *17*(2), 81–83. https://doi.org/10.1177/15394492970170020

Iwama, M. (2003). Toward culturally relevant epistemologies in occupational therapy. *American Journal of Occupational Therapy*, *57*(5), 58–588. https://doi.org/10.5014/ajot.57.5.582

Lune, H., & Berg, B. L. (2017). *Qualitative research methods for the social sciences* (9th ed.). Pearson.

Manohar, N., Liamputtong, P., Bhole, S., & Arora, A. (2017). Researcher positionality in cross-cultural and sensitive research. In P. Liamputtong (Ed.), *Handbook of research methods in health social sciences* (pp. 1–15). Springer.

Mills, J., & Birks, M. (2014). *Qualitative methodology: A practical guide*. SAGE.

Morrison, R. (2016). Pragmatist epistemology and Jane Addams: Fundamental concepts for the social paradigm of occupational therapy. *Occupational Therapy International*, *23*(4), 295–304. https://doi.org/10.1002/oti.1430

Morse, J. (1994). *Critical issues in qualitative research methods.* SAGE.

Myerhoff, B., & Ruby, J. (1982/1992). A crack in the mirror: Reflexive perspectives in anthropology. In B. Myerhoff (Ed.), *Remembered lives: The work of ritual, storytelling, and growing older* (pp. 307–340). University of Michigan Press.

Nayar, S. (2011). Settling in New Zealand: The wellbeing of Indian immigrant women as shaped by their children. *Diversity in Health and Care, 8*(2), 93–102.

Nayar, S., Hocking, C., & Giddings, L. (2012). Using occupation to navigate cultural spaces: Indian immigrant women settling in New Zealand. *Journal of Occupational Science, 19*(1), 62–75. https://doi.org/10.1080/14427591.2011.602628

Nayar, S., & Stanley, M. (2014). Occupational adaptation as a social process in everyday life. *Journal of Occupational Science, 22*(1), 26–38. https://doi.org/10.1080/14427591.2014.882251

Nayar, S., & Wright St. Clair, V. (2018). Strengthening community: Senior Asian immigrants contributing to New Zealand society. *Journal of Cross-Cultural Gerontology, 33*(4), 355–368. https://doi.org/10.1007/s10823-018-9357-5

Nayar, S., & Wright-St Clair, V. (2020). Multiple cultures – one process: Undertaking a cross cultural grounded theory study. *American Journal of Qualitative Research, 4*(3), 131–145. https://doi.org/10.29333/ajqr/9310

Nicholls, D. (2009a). Qualitative research: Part two – methodologies ... second in a three part series. *International Journal of Therapy and Rehabilitation, 16*(11), 586–592. https://doi.org/10.12968/ijtr.2009.16.12.45433

Nicholls, D. (2009b). Qualitative research: Part three – methods. *International Journal of Therapy and Rehabilitation, 16*(12), 638–647. https://doi.org/10.12968/ijtr.2009.16.11.44939

Ryan, A., Gilroy, J., & Gibson, C. (2020). #Changethedate: Advocacy as an on-line and decolonising occupation. *Journal of Occupational Science, 27*(3), 405–416. https://doi.org/10.1080/14427591.2020.1759448

Schwartz-Shea, P., & Yanow, D. (2020). Intepretivism. In P. Atkinson, S. Delamont, A. Cernat, J. W. Sakshaug, & R. A. Williams (Eds.), *SAGE research methods foundations.* SAGE. https://doi.org/10.4135/9781526421036915455

Shoredike, A., Hocking, C., Pierce, D., Wright-St Clair, V., Vittayakorn, S., Rattakorn, P., & Bunrayong, W. (2010). Respecting regional culture in an international multi-site study: A derived eticmethod. *Qualitative Research, 10*(3), 333–355. https://doi.org/10.1177/1468794109369145

Shoredike, A., & Pierce, D. (2005). Cooking up Christmas in Kentucky: Occupation and tradition in the stream of time. *Journal of Occupational Science, 12*(3), 140–148. https://doi.org/10.1080/14427591.2005.9686557

Thomas, Y., Gray, M., & McGinty, S. (2012). An exploration of subjective wellbeing among people experiencing homelessness: A strengths-based approach. *Social Work in Health Care, 51,* 780–797. https://doi.org/10.1080/00981389.2012.686475

Tuhiwai Smith, L. (2012). *Decolonizing methodologies: Research and indigenous peoples* (2nd ed.). Zed Books.

Wilkerson, J.M., Iantaffi, A., Grey, J. Bockting, W., & Rosser, B.R.S. (2014). Recommendations for internet-based qualitative health research with hard-to-reach populations. *Qualitative Health Research, 24*(4), 561–574. https://doi.org/10.1177/1049732314524635

Willig, C. (2009). *Introducing qualitative research in psychology.* McGraw Hill.

Willis, J. W. (2007). *Foundations of qualitative research: Interpretive and critical approaches.* SAGE.

Wilson, L. (2010). Occupational consequences of weight loss surgery: A personal reflection. *Journal of Occupational Science, 17*(1), 47–54. https://doi.org/10.1080/14427591.2010.9686672

Wright-St Clair, V., Bunrayong, W., Vittayakorn, S., Rattakorn, P., & Hocking, C. (2004). Offerings: Food traditions of older Thai women at Songkran. *Journal of Occupational Science, 11*(3), 115–124. https://doi.org/10.1080/14427591.2004.9686539

Wright St. Clair, V., & Nayar, S. (2018). Late-life Asian immigrants managing wellness through contributing to socially embedded networks. *Journal of Occupational Science, 25*(1), 51–64. https://doi.org/10.1080/14427591.2017.1370607

Wright St. Clair, V., Pierce, D., Bunrayong, W., Rattakorn, P, Vittayakorn, S., Shoredike, A., & Hocking, C. (2013). Cross-cultural understandings of festival food-related activities for older women in Chiang Mai, Thailand, Eastern Kentucky, USA, and Auckland, New Zealand. *Journal of Cross Cultural Gerontology, 28*(2), 103–119. https://doi.org/10.1007/s10823-013-9194-5

Yalmambirra. (2000). Black time … white time: My time … your time. *Journal of Occupational Science, 7*(3), 133–137. https://doi.org/10.1080/14427591.2000.9686476

Additional Resources

Denzin, N., & Lincoln, Y. (Eds.). (2005). *The SAGE handbook of qualitative research* (3rd ed.). SAGE.

Finlay, L., & Gough, B. (2003). *Reflexivity: A practical guide for researchers in health and social sciences.* Blackwell Science.

Patel, S. (2020). *The research paradigm – methodology, epistemology and ontology – explained in simple language.* https://salmapatel.co.uk/academia/the-research-paradigm-methodology-epistemology-and-ontology-explained-in-simple-language/

Patton, M. Q. (2002). *Qualitative research and evaluation methods* (3rd ed.). SAGE.

SLAC. (2022). *The key role of sponsorship.* https://inclusion.slac.stanford.edu/sites/default/files/The_Key_Role_of_a_Sponsorship_for_Diverse_Talent.pdf

The Qualitative Report. (2022). *Where the world comes to learn qualitative research.* www.nova.edu/ssss/QR/qualres.html

3 Connections, Disruptions, and Transformations

Decolonizing Qualitative Research

Isla Emery-Whittington, Lana Draper and Chontel Gibson

We introduce this chapter with a poem called "Decolonisation" by Ambelin Kwaymullina. Ambelin is an Aboriginal writer and illustrator from the Palku people, who belongs to the Pilbara region of Western Australia. The poem highlights the insidious and systematic nature of colonization. It centers decolonization as a journey—a journey embedded in Indigenous sovereignties and born from genuine relationships with local Indigenous peoples.

Decolonisation

> Settler-colonial lands
> will only be decolonised
> when structures of settler-colonialism
> have been replaced
> by structures grown out of respectful
> relationships
> with Indigenous sovereignties
>
> The structures of settler-colonialism
> are everywhere
> in governments
> corporations
> educational institutions
> in every place
> where something was founded
> developed
> sustained
> in the absence of respect
> for Indigenous sovereignties
>
> Decolonisation requires
> that settlers
> continually identify
> challenge
> disrupt
> the structures of settler-colonialism
> including those patterns embedded

DOI: 10.4324/9781003456216-3

in minds and hearts
and in ways of relating
to Indigenous peoples

Decolonisation
is a process
it is journeys
not destinations
a series of transformations
which can only be born out of
and be answerable
to locally based relationships
with the sovereign Indigenous peoples
in whose homelands
settlers live
work
play
   (Kwaymullina, 2020, pp. 15–16)

Background

Colonization is often heralded by research, the oft-cited example in the South Pacific being British Captain James Cook and his crew of market researchers who recorded, measured, counted, and chartered their way around Indigenous territories (L. T. Smith, 2012). Indigenous peoples have responded in a myriad of ways to the multiple and far-reaching impacts of the early researchers and the subsequent settler systems. Indeed, for over 40 years, Indigenous peoples across the globe have created, developed, and implemented explicit and written research that directly engages and transforms colonial legacies in research methodologies, designs, and methods. Indigenous scholars work alongside their communities, either within or outside of colonial institutions, to both analyze and critique 'dominant' paradigms, while also "valuing and revitalizing" (Cull et al., 2018, p. 7) Indigenous ways of knowing, doing, and being.

For occupational scientists and occupational therapists, decolonial research is really an extension of a decolonial approach to everyday life. In settler colonial spaces, especially, everyday life and the occupations that make up the everyday, are sites of struggle. The question 'how can qualitative research be decolonial?' is answered with another question, 'how is your everyday life decolonial?' That is, the spaces you inhabit and cohabit, your commute, your food and medicines, shopping choices, conversations, lecture reading lists, marking rubrics, faculty meetings, clinics, schedules, workshop series, blogs, podcasts, and so on. In this way, decolonial research is not just a good match for occupational scientists and occupational therapists who undertake research; but it is perhaps one of the most important and well-fitted contributions that this profession of occupation aficionados can make.

In addition, colonial harms are already well established, monitored, and reported on in a plethora of ways, while inequity impacts all parts of society (Commission on Social Determinants of Health, 2007; Wilkinson & Pickett, 2010). So then, why is not all research decolonial? We assert that research in the profession is too slow to move away from being a function of coloniality to becoming a tool for equity and justice. Certainly, Indigenous Knowledge production and sharing is beyond coloniality. As discomforting, novel, and uncertain as decolonial research might initially seem—depending on your position—research and every aspect of research is already being decolonized and becoming decolonial.

This chapter aims to center and privilege Indigenous worldviews and decolonial scholarly practices. We, the authors, write in the spirit of collegiality and in solidarity with all researchers who understand the urgency of decolonial approaches and those who still lean in despite discomfort, inconvenience, and sometimes isolation from others in the profession who are yet to undertake a decolonial journey. We now share our positionality as the Indigenous authors of the chapter.

Authors' Positionality

Isla is a Māori cis wahine (woman) from Ngāti Unu, Ngāti Kahu hapū (kinship group, tribe) and uses she/her/ia pronouns. Having completed qualitative research from both Indigenous and non-Indigenous lens I am convinced that decolonial research can displace or embed coloniality. To be curious; to refuse status quo; to carve and create spaces to imagine, wonder, and design research that privileges Indigenous epistemologies, is to engage in decolonial research. I acknowledge and thank the researchers, practitioners, educators, and learners who locate themselves in the struggle to design and enact transformational decolonial research despite risk and backlash.

Lana is a Ngiyampaa winarr (woman) with ancestral ties to Gundabooka Mountain through her Murphy and Wilson family connections. I am cisgender and use she/her pronouns. With client centered work being the foundation of occupational therapy intervention, it makes sense that researchers, therapists, and human beings should be doing better to have Indigenous voices heard, honored, and translated into action. The work to decolonize starts with critical self-reflection and moves towards an evolving state of cultural responsiveness. Working as an occupational therapist for over 20 years across a range of industries, my energies are now focused on moving towards the north star to decolonize the child protection system and to embed Indigenous ways of knowing, doing, and being in all aspects of policy, intervention, and decision making.

Chontel is a Kamilaroi yinarr (woman) with family ties to the Weatherall, Thorne, and Kennedy families. I use she/her pronouns. My positioning in research commenced in childhood. I was nurtured to actively seek out knowledge and to critique it, like uncovering whose truth exists in the spaces that I engaged in. I was encouraged to keep my eyes, ears, and voice open to injustices that unfolded, not just the injustices in front of me, but to injustices that occurred before my time or out of my sight. I learnt more about advocacy from my family and other Indigenous people than what I have learnt at university or any other Western system. It is not surprising that my advocacy is considered unorthodox by some non-Indigenous people who are yet to understand that my work is nothing more than being decolonial in nature.

Indigenous Peoples and Terminology

Amnesty International (n.d.) recognizes over 5,000 Indigenous Peoples globally, who hold over 4,000 languages and dialects, spanning 90 countries. As three Indigenous researchers who chose to study and practice in occupational therapy, we desire to share decolonial approaches from our work and work of other Indigenous people, and to support colleagues to use their research platforms and privilege in ways that disrupt colonialism. Certainly, occupational science and occupational therapy have a unique contribution and framing with regards to oppression (Emery-Whittington, 2021; Johnson & Lavalley, 2021), and Indigenous colleagues have much to offer to that work.

Importantly, the term 'Indigenous' is political, and not universally accepted or used. For example, Chontel does not identify as an Indigenous person within local communities she is connected to as it is not a well-accepted term and carries many connotations; further, if used in certain places it can cause grief and harm. The terms 'Indigenous people' or 'Indigenous peoples' are used when referring to Indigenous communities with some communities and researchers opting to include the 's' on the end of the term Indigenous peoples, to remind readers of the diversity that exists in Indigenous communities. We aim to use terminology that makes sense to us as authors, as well as terminology that is consistent with platformed literature.

To that end, sometimes the word knowledge is capitalized and at times it is not. When the word knowledge is capitalized, we are referring to knowledge/s as a pronoun and as a discrete entity. Indigenous Knowledges are sometimes viewed as an abstract and a 'type' of knowledge, almost a sub-set of expanded but still western notions of knowledge. For some Indigenous peoples, knowledge is not an entity in and of itself; rather, it is woven into the fabric of living. Indigenous Knowledges are not always able to be grasped or understood using a western view of knowledge and, therefore, there are times when we are using the term as a discrete entity without reference to coloniality. Finally, Indigenous Knowledges are a way of life, a science, and context specific.

Coloniality is recognizable by its need to name, delineate, define exactly, and mark progress (especially using time). Hence, decolonial research refrains from applying labels and 'standard' measures of 'progress' and, instead, spends time building trusting relationships, seeking understanding and agreement for names, vocabulary, and language. Indigenous languages are contextual. They are not only related to lands and territories but arise from lands and territories. Therefore, agreements of a shared vocabulary, carefully ascertained at the outset of and throughout the relationship, is a unique opportunity to learn to be in place anew.

The terms decolonization and decoloniality are both used in this chapter. Botswanan scholar Bagele Chilisa (2019) defined decolonization as a process that honors Indigenous people by sharing their voices in a way that promotes Indigenous people's worldviews, values, and beliefs. The central aim is to restore, develop, and maintain cultural practices that were lost or left dormant due to colonial processes (Chilisa, 2019). Pat Dudgeon (2008), a Bardi woman from the Kimberly area in Western Australia, highlighted how a decolonizing standpoint aims to both challenge colonization and creates respectful spaces to highlight cultural differences. Dudgeon added that diversity and exploring the power relationships that exist between the colonizer and colonized is at the heart of that approach. Dudgeon and her peers have gone on to decolonize psychology and center Indigenous psychology in practice, policy, and research. Examples of both decolonizing psychology and centering Indigenous psychology can be found in the following literature: Dudgeon and Walker (2015), Dudgeon et al. (2014), Dudgeon et al. (2023), Milroy et al. (2022), and, finally, Wright et al. (2021).

South African activist scholar, occupational therapist, and occupational scientist Elelwani Ramugondo (2018) has referred to the failure of decolonization efforts in some spaces to move beyond discourse. Decoloniality, she argued, shifts attention and actions to long-term thinking and epistemological concerns whereby decoloniality is, in essence, the 'doing as healing work' aspect of decolonization (Ramugondo, 2018). Either way, decolonization and decoloniality feel whole heartedly different from usual research approaches because of where the research emerges.

Research with Indigenous communities ideally begins within Indigenous communities and the intentional practiced care for them and their lands, as lands and Indigenous communities are one and the same. Serving Indigenous communities and lands is characterized by good relations over time and in place. Being seen and known in communities grows alignment and genuine deep belief in a community's right to epistemological freedom (L. T. Smith, 2012). Hence, research questions that emerge from such shared spaces rarely conform to tidy delineations between qualitative and quantitative research (C. Smith, 2013). Instead, research methods that converge to suit the research questions posed by Indigenous communities are decolonial in approach. For too long, research has been a tool for colonization with many disastrous 'first contact' experiences; therefore, Indigenous communities are rightly wary of researchers from outside the community (L. T. Smith, 2012). Non-Indigenous researchers, who desire to research with Indigenous peoples, would do well to examine and interrogate their positioning alongside trusted mentors, and understand the shape of their contribution to the community's research priorities.

Epistemology, Ontology, Axiology

Epistemology is concerned with the nature of what is known and how knowledge is created. Many, if not most, people construct theories to understand and explain the world, and such epistemological construction draws from the known world and the contexts that hold lifetimes of knowledge (Royal, 2011). However, Western notions, language, and research methods have tended to view Indigenous peoples as 'producers of culture' instead of 'producers of knowledge' (Cooper, 2012). Such colonial viewpoints arose from early ethnographic methods of viewing, 'obtaining,' and interpreting 'culture,' as well as supremacist ideologies that assume knowledge arises only from particular geographies and bodies (L. T. Smith, 2012). In addition, neoliberalism, which is a direct descendent of imperialism, tends to view Indigenous peoples' Knowledges as spaces to find novel, commodifiable resources that cross borders, are chapter-able, and profitable. Hence, understanding Indigenous peoples as active and vital 'producers of knowledge' supports epistemological justice and decolonial research (Cooper, 2012).

Ontology refers to the assumptions of reality or the ways in which people exist and be in the world (Chilisa, 2012; Moreton-Robinson, 2013). For many Indigenous people, growth and maintenance of cultural connections are an essential way of being, occurring, in part, through collaborations with community members. Indigenous people view knowledge as being produced inside relationships and it is the relationship dynamics, as well as cultural connections, that frame what is to be known and how it is to be known (Royal, 2011). Without relationships it is tricky to understand the nature of knowledge and how knowledge is produced. Therefore, relationships are the ethical frameworks that both hold responsibility, and demonstrate value and care, for knowledge. For research purposes, and especially research in spaces where profound damage to Indigenous peoples has occurred, serious attention needs to be given to how multiple relationships can be fostered and respectfully maintained. Certainly, discussions about Indigenous Knowledges are really a discussion about ethical behavior. Indigenous researchers understand that change moves at the speed of trust (Y. Paradies, personal communication, March 24, 2022) and that trust underscores every research relationship, every obligation and responsibility as knowledge bearers and producers.

A key tenet of decolonial research is privileging voices. When it comes to the Australian context, allowing Aboriginal and Torres Strait Islander people to explore, elevate, and voice experiences, knowledge, and understanding in the research process is a core value guiding how research is done (Fredericks, 2008; Nakata, 2007; Rigney, 1999). Axiology refers to the values and beliefs guiding actions or the ways of doing research (Chilisa, 2012; Moreton-Robinson, 2013). Decolonial research allows for Indigenous ways of doing to extend beyond Western research and science understanding of knowledge and research practices. Indeed, Indigenous decolonial studies exist within a paradox of centering epistemologies of our own communities, and the struggle to disrupt western spaces (Cooper, 2012). Hence, research is simultaneously a site of struggle and opportunity, as well as a site of resistance and transformation. Indigenous researchers also bring a sense of responsibility and shared obligation to ensure the research approach is experienced by Indigenous communities as culturally safe and as "a series of transformations" (Kwaymullina, 2020, p. 16).

In settler–colonial nations, epistemological dominance in research is status quo, as seen in the choice of research questions and funding decisions of ethical approval applications (Moewaka Barnes et al., 2009). Indeed, "Māori epistemological and ethical schemata are essentially other and, despite advances and ambiguities, remain add-ons, widely seen as politically forced rather than critical and vital alternatives to the status quo" (Moewaka Barnes et al., 2009, p. 5). Sachindri Wijekoon and Nedra Peters (2022) called for research that is epistemically antiracist while noting that barriers to such research are not small. The two barriers we outline next are unexamined privilege and critical reflexivity as a primarily individualized task.

Privilege is, itself, a formidable barrier to epistemic justices because it shapes what is valued, held, and cared for. For example, the framing and posing of research questions are considered a community or collective-based task for Indigenous communities. Therefore, when ethics committees have approved studies from individuals newly acquainted to centuries and sometimes millennia old collectives, it is highly problematic and signals privilege. Certainly, privilege underscores ethics which is the foundation of good relationships across all aspects of research and, as such, privilege is discussed further throughout the chapter.

The second barrier to epistemic, ontological, and axiological justice is critical reflexivity when undertaken as an individual pursuit. We argue that the benefits of critical reflexivity as sound scholarly practice have been overstated and underutilized. Critical reflexivity has, for too long, been treated as an individual-centric tool (even for social justice efforts) where an individual's ethics, motivations, competencies, and capabilities are examined to various degrees. Locating this task in the individual weakens its power and potential as learnings can easily be put aside for more pressing tasks, moved on from if difficult feelings or tensions arise, or discarded completely when the project is completed. Instead, Indigenous and activist scholars have argued for critical reflexivity that is accountable to teams, groups, and communities, resulting in organized and effective actions (Beagan et al., 2023; Ryan et al., 2020). Amongst researcher groups, Park and Zafran (2018) argued for team reflexivity as a way to hold the various epistemological orientations that necessarily arise within human collectives. Using metaphors to theorize 'epistemological bumps,' researchers were able to deeply understand the ethical, moral, and epistemological orientations that impacted analysis and discussions of findings.

Topics and Questions Best Suited for Decolonial Methodologies

Decolonial approaches necessarily reach far, think deep, and always change an oppressive situation for the better. Topics and questions suited to decolonizing and decolonial methodologies such as Indigenous Standpoint Theory and Kaupapa Māori methodologies are accordingly structural and aim to counter coloniality as an invisible and taken for granted way of doing life. Examining colonial structures, systems, theories, notions, and subsequent techniques for maintaining oppression also suit decolonial methodologies (Marsh et al., 2015; Murrup-Stewart et al., 2022; H. Smith, 2019). For example, Isla is completing research using Kaupapa Māori methodology and the research question is 'In what ways do everyday occupations maintain and transform colonialism?' As well, Indigenous Women's Standpoint Theory, which was developed as a means to exercise Indigenous women's sovereignty in the academy, addresses the privileged relationships of Indigenous women to the nation's sovereignty, underpinning their social situation and considering the process of a colonized history of Australia (Moreton-Robinson, 2013). Certainly, Aboriginal and Torres Strait Islander methodologies, like other Indigenous methodologies, are founded on connections to countries, communities, and ancestors, and reflect cultural protocols (Moreton-Robinson, 2013).

Research that centers Indigenous peoples as knowledge holders and producers (Chilisa, 2019; Geia et al., 2013) while utilizing Indigenous ways of knowing, doing, and being in the design, methods, and analysis, demonstrate a decolonizing methodology. Moreover, questions and topics that recognize and platform Indigenous strengths-based responses to colonialism are good examples of decolonial studies (Gibson, 2020; L. T. Smith, 2012). Research questions that examine systems and structures causing harm, buck the trend of research that determinedly searches for and locates problems and issues within an Indigenous individual and/or collective. Certainly, decolonial research would also be aligned with well-established evidence that social factors determine health (Commission on Social Determinants of Health, 2007) while aiming to directly address those social factors. Finally, Indigenous peoples are diverse—both across Indigenous nations and within Indigenous nations. Therefore, research designs, and topics and questions, that seek to capture bespoke, local, land-based approaches co-developed with the community are fine examples of decolonial approaches.

Recruitment and Sampling

Where a research need arises from within a community, a natural next step for the community is to identify who is to be involved and to what extent. Social norms of encounter, growing, and maintaining relationships ought to guide the recruitment and sampling processes (L. T. Smith, 2012). Indeed, where the community actively guide and feel in control of the study, it is not unusual for recruitment and sampling to occur by way of being told who the researcher must speak to (Moewaka Barnes et al., 2009). As such, snowball sampling is an example of a method that ensures the community is in control of steering towards mandated Knowledge Keepers.

Where the 'community of interest' is not known to the researcher, we strongly suggest some tough questions are worked through. In this kind of scenario, research has the potential to cause lasting harm to Indigenous communities and especially Indigenous advisors and assistants. L. T. Smith (2012) discussed the importance of researcher self-audit; which includes questioning, why you? Are you the best person to support the community's search for knowledge? Why this research question? And why this methodology? In addition, background information, such as who has identified the research need and how they came to that knowledge, is important for the community to assess the rigor and ethics of the research (C. Smith, 2013). Unless specifically invited by the 'community of interest' for research expertise or relationship with the community, it is not a given that research is a priority for the community at that time. We contend that colonial habits die hard, and research with Indigenous communities that is uninvited and benefits the researcher more than the community is unlikely to be decolonial in approach nor lead to transformative benefits. Worse still, it may lead to further harm.

Data Collection

Data collection methods that are decolonizing in nature are obvious in that direct and measurable benefits are experienced and reported by the community because of their engagement with and support of the study. There are many ways that Indigenous researchers and critical allies have co-designed studies that are transformative in nature and lighten the colonial load, so to speak. Examples include data collection processes being designed around the fulfilment of a desired community goal such as writing a children's book of ancient stories and walking ancestral journeys, through to holding gatherings that privilege co-theorizing of a theory, framework, or model. Sound decolonial research design founded on mutually beneficial relationships allows the research process itself to suggest and guide data collection and, in so doing, uphold the data sovereignty of the community.

Kamilaroi woman, Cheree Dean, described yarning as a culturally respectful communication tool which is reliant on relationships and cultural protocols (Dean, 2010). It not surprising that yarning has become a research method of choice for many Indigenous researchers. For example, Dawn Bessarab from the Bardi and Yjindabandi nations in Western Australia; Brigit Ng'andu from Botswana; Aboriginal woman, Bronwyn Fredericks; and Kamilaroi woman, Kyly Mills, all find yarning a flexible, adaptable, and feasible research method to use with Indigenous communities (Bessarab & Ng'andu, 2010; M. Walker et al., 2013). There are six types of yarning identified in research. Bessarab and Ng'andu (2010) identified the first four, including social yarning, research topic yarning, collaborative yarning, and theraputic yarning. M. Walker, Fredericks, Mills, and Anderson (2013) identified a further two types—family yarning and cross cultural yarning. Thus, it is not about simply saying that 'yarning' is being used as a tool for data collection. We encourage researchers to become familiar with the different types of yarning and how to apply them in the research to ensure the intention of the research and the voices of the community are upheld.

Yarning is decolonizing in nature, as it:

- centres Aboriginal ways of knowing, being, and doing,
- promotes Indigenous soveriegnties and Indigenous theorizing
- supports self-determiation, shifting the oppressive nature of Western research

(Walker et al., 2013)

More recently, a team of researchers, including Wiradjuri woman Michelle Kennedy; Noongar woman Siam Maidment; Raglan Maddox, from the Bagumani (Modewa) Clan in Papua New Guinea; and Catherine Chamberlain, a Palawa woman from the Trawlwoolway clan, along with Dawn Bessarab, investigated how researchers apply yarning, and made recommendations for how to report yarning in research articles (Kennedy et al., 2022). If researchers choose yarning as a method, or perhaps even as a methodology, we suggest consideration of these recommendations.

In the next section, we describe the global movement that is Indigenous Data Sovereignty (IDS). This vital topic could equally fit in the 'Rigor and Ethics' section of the chapter as it is broad and encompasses the entire research venture.

Indigenous Cultural Intellectual Property

Indigenous data refer to any knowledge or information, in any format, that are about Indigenous people and how it impacts Indigenous people at an individual and/or collective level (Walters & Carrol, 2021). IDS is founded on "the rights of Indigenous Peoples to control the collection, access, analysis, interpretation, management, dissemination and reuse of Indigenous data" (Walters & Carrol, 2021, p. 3). Eight common principles relating to IDS have been identified by Skye Trudgett, Gamilaroi woman, et al. (2022) using information from Australia, Aoteaora New Zealand, and Canada. These principles are described by way of conversations that, as the chapter authors, we engaged in as part of the process of thinking, discussing, and writing this chapter together, and are bracketed and italicized as they occur.

Decolonial research topics are typically identified, discussed and prioritized by Indigenous collectives (IDS: *Ownership; Sustainability and suitability*) with power and decision-making resting within Indigenous collectives (IDS: *Control*). Holding stewardship of the methodology, collected data and collection processes, analysis methods, and dissemination are demonstrating deep and complex levels of care (IDS: *Custodianship*). This can manifest in Indigenous communities seeking full Intellectual and Cultural Property Rights of all data collected in a research project (IDS: *Ownership*). There are multiple ways in which Indigenous people connect with each other, to country, and to culture (IDS: *Sustainability and suitability*). Therefore, using appropriate ways to ensure research directly and tangibly benefits the community is a basic tenet of decolonial research (IDS: *Access*). In addition, decolonial research includes truth telling and can sometimes be the first time some truths are told (IDS: *Accountable to First Nations; Amplifies voices of First Nations*). Finally, for some Indigenous communities, knowledge and wisdom are not separate from deed nor context; therefore, knowledge needs to be practiced in context with relevant others (IDS: *Relevant and reciprocal; Sustainability and suitability*).

In addition, Janke (2021) proposed an Indigenous Cultural and Intellectual Property (ICIP) Framework consisting of 10 principles specifically designed to provide knowledge holders with control over what, who, how, when, where, and why their Indigenous Knowledge may be used. These ICIP principles are similar to the core principles involved in IDS. ICIP principles, in most instances, do not hold any legal rights in their local/ national jurisdictions. Thus, although some universities are moving towards protecting ICIP and developing policies and procedures to protect ICIP from their own internal intellectual property rights, every researcher should be clear on what their workplace's intellectual property protocols are and any discrepancies with ICIP.

Having clarified how ICIP is viewed in the research institution or workplace, clear, direct conversations with Indigenous key stakeholders about how ICIP rights should be protected are an important next step. There are instances where universities and communities engage legal advice to help clarify their position with regards Indigenous data. For certain, the landscape of claiming and collecting data from Indigenous people is changing, and all researchers conducting Indigenous research are demonstrating best and wise practice by making themselves aware of their local ICIP.

Decolonial approaches value active facilitation of relationships amongst all members of the research, including decisions about the data collection methods. Where an Indigenous researcher is from the community of interest, then 'data collection' can be treated as a mere continuation of often years-long conversation (Gibson et al., 2020a, 2020b). As research is formal business, some formalities in the data collection methods are required to delineate 'data collection moments' (Gibson et al., 2020a, 2020b). Again, trusted relationships built over time go a long way to ensuring safe and transformative research occurs.

Data Analysis

Indigenous occupational scientists and occupational therapists who research with their own communities have begun to develop and implement Indigenous data analysis methods. For example, Chontel's doctoral research, with older Aboriginal people, utilized a framework and concept of data analysis that had been discussed and agreed with community at the very beginning of the research (Gibson et al., 2020a, 2020b). In addition, thematic analysis was adapted to center and value older Aboriginal people's voices and perspectives across the entire research journey (Gibson et al., 2020a, 2020b). Wiradjuri and Bundjalong woman Ashley Ryan conducted an occupational therapy honors research, using Indigenous Standpoint to provide the foundation of a decolonizing document analysis (Ryan et al., 2020). Georgina Davis (Ngā Puhi, Ngāi Tai, Ngāti Porou) utilized a Kaupapa Māori (Māori philosophical) framework of Pū-Rā-Ka-Ū, which drew on traditional Māori Mātauranga (knowledges) to frame and scaffold student stories of Māori occupational therapists (Davis & Came, 2022).

These decolonial approaches exemplify how Indigenous researchers and communities centered across the entire project bring both scientific and cultural rigor. In addition, the data analysis processes show how Indigenous researchers connect key pieces of information in the data. For Indigenous communities, rigor and ethics in data analysis is about discerning which connections and relationships amongst and between data are important to highlight and share widely, and which are held more closely. Similarly, Indigenous researchers can discern which 'data' are not meant for inclusion in the research, versus stories and knowledge shared to build relationships.

Rigor and Ethics

Ethics—principles and practices—are not universal; yet, they are often treated as if they are. Just as every society theorizes and produces knowledge, so too does every society have ethical guidelines and processes for the production, sharing, and safe storage of knowledge. However, as for many aspects of colonial life, western research ethics guidelines and processes are treated as universal research ethics no matter the country, peoples, jurisdiction. As aforementioned, ethical approaches are informed by epistemology and worldview; and for Indigenous peoples, often our origin stories guide who we are to one another and nature (C. Smith, 2013). This means that research ethics are—as in life—about connection and responsibility to each other (Cram & Kennedy, 2010). In this way, ethical behavior is closely linked to identity and contribution to the wider social group and is, therefore, always in play. For example, practices of anonymity in research can clash directly with communities that wish to have their contribution accurately remembered to them. In contrast, some communities may use the research to share their stories that they cannot share in families or communities; as such, anonymity should be upheld. At times, varied approaches are put down to 'cultural difference' or individual personality, rather than different sets of ethics being accommodated as best as can be.

Founded upon western notions of ethics, many research ethics committees are shaped by local, historical research misdeeds and institution (neo-liberal) guidelines, especially regarding resourcing, and sometimes Indigenous or 'minority group' interests (Moewaka Barnes et al., 2009). The latter voices tend to also number in the minority so can be easily outnumbered in matters of vote. Thus, ethics approval from research ethics committees is by no means a signal of researcher ethical behavior. Like critical reflexivity, the onus and responsibility for ethical behavior is with an individual or team that rarely has a feedback loop of accountability to the community built into the study. It is not unusual for negotiation and education of ethics committees to ensure that all sets of ethics are being considered as part of a study's application, not just western ones (Moewaka Barnes et al., 2009). Too often, the realization that Indigenous involvement is required for ethical approval comes long after the point where a meaningful shared ethical process can be co-created. In these instances, it is almost a guarantee that the 'ethical' approach employed is exclusively a colonial one. Further, as much as western ethical approval might be gained, it is not a given that the research designed along 'usual' colonial lines is safe or decolonial.

Recognizing that working well with communities takes time, ethics applications might even factor in and reflect extra time across all documentation, not just proposals. Such applications that have accounted for the time needed to build and nurture trusting relationships with communities, are demonstrating decolonizing approaches. Where studies do not explicitly address needs of Indigenous or any historically excluded communities, it is tempting to assert that particular decolonial considerations are not necessary. In these cases, we would argue for deep consideration of why research time and funding, in this day and age, are not addressing the needs of historically excluded communities facing growing inequities, given the well-established evidence of need.

Certainly, there are a number of bespoke, contextual, and clever publications to guide ethical research with Indigenous peoples. In Aotearoa New Zealand, the Health Research Council published *Te Ara Tika guidelines for Māori research ethics: A framework for researchers and ethics committee members* (Hudson et al., 2010). The authors noted that the United Nations Declaration on the Rights of Indigenous Peoples guides the ethical framework and intellectual property concerns of all studies related to Indigenous research in Aotearoa New Zealand. Building on Te Ara Tika, the SHORE Whariki Research Institute at Massey University has explored the role of privilege when it comes to research and research ethics (Borell, 2014; Moewaka Barnes et al., 2009). In some jurisdictions, Indigenous specific ethics committees exist to guide and uphold Indigenous ethics in research while providing sound feedback.

To acknowledge that there are multiple sets of ethics in play and to move between, understand, and value each, is absolutely the role of occupational scientists and occupational therapists. Ethics are constructed from within societies and put into practice—or not—every day. Moreover, research is formal business, so great care is required; and, without experience, situations can quickly become culturally unsafe and unethical. For some non-Indigenous academics, embarking on research involving Indigenous peoples is the first time they are learning about Indigenous knowledge systems or sets of ethics, let alone having a requirement and expectation to design and conduct ethical research. Hence, one of the most ethical practices that non-Indigenous researchers can undertake when considering research with Indigenous communities is to question oneself, including one's motivation, skills, and expertise (C. Smith, 2013; L. T. Smith, 2012)—see Textbox 3.1.

Textbox 3.1   Questions to Ask Oneself When Considering Research with Indigenous Communities

- Who am I in relation to this work?
- Why me, and why now?
- Why in this way?

Supporting rigor in research is knowing one's social positioning. Social positioning necessitates a critical self-awareness and speaking out loud, and in text, one's motivations for engaging with the research. Knowing one's privilege, identities, and epistemological orientations aligns and supports critical reflexivity. More recently, researchers' positionality is becoming an expected part of sound academic and scholarly conduct. The number of thoughtful and meaningful examples of non-Indigenous people sharing their positioning can be leaned into when crafting and shaping positioning statements (see Additional Resources section). Social positioning statements must be emotionally honest, ring true, be updated frequently, and clarify authority and relationships to the communities of interest. Refusal and hesitation to engage in understanding one's social positioning needs careful management, as social positioning is often the first building block for trustworthiness and any absence might indicate hidden agendas. Lerner (2022) argued that it is necessary to understand "how a culture of 'whiteness'" (p. 605) influences ways of knowing, doing, and being; but also, how quiet complicity in systems perpetuates reproduction of oppressive social determinants of health.

We have sometimes been asked, 'Can non-Indigenous peoples lead decolonial research?' This really depends on the context and wishes of the Indigenous community and relationships of the researcher to their privilege and social positioning. Either way, it is always fitting that non-Indigenous peoples use their influence, platforms, and privileges to tightly scaffold the research, whether or not in the position of research lead.

For Indigenous researchers, often the ethical equation being worked out is both 'what do I need to know and do that is ethical' and 'in what ways could my conduct reflect on my family, tribe, and elders beyond the end of this project?' Importantly, Indigenous researchers are aware that health, career, and standing in the community can be impacted by ethical conduct during research (L. T. Smith, 2012). It is a long-standing understanding in Indigenous communities that formal qualifications, titles, and power within a university or profession are meaningless unless, of course, researchers can connect with community. Despite, and in spite of, the terrain of the neoliberal academy, Indigenous researchers strive to innovate and implement safe, meaningful, and transformative research with their communities and beyond (Borell, 2014; Cram & Kennedy, 2010).

Best Practice

Best practice is about consensus on whatever is the best thing to do in a given context and time. Often best practice includes resource efficiencies like human resource, time, and money which, in decolonial contexts, can be detrimental, given the allocation of human resource is paramount for building effective and long-lasting relationships with Indigenous people. Therefore, best practice with regards to decolonial research must be agreed, co-developed, and sustained for its local context as projects in decoloniality in the metropole are wildly different compared to, for example, an ex-colony. We can use the recent drive to decolonize occupation studies curricula. In an imperial nation, for instance, there will not be a need to necessarily design and implement social justice projects that support theorizing and praxis of reparations and landback. But reparations and landback must be core and central to decolonizing and social justice curricula in ex-colonies. Furthermore, it is not uncommon to hear about wise practice as opposed to best practice in Indigenous research. Wise practice, as conceptualized by Goodfellow (2003), is about making ethical and philosophical choices, and doing so with your partners. Choices then result in actions which, in a decolonial context, need to be transformative by nature.

Wise and best practice regarding decolonial methodologies encompasses good relations nurtured and maintained over time, through adversity or difficulty, and with measurable and direct benefits to Indigenous communities. Giving due recognition of labor and skill is a great example of good relations being nurtured and strengthened. Crucially, wise and best practice of decolonial research is about where power and control sit. Figure 3.1 is an image of a continuum of control of research and is written from the perspective of Indigenous power and control. The purpose of the continuum is to help occupational science and occupational therapy researchers to gauge the level of power and control that research can and does afford. The presence of Indigenous peoples in research alone is not a fair representation of the experience of cultural safety, antiracism, nor transformation. Mere presence is not control, mere mention is not engagement; and it is our experience that researchers have celebrated minor representation as a reflection on themselves as opposed to the benefits for community. In addition, we encourage all researchers to use a suitable method for upholding IDS in their own research projects.

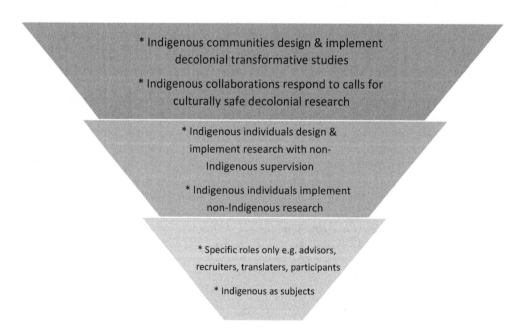

Figure 3.1 A continuum of Indigenous control in occupational science and occupational therapy research. Author created.

Colonization severs ties to Indigenous Knowledges through cultural genocide and the implementation of policies and practices that displace Indigenous cultural identity (Short, 2016; Van Krieken, 1999). Indigenous cultures and knowledges have been passed on from generation to generation with a level of fidelity that existed before the establishment of Western civilization. Vital knowledge about medicines, agriculture, food harvesting, ecology, biodiversity, cosmology, and technology has been developed and maintained through oral narrative and a 'practice-base' that has seen the Aboriginal culture survive for 60,000 years (Charles, 2020). In this way, knowledge holders are the knowledge implementers, which is the community, and this means that knowledge cannot be amassed for the purpose of positioning individuals with power over others.

Best practice requires long term commitment to relationships and for Indigenous communities this means community-led, land-based research design. In addition, due to the high value placed on facilitating good relationship with community in their contexts, where tension or conflict arises in research it is important to understand causes from multiple perspectives. Sometimes Indigenous researchers are called on to help repair and rebuild relationships that have gone awry between Indigenous communities and non-Indigenous researchers (Moewaka Barnes et al., 2009). We strongly encourage non-Indigenous researchers to stay with the tension, work through any issues of privilege and power, and refrain from seeking alternative (perhaps more palatable) Indigenous perspectives. Staying with tension includes the full expectation of it, agreeing early in the relationship how tension is perceived by each person and then agreeing how it might be navigated together. For some Indigenous communities, feelings, like love, are also expressed by impassioned work and expression. Hence, what can sometimes be perceived as tension, may be a usual and expected part of engagement in a crucially important project.

Application to Occupational Science

Because of the structural and systems level perspective, and reach of decolonial methodologies and approaches, many decolonial studies span both foundational knowledge (occupational science) and application to therapeutic practice. Therefore, some of the examples of decolonial studies mentioned in the current section also apply to the following section and vice versa. Importantly, there is a correlation between colonial institutions' infrequent and slow uptake of decolonial research and low numbers of decolonial studies in occupational science and occupational therapy. For example, Isla used a decolonial methodology and methods to develop a theory and practice model; yet, completed her study outside of occupation studies training programs. This situation speaks directly to cultural safety, capacity, and expertise of training programs across the profession to nurture and grow decolonial research. Bridging the gaps between health care needs of Indigenous peoples and training programs is exactly why decolonial methodologies and research are needed.

Indigenous occupational science and occupational therapy scholars are developing and/or identifying theories and processes they use to decolonize research. Elelwani Ramugondo (2015) developed the theoretical framework occupational consciousness, whereby everyday doing is potentially a liberating response to oppressive social structures. Isla examined links between colonization and occupation through the theorizing of occupational stages of colonization and highlighted how everyday business of occupational scientists and occupational therapists is tied up with colonization (Emery-Whittington, 2021). Alejandro Guajardo Cordoba, Frank Kronenberg, and Elelwani Ramugondo (2015) illustrated how the historical context of occupational therapy creates a contemporary space for exclusion, individualistic views of human occupations, and a lack of inclusion for diverse ways of knowing being and doing.

Application to Occupational Therapy

Carly Hunter and Tara Pride (2021) examined a popular occupational therapy model and demonstrated how white power and privilege is enacted in everyday language of occupational therapists. Indeed, health care is underpinned by historical inequities that perpetuate institutional racism resulting in inequitable health care for Indigenous people (Hunter & Pride, 2021). However, decolonial research methodologies and approaches can identify "how, where and when racism occurs within occupational therapy's structures" (Ahmed-Landeryou et al., 2022, p. 14). Decolonial research methodologies and approaches can also carve space for Indigenous theorizing and innovation (H. Smith, 2019). For example, Ramugondo's (2015) aforementioned research examined occupational consciousness and human occupation within the constructs of "occupational possibilities, occupational choice, occupational apartheid, and collective occupation" (p. 488). Further, her decolonial research expanded the way everyday acts could be constructed to decolonize systems that preserve an imbalance of power that favors the non-Indigenous (Ramugondo, 2015).

Because decolonial approaches are still fledgling across the profession, the role of the decolonial researcher frequently and necessarily extends beyond research into advocacy, promotion, and antiracist praxis. Guajardo et al. (2015) listed six key steps that could support institutional reflexivity for occupational therapy, which we believe are also relevant for occupational science: Step 1) Centering communities that are ostracized and/or excluded in occupational science (and societies more broadly). Noting, that the process of centering will lend itself to uncovering the plurality of life. Step 2) Disrupting dominant ways of thinking, including epistemologies, ontologies, and axiologies. Step 3) Confronting pragmatic biases, such as the inability to imagine that plurality of life and science exist. Step 4) Tapping into historical existence, including the ongoing act of colonization and racism, to ensure that the institution and its practices are relevant for communities, including those ostracized by the profession and/or society. Step 5) Moving beyond the single story; and, finally, Step 6) Challenging institutional monoculturalism, which we believe involves taking an anti-racist praxis. Indeed, the decolonizing literature and now the anti-racist literature in occupational therapy contributes to sophisticated approaches that expand, deviate from, and/or strengthen occupational therapy practices.

Critiquing Literature

Indigenous researchers have created and shared standards for appraisal of decolonial and transformative research. In Australia, Ferguson et al. (2023) illustrated two tools to support co-design and a strength-based approach in their research. The first such tool is the Lowitja Institute's Research for Impact Tool, which provides a process for planning, implementing, translating, and evaluating research with Aboriginal and Torres Strait Islander peoples. Second, the Centre of Research Excellence in Aboriginal Chronic Disease Knowledge Translation and Exchange Tool (CREATE Tool) includes checking that communities chose if, when, and how to engage in Indigenous research, set research priorities, and directed research approaches and methods (Ferguson et al., 2023). Although both tools can be used by researchers to plan their research with Indigenous peoples, they can also be used to critique the literature. For example, the CREATE Tool lists 14 questions (CREATE, 2023; Harfield et al., 2020), which are highlighted in Table 3.1. The CREATE Tool has been used to assess the cultural integrity of Indigenous research (c.f. Biles et al., 2022; Esgin et al., 2023).

Table 3.1 Questions from the CREATE Tool

Question	Yes	Partially	No	Unclear
1 Did the research respond to a need or priority determined by the community?				
2 Was community consultation and engagement appropriately inclusive?				
3 Did the research have Aboriginal and Torres Strait Islander research leadership?				
4 Did the research have Aboriginal and Torres Strait Islander governance?				
5 Were local community protocols respected and followed?				
6 Did the researchers negotiate agreements in regard to rights of access to Aboriginal and Torres Strait Islander peoples' *existing* intellectual and cultural property?				
7 Did the researchers negotiate agreements to protect Aboriginal and Torres Strait Islander peoples' ownership of intellectual and cultural property *created* through the research?				
8 Did Aboriginal and Torres Strait Islander peoples and communities have control over the collection and management of research materials?				
9 Was the research guided by an Indigenous paradigm?				
10 Does the research take a strengths-based approach, acknowledging and moving beyond practices that have harmed Aboriginal and Torres Strait Islander peoples in the past?				
11 Did the researchers plan and translate the findings into sustainable changes in policy and/or practice?				
12 Did the research benefit the participants and Aboriginal and Torres Strait Islander communities?				
13 Did the research demonstrate capacity strengthening for Aboriginal and Torres Strait Islander individuals?				
14 Did everyone involved in the research have opportunities to learn from each other?				

Source: (CREATE, 2023; Harfield et al., 2020) Author created

In addition, Canadian Indigenous and activist scholars Angie Phenix, Kaarina Valavaara, and Gayle Restall have applied ethical research considerations of local Indigenous communities to guidelines for publication in the *Canadian Journal of Occupational Therapy* (Restall et al., 2019). These guidelines are decolonial because the social positioning is upfront and evident; that is, they are unapologetically Canadian. Instead of universal suggestions or subtle nods to being *the* standard, Phenix and colleagues have stated and claimed their standard as theirs, thus leaving room for international colleagues to work out for themselves and their contexts, their own guidelines.

Reflections and Journeys

As a trio of Indigenous researchers who have studied, practiced, taught, and researched in occupational science and occupational therapy, we have reflected in depth about our journeys and connections during the collaboration for writing this chapter. Two aspects of this journey became apparent. First, that Indigenous and non-Indigenous researchers' roles and responsibilities in relation to qualitative research share some similarities as well as some important differences. We have been both terrified by unexamined privilege and greatly heartened by the critical actions of past colleagues' processes and relationships to research. Second, that we use this opportunity of writing together to fashion our various highlights and lowlights as Indigenous researchers to explicate actionable decolonial steps that researchers can take based on our collective reflections and journeys to date (see Table 3.2).

Conclusion

Privilege is knowing what is the right thing to do, knowing what persons most in need require, and then doing something else, with impunity. But a rarely noted drawback to privilege is that skills, knowledge, and expertise in doing what is right by and with the most needed, are kicked down the path and left for the next generation of scholars, learners, and researchers to address. Decoloniality is saying, in my lifetime and my career, and especially in my research, I will do my best to make this world better for future generations. Decolonial research is, after all, really just an extension of decolonial study practices and, more broadly, knowledge seeking, holding, and sharing.

Certainly, every time Indigenous peoples choose and stay in the discipline of occupational science and the profession of occupational therapy it is a time for celebration. Celebration is warranted because Indigenous peoples are community minded, with epistemological advantage that expands the boundaries of both occupational science and occupational therapy. Epistemological advantage is being able to live with paradox, with more than one 'truth' simultaneously (i.e., that both Māui and Grandmother Spider brought fire to the world). Epistemological advantage means that knowledge is understood to be from somewhere, from someone, and for good reason. Understanding knowledge 'as context' and that centuries-old wisdom dwells in context is not dissimilar from the aims of qualitative research. However, qualitative research occurs in the global context of knowledge as profit and power. Knowledge 'as context' can still be the nourishment from ancestors carefully honed and handed down as it always was. However, colonial contaminants need to be anticipated and reckoned with in the careful design and caring implementation of decolonial qualitative research.

Table 3.2 Roles and responsibilities of researchers in Indigenous research

Indigenous researchers	Non-Indigenous researchers
• Always center Indigenous ways of knowing being and doing. • Continue to grow and strengthen connections in your communities. • Make seeking advice from community and senior Indigenous researchers routine. • Grow critical consciousness and strengthen your own cultural ways of doing, knowing and being. • Gather regularly with other Indigenous researchers studying different topics. • Understand how internalized oppression maintains colonial harm. • Guard cultural knowledge. • Build your method if the best one for your research doesn't exist. • Identify critical allies and co-conspirators. • Avoid being 'collected.'	• Listen to Indigenous advice, especially when you have requested it. • Seek Indigenous advice from the correct places, not the easy places. • Find a senior researcher who can help you reflect on white power and privilege as a researcher. • Understand and grow language of decoloniality. • Understand that until trust is established, for some Indigenous people, you represent trauma and harm. • Check before using language or any cultural knowledge– preferably do not use unless asked by Indigenous people to do so. • Publish with and cite Indigenous researchers. • Follow guidance carefully for working with Indigenous Knowledges.

Responsibilities of both Indigenous and non-Indigenous researchers

• Find and map your internalized oppression and racism and make plans to manage every time they are noticed.
• Know your own cultural identity and how that informs the way that you work and connect with people, country, and history.
• Know what you are good at, know your sphere of influence and what you can contribute.
• Anticipate that collective and individual trauma can resurface as part of decolonizing process.
• Understand the flipside of historical trauma (i.e., historical privilege).
• Let emotions guide connection to understanding filters.
• Explore and move through discomfort—act—reflect—act.
• Ensure transformative actions occur during and beyond the research.
• Find or start a trusted affinity and/or antiracism group that balances support *and* accountability.
• Remember that good intentions rarely equate to just actions, but just actions spark just actions.
• Think and plan big and long projects that can care for Nature.

Author created

References

Ahmed-Landeryou, M. J., Emery-Whittington, I., Ivlev, S. R., & Elder, R. (2022). Pause, reflect, reframe: Deep discussions on co-creating a decolonial approach for an antiracist framework in occupational therapy. *Occupational Therapy Now*, 25, 14–17. www.caot.ca/document/7758/OT%20Now_Mar_22.pdf

Amnesty International. (n.d.). *Indigenous peoples rights are human rights.* Retrieved March 12, 2023, from www.amnesty.org/en/what-we-do/indigenous-peoples

Beagan, B. L., Bizzeth, S. R., Pride, T. M., & Sibbald, K. R. (2023). Racism in occupational therapy: "It's part of who we are …" *British Journal of Occupational Therapy*, https://doi.org/10.1177/03080226231153345

Bessarab, D., & Ng'Andu, B. (2010). Yarning about yarning as a legitimate method in Indigenous research. *International Journal of Critical Indigenous Studies*, 3(1), 37–50. https://doi.org/10.5204/ijcis.v3i1.57

Biles, B., Biles, J., Friere, K., Deravin, L., Lawrence, J., & Yashadhana, A. (2022) Appraising community driven health research with Aboriginal and Torres Strait Islander communities: A scoping review using the Aboriginal and Torres Strait Islander Quality Appraisal Tool. *Health Promotion International*, 37(5), daac077. https://doi.org/10.1093/heapro/daac077

Borell, B. (2014). When the marginalised research the privileged: One Māori group's experience. *International Journal of Critical Indigenous Studies*, 7(2), 1–11. https://doi.org/10.5204/ijcis.v7i2.112

Centre for Research of Excellence in Aboriginal Chronic Disease Knowledge Translation and Exchange (CREATE). (2023). *Introducing the CREATE tool.* CREATE. https://create.sahmri.org/create-critical-appraisal-tool/

Charles, J. A. (2020). The survival of Aboriginal Australians through the harshest time in human history: Community strength. *International Journal of Indigenous Health*, 15(1), 5–20. https://doi.org/10.32799/ijih.v15i1.33925

Chilisa, B. (2012). *Indigenous research methodologies.* SAGE.

Chilisa, B. (2019). *Indigenous research methodologies* (2nd ed.). SAGE.

Cooper, G. (2012). Kaupapa Maori research: Epistemic wilderness as freedom? *New Zealand Journal of Educational Studies*, 47(2), 64–73.

Cram, F., & Kennedy, V. (2010). Researching with whānau collectives. *Mai Review*, 3(1), 1–12.

Commission on Social Determinants of Health. (2007). Achieving health equity: From root causes to fair outcomes. *The Lancet*, 370(9593), 1153–1163. https://doi.org/10.1016/S0140-6736(07)61385-3

Cull, I., Biin, D., Simcoe, J., Erickson, M., Hancock, R. L., McKeown, S., Pidgeon, M., & Vedan, A. (2018). *Pulling together: A guide for front-line staff, student services, and advisors.* BCcampus.

Davis, G., & Came, H. (2022). A pūrākau analysis of institutional barriers facing Māori occupational therapy students. *Australian Occupational Therapy Journal*, 69(4), 414–423. https://doi.org/10.1111/1440-1630.12800

Dean, C. (2010). A yarning place in narrative histories. *History of Education Review*, 39(2), 6–13. https://doi.org/10.1108/08198691201000005

Dudgeon, P. (2008). Empowering research with Indigenous communities. *Ngoonjook: A Journal of Australian Indigenous Issues*, 32, 8–26.

Dudgeon, P., Milroy, H., & Walker, R. (Eds.). (2014). *Working together: Aboriginal and Torres Strait Islander mental health and wellbeing principles and practice.* Commonwealth of Australia.

Dudgeon, P., Bray, A., & Walker, R. (2023). Mitigating the impacts of racism on Indigenous wellbeing through human rights, legislative and health policy reform. *Medical Journal of Australia*, 218(5), 203–205. https://doi.org/10.5694/mja2.51862

Dudgeon, P., & Walker, R. (2015). Decolonising Australian psychology: Discourses, strategies, and practice. *Journal of Social and Political Psychology*, 3(1), 276–297. https://doi.org/10.5964/jspp.v3i1.126

Emery-Whittington, I. G. (2021). Occupational justice—Colonial business as usual? Indigenous observations from Aotearoa New Zealand: La justice occupationnelle: Sous régime colonial comme d'habitude? Observations d'autochtones d'Aotearoa en Nouvelle-Zélande. *Canadian Journal of Occupational Therapy*, *88*(2), 153–162. https://doi.org/10.1177/00084 174211005891

Esgin, T., Macniven, R., Crouch, A., & Martiniuk, A. (2023). At the cultural interface: A systematic review of study characteristics and cultural integrity from twenty years of randomised controlled trials with Indigenous participants. *Dialogues in Health*, *2*, Art. 100097. https://doi. org/10.1016/j.dialog.2023.100097

Ferguson, M., Tonkin, E., Brimblecombe, J., Lee, A., Fredericks, B., Cullerton, K., Mah, C. L., Brown, C., McMahon, E., & Chatfield, M. D. (2023). Communities setting the direction for their right to nutritious, affordable food: Co-design of the remote food security project in Australian Indigenous communities. *International Journal of Environmental Research and Public Health*, *20*(4), 2936. https://doi.org/10.3390/ijerph20042936

Fredericks, B. (2008). Researching with Aboriginal women as an Aboriginal woman researcher. *Australian Feminist Studies*, *23*(55), 113–129. https://doi.org/10.1080/08164640701816272

Geia, L. K., Hayes, B., & Usher, K. (2013). Yarning/Aboriginal storytelling: Towards an understanding of an Indigenous perspective and its implications for research practice. *Contemporary Nurse*, *46*(1), 13–17. https://doi.org/10.5172/conu.2013.46.1.13

Gibson, C. (2020). When the river runs dry: Leadership, decolonisation and healing in occupational therapy. *New Zealand Journal of Occupational Therapy*, *67*(1), 11–20.

Gibson, C., Crockett, J., Dudgeon, P., Bernoth, M., & Lincoln, M. (2020a). Sharing and valuing older Aboriginal people's voices about social and emotional wellbeing services: A strength-based approach for service providers. *Aging & Mental Health*, *24*(3), 481–488. https://doi.org/10.10 80/13607863.2018.1544220

Gibson, C., Dudgeon, P., & Crockett, J. (2020b). Listen, look & learn: Exploring cultural obligations of Elders and older Aboriginal people. *Journal of Occupational Science*, *27*(2), 193–203. https://doi.org/10.1080/14427591.2020.1732228

Goodfellow, J. (2003). Practical wisdom in professional practice: The person in the process. *Contemporary Issues in Early Childhood*, *4*(1), 48–63. https://doi.org/10.2304/ciec.2003.4.1.6

Guajardo, A., Kronenberg, F., & Ramugondo, E. L. (2015). Southern occupational therapies: Emerging identities, epistemologies and practices. *South African Journal of Occupational Therapy*, *45*(1), 3–10. https://doi.org/10.17159/2310-3833/2015/v45no1a2

Harfield, S., Pearson, O., Morey, K., Kite, E., Canuto, K., Glover, K., Gomersall, J. S., Carter, D., Davy, C., Aromataris, E., & Braunack-Mayer, A. (2020). Assessing the quality of health research from an Indigenous perspective: The Aboriginal and Torres Strait Islander quality appraisal tool. *BMC Medical Research Methodology*, *20*(1), 79. https://doi.org/10.1186/s12874-020-00959-3

Hudson, M., Milne, M., Reynolds, P., Russell, K., & Smith, B. (2010). *Te Ara Tika: Guidelines for researchers on health research involving Māori*. Health Research Council of New Zealand. www.hrc.govt.nz

Hunter, C., & Pride, T. (2021). Critiquing the Canadian model of client-centered enablement (CMCE) for indigenous contexts. *Canadian Journal of Occupational Therapy*, *88*(4), 329–339. https://doi.org/10.1177/00084174211042960

Janke, T. (2021). *True Tracks: Respecting Indigenous knowledge and culture*. University of New South Wales Press.

Johnson, K. R., & Lavalley, R. (2021). From racialized think-pieces toward anti-racist praxis in our science, education, and practice. *Journal of Occupational Science*, *28*(3), 404–409. https://doi. org/10.1080/14427591.2020.1847598

Kennedy, M., Maddox, R., Booth, K., Maidment, S., Chamberlain, C., & Bessarab, D. (2022). Decolonising qualitative research with respectful, reciprocal, and responsible research practice: A narrative review of the application of Yarning method in qualitative Aboriginal and Torres Strait Islander health research. *International Journal for Equity in Health*, *21*(1), 1–22. https://doi. org/10.1186/s12939-022-01738-w

Kwaymullina, A. (2020). *Decolonisation. Living on stolen land*. Magabala Books.

Lerner, J. E. (2022). Social work the 'white way': Helping white students self-reflect on a culture of whiteness in the classroom and beyond. *Social Work Education*, *41*(4), 605–624. https://doi.org /10.1080/02615479.2020.1868422

Marsh, T. N., Cote-Meek, S., Toulouse, P., Najavits, L. M., & Young, N. L. (2015). The application of two-eyed seeing decolonizing methodology in qualitative and quantitative research for the treatment of intergenerational trauma and substance use disorders. *International Journal of Qualitative Methods*, *14*(5). https://doi.org/10.1177/1609406915618018

Milroy, H., Kashyap, S., Collova, J., Mitchell, M., Derry, K. L., Alexi, J., Chang, E. P., & Dudgeon, P. (2022). Co-designing research with Aboriginal and Torres Strait Islander consumers of mental health services, mental health workers, elders and cultural healers. *Australian Journal of Rural Health*, *30*(6), 772–781. https://doi.org/10.1111/ajr.12945

Moewaka Barnes, H., McCreanor, T., Edwards, S., & Borell, B. (2009). Epistemological domination: Social science research ethics in Aotearoa. In D. M. Mertens & P. E. Ginsberg (Eds.), *The handbook of social research ethics* (pp. 442–457). SAGE. https://doi.org/10.4135/9781483348971

Moreton-Robinson, A. (2013). Towards an Australian Indigenous women's standpoint theory. *Australian Feminist Studies*, *28*(78), 331–347. https://doi.org/10.1080/08164649.2013.876664

Murrup-Stewart, C., Atkinson, P., & Adams, K. (2022). Storying ways to reflect on power, contestation, and yarning research method application. *The Qualitative Report*, *27*(3), 777–791. https://doi.org/10.46743/2160-3715/2022.5173

Nakata, M. (2007). *Disciplining the savages: Savaging the disciplines*. Aboriginal Studies Press.

Park, M., & Zafran, H. (2018). View from the penthouse: Epistemological bumps and emergent metaphors as method for team reflexivity. *Qualitative Health Research*, *28*(3), 408–417. https:// doi.org/10.1177/1049732317746379

Ramugondo, E. L. (2015). Occupational consciousness. *Journal of Occupational Science*, *22*(4), 488–501. https://doi.org/10.1080/14427591.2015.1042516

Ramugondo, E. L. (2018). Healing work: Intersections for decoloniality. *World Federation of Occupational Therapists Bulletin*, *74*(2), 83–91. https://doi.org/10.1080/14473828.2018.1523981

Restall, G., Phenix, A., & Valavaara, K. (2019). Advancing reconciliation in scholarship of occupational therapy and Indigenous peoples' health. *Canadian Journal of Occupational Therapy*, *86*(4), 256–261. https://doi.org/10.1177/0008417419872461

Rigney, L.-I. (1999). Internationalization of an Indigenous anticolonial cultural critique of research methodologies: A guide to Indigenist research methodology and its principles. *Wicazo Sa Review*, *14*(2), 109–121. https://doi.org/10.2307/1409555

Royal, C. T. A. (2011). *Wānanga: The creative potential of Mātauranga Māori* (Monograph 4). Mauriora-ki-te-Ao/ Living Universe Ltd. http://www.charles-royal.nz/

Ryan, A., Gilroy, J., & Gibson, C. (2020). #Changethedate: Advocacy as an on-line and decolonising occupation. *Journal of Occupational Science*, *27*(3), 405–416. https://doi.org/10.1080/144 27591.2020.1759448

Short, D. (2016). *Redefining genocide: Settler colonialism, social death and ecocide*. Bloomsbury Publishing.

Smith, C. (2013). Becoming a Kaupapa Māori researcher. In D. M. Mertens, F. Cram, & B. Chilisa (Eds.), *Indigenous pathways into social research: Voices of a new generation* (pp. 89–100). Left Coast Press.

Smith, H. (2019). Whatuora: Theorizing 'new' Indigenous research methodology from 'old' Indigenous weaving practice. *Art/Research International: A Transdisciplinary Journal*, *4*(1), 1–27 https://doi.org/10.18432/ari29393

Smith, L. T. (2012). *Decolonizing methodologies: Research and Indigenous peoples* (2nd ed.). Zed Books.

Trudgett, S., Griffiths, K., Farnbach, S., & Shakeshaft, A. (2022). A framework for operationalising Aboriginal and Torres Strait Islander data sovereignty in Australia: Results of a systematic literature review of published studies. *EClinicalMedicine*, *45*, 101302. https://doi.org/10.1016/j. eclinm.2022.101302

Van Krieken, R. (1999). The barbarism of civilization: Cultural genocide and the 'stolen generations'. *The British Journal of Sociology, 50*(2), 297–315. https://doi.org/10.1111/j.1468-4446.1999.00297.x

Walker, M., Fredericks, B., Mills, K., & Anderson, D. (2013). 'Yarning' as a method for community-based health research with Indigenous women: The Indigenous Women's Wellness Research Program. *Health Care for Women International, 35*(10), 1216–1226. https://doi.org/10.1080/07399332.2013.815754

Walters, M., & Carrol, S. R. (2021). *Indigenous data sovereignty, governance and the link to Indigenous policy*. Routledge.

Wijekoon, S., & Peter, N. (2022). Examining racial, ethnic, and cultural diversity in occupational science research: Perspectives of persons of color. *Journal of Occupational Science*, 1–20. https://doi.org/10.1080/14427591.2022.2119269

Wilkinson, R. G., & Pickett, K. (2010). *The spirit level: Why greater equality makes societies stronger*. Bloomsbury Press.

Wright, M., Getta, A. D., Green, A. O., Kickett, U. C., Kickett, A. H., McNamara, A. I., & O'Connell, M. (2021). Co-designing health service evaluation tools that foreground first nation worldviews for better mental health and wellbeing outcomes. *International Journal of Environmental Research and Public Health, 18*(16), 8555. https://doi.org/10.3390/ijerph18168555

Additional Resources

For examples of social positioning in journal article form see:

Ahmed-Landeryou, M. J. (Ed.). (2023). *Anti-racist occupational therapy: Unsettling the status quo*. Jessica Kingsley Publisher.

Hammell, K. W. (2021). Building back better: Imagining an occupational therapy for a post-COVID-19 world. *Australian Occupational Therapy Journal, 68*(5), 444–453. https://doi.org/10.1111/1440-1630.12760

4 Qualitative Descriptive

A Very Good Place to Start

Mandy Stanley

In this the first methodology specific chapter, I begin with the most exploratory generic approach to qualitative research: qualitative descriptive. It is the least sophisticated approach with regards to epistemological stance as there is no alignment to a particular theoretical orientation. However, just because it is generic and the least theoretically sophisticated do not mistakenly think it is simple! When novice researchers begin their foray into the world of qualitative research this is often the approach chosen as there is possibly a less steep learning curve than some of the methodological approaches that follow in later chapters. However, the elegant simplicity of a quality study belies the thinking and planning required for data collection, analysis, and presentation of the findings.

A descriptive qualitative approach is a good place for novices to 'cut their teeth' with a generic approach to the design and conduct of a qualitative study. Equally, more experienced researchers find the approach meets their needs for a pragmatic design that yields rich data and the ability to reveal taken for granted ideas. Many of the techniques used in descriptive qualitative studies are employed in other methodological approaches, as you will see in later chapters, but with greater attention paid to the theoretical underpinnings of the methodology. In this chapter, I utilize my experience of conducting numerous studies employing a descriptive qualitative methodology, drawing on a funded study with a team of researchers in which we explored older people's perceptions of driverless cars.

I use this particular methodological approach frequently in my own work and with occupational therapy honors and higher degree students. However, often students report their struggle to find literature that guides how to go about planning and conducting a rigorous qualitative descriptive study—a frustration which I share. Therefore, my aim in this chapter is to contribute to the literature on descriptive qualitative methodology and provide guidance to researchers, particularly novices, in utilizing the approach.

Background

According to Strecker and Hitch (2021), the methodology is most often attributed to Sandelowski (2000) after the publication of her article "Whatever happened to qualitative description?". However, in 2010, Sandelowski wrote to clarify that it was not *her* methodology (Sandelowski, 2010); rather, the intent of the 2000 article was to outline the approach. She claimed to have been misinterpreted as she was not arguing that it is purely descriptive without any interpretation: in the act of describing the researcher is already adding interpretation. Thus, the term qualitative descriptive is used to refer to a range of approaches varying in the amount of interpretation in the analysis. Approaches to enacting a qualitative descriptive study could be placed along a continuum of interpretation from

DOI: 10.4324/9781003456216-4

low to high levels of interpretation. My work, and the study referred to in this chapter, is towards the more interpretive (high) end of the continuum. Wherever a study is located along that continuum the level of interpretation needs to be understood by the researcher and made explicit to the reader. The outcome will be a description of the phenomenon studied, with highly interpretive studies providing rich in-depth descriptions.

Sandelowski's intention in writing the 2000 article was to address the issue of researchers stating that they were using methodologies such as grounded theory or narrative or phenomenology, when clearly this was not the case. While this critique was leveled at nursing research, it could equally have applied to occupational science and occupational therapy. Some of the earliest occupational therapy qualitative studies published claim to draw on phenomenology (Kibele & Llorens, 1989) or do not state the research design (Merrill, 1985); however, they appear to be qualitative descriptive studies.

Epistemology, Ontology, Axiology

Qualitative descriptive is a methodological approach commonly used by occupation-focused researchers; yet, it is the least well-articulated in the research texts. While there is no specific philosophy or theory guiding the approach, it is not atheoretical (Braun & Clarke, 2021a), and the occupational science or occupational therapy researcher can look to authors such as Sandelowski (2000) who convincingly argued for the place of qualitative descriptive studies in health research, or Thorne (2013) referring to interpretive description in nursing research, rather than it being considered as 'the poor cousin' to other methodologies with philosophical underpinnings (Neergaard et al., 2009).

Aside from any debates about the amount of interpretation, a qualitative descriptive methodology fits within an interpretive paradigm (Denzin & Lincoln, 2005). The methodology provides a way of studying people in their context and how they make sense of the world with a subjectivist epistemology; that is, that knowledge is filtered through the lens of the researcher. The ontology is relativist (Guba & Lincoln, 2005) where reality is constructed within the human mind such that it is an intangible mental construction which does not exist outside of the person. The research design is an approach which is a good fit for many occupational scientists and occupational therapists who value the perspective of the person with lived experience. The axiology is balanced with the interpreted account ensuring that the participant's experience is foregrounded and can be supported by the data. Consistent with my professional background, I hold the belief that participants are the experts of their own lives and occupational experiences, and I value their perspective.

Author Positioning

In keeping with best practice, before I go any further, I position myself as a qualitative researcher and how I came to the 'driverless cars' study so that the reader has a context for my writing. The university where I was employed at the time had taken a strategic approach to developing research aligned with grand themes and a related funding round in support of those themes. I was invited to join a team submitting a grant application to better understand older people's perspectives on driverless cars. I came to the study with expertise in the use of qualitative research methodologies with older people, a strong clinical background in all aspects of aged care, a passion for researching what enables older people to live well, and very little knowledge of driverless cars. The other members of the research team were engineers and experts in the built environment or transport, and we had an industry partner from the motoring industry with an interest in enabling its members to be mobile within the community. The study had two phases with the first phase utilizing a qualitative descriptive study design and the second phase discrete choice experiments; in this chapter, I will only focus on the first phase.

Topics and Questions Best Suited for Qualitative Descriptive

There is much debate about the place of the literature in a qualitative study and the extent to which a literature review is conducted prior to doing the study. Some authors argue that doing an extensive literature review has too much influence on the data collection and the analysis, so there is a danger that the researcher will find what is already known and not be open to the unknown or unexpected (Creswell, 2007). However, granting bodies and research ethics committees will not approve studies that do not have a review of literature which clearly establishes the need for the proposed study, and a strong rationale for why a qualitative approach is the right choice for the study. Therefore, the literature review is important. The researcher needs to be able to situate their study within the literature and be sensitized to what is already known but be open to new unforeseen or unexpected data.

Gaining 'real' collaboration with the industry partner and 'buy in' to conduct the study with genuine interest and collaboration is facilitated by working on a 'real' problem in the everyday world of the industry partner. In the case of our study, the industry partner was a community motoring organization. When we turned to the literature about older people and driverless cars we found that the perspective of the older person was largely absent, with much of the literature focusing on loss of a driver's license and the implications for community access, and assumptions that older people are reluctant to accept technological advancement. These key points provided a very strong argument for the study, and for using a descriptive qualitative approach. Therefore, the study sought to answer the research question "What are older people's perspectives on driverless cars?". Other examples of research questions from published occupational science and occupational therapy studies are included in Table 4.1.

According to Patton (2002), a qualitative descriptive approach is well suited to program evaluation research. Correspondingly research questions might be: "What do the clients think of this service?" or "What are service users' perspectives?". The aim is to seek the view or perspective of a sample group, such as occupational therapists' descriptions of their occupation based practice in tertiary hospitals (Hess-April et al., 2017) or occupational therapists' perceptions of their participation in different modalities for maintenance of professional currency (Murray & Lawry, 2011). For occupational scientists, the approach

Table 4.1 Examples of research questions studied with a qualitative descriptive methodology

Author	Research question
Hess-April et al. (2017)	What are the perspectives and experiences of occupation-based practice of South African therapists in a tertiary hospital?
Peoples et al. (2021)	How do people with advanced cancer who live at home perceive their quality of life?
McCarthy et al. (2022)	What are the occupational experiences of nonbinary people?

Author created

is useful for very exploratory studies such as "What are the perspectives of people living in rural areas on occupational balance?" or "What are the perspectives of graduate occupational therapy students on time use during the pandemic?" (Werner & Jozkowski, 2022).

Recruitment and Sampling

The researcher can draw on different types of purposive sampling, depending on the topic and question, as well as pragmatics of whom one can access, time, finances, and location. Furthermore, it is important to remember that this type of research does not require a representative sample. Given the broad scope for sampling in this approach, it is important that the researcher provide specific details of the type of sampling used. Traditionally, Patton (2002) had described 15 different approaches to sampling—different types of purposive sampling and the logic behind them—which provide guidance to the researcher about the type of purposive sampling to suit the purpose of their study. In the fourth edition of his seminal text, *Qualitative Research & Evaluation Methods*, Patton (2015) has expanded the choices of sampling approaches to 40 within eight categories of options. Making a considered choice about sampling will help enhance the rigor of the study.

In the driverless car study, we used maximum variation sampling. Our rationale for the decision was that 'older people' are a very large population and they are not a homogenous group. We were looking to explore the variation around the phenomenon of interest. Therefore, we wanted to recruit men and women, as driving is probably a gendered experience; both drivers and non-drivers; a range of geographical locations; and a range of ages. It can be helpful to outline a sampling frame to ensure that any potential sample shows variation in the experience of the phenomenon. For instance, we were not after equal numbers and a sampling frame (see Table 4.2) ensured we attended to all aspects in our recruitment. The older people were not required to have any experience with driverless cars but needed to be able to talk about their perceptions of them.

Table 4.2 Sampling frame for 'driverless car' study

Age	Gender	Driver status	Geographical location
65 years through to 90+	Male Female	Drives own car Drives and uses public transport Non-driver	Metropolitan Hills region Rural area

Author created

It is important also to think about the sites for data collection and sampling in relation to those sites. Guided by purposive sampling, and in consultation with our industry partner, we chose a regional and a rural site for two of the focus groups as information rich sites for the study because of their rapid growth or large numbers of people aged 65 years and over (Council of the Aging South Australia, 2020). The industry partners in each State are large providers of care and services to older people, including retirement living, long-term and community care in their respective States, and were selected using the strategy of typical site purposive sampling, in that they are "not in any major way atypical, extreme, deviant, or intensely unusual" (Patton, 2002, p. 236).

Participants were recruited through advertising in newsletters and flyers as well as using key contacts within each of the industry partner organizations. In total, 60 older people participated in in-depth interviews. Key contacts also recruited support and service providers for the focus groups from within their aged care organizations as well as from the local community. Focus groups were held in both metropolitan and rural areas with approximately ten people attending each group. The rural areas were chosen for being regional centers and having high numbers of older people, with one of those rural areas being known for its reputation as a retirement destination.

Determining sample size is influenced by the pragmatics of the funding available and the size of the population from which the sample can be drawn. Researchers' decisions about the appropriate sample size can be guided by exemplars in the literature of published studies that have undergone peer review drawing on similar populations. The notion of saturation is posited as a guide to sample size; that is, the researcher keeps collecting data until a point where they are not hearing or seeing anything new. Alternatively, it is a point of analytic saturation where analysis does not reveal any new codes, categories, or themes. The researcher needs to be aware that saturation is a contested concept (Braun & Clarke, 2021b) and that it is better to work towards a rich reflexive analysis rather than a point of data redundancy.

Data Collection

The primary sources of data in a qualitative descriptive study are likely to be semi-structured in-depth interviews or focus groups; however, it is also possible to use the methods of observation and document analysis in this approach. Interview questions are broad and open-ended to elicit a rich response, but it is surprising how easy it is to slip back into asking closed questions. Many readers will be familiar with asking focused questions in their work with people to access accurate information in as short a time as possible; however, research interviewing is quite different. One line of questioning I have found to be helpful is to encourage participants to think about someone outside of themselves; for instance, an interview question might be: "If you were talking to your daughter on the phone, how would you describe the service?" It is a good idea to have a concluding question such as "Is there anything I have not asked about with regard to X that you would like to tell me about?" to elicit material that was not anticipated.

The researcher may also benefit from having a store of probing questions at the ready to extend responses and to assist participants to articulate their experience. Examples of probing questions are provided in Textbox 4.1.

Textbox 4.1   Examples of the Types and Format of Probing Questions (Gillham, 2000)

Clarifying: I don't quite understand that, can you explain it to me?
Showing understanding: How did you feel about that?
Justifying: What makes you say that?
Relevance: You've lost me, how do those two things connect?
Asking for an example: What do you mean by …? Can you give me an example?
Extending the narrative: Tell me more about that.
Accuracy: Now, let me see if I've got things in the right order?

Textbox 4.2   Focus Group Question Guide

1 When you think about driverless cars what are some of the thoughts that come to mind?
2 What is appealing to you in thinking about the possibility of a driverless car?
3 What are the reasons why you might want to use a driverless car?
4 If a friend told you that they were planning to use a driverless car as soon as they were available what would be your concerns?
5 What would need to change for driverless cars to be highly appealing to you personally?
6 What information would you need in order for you to consider using a driverless car?
7 Is there anything else about driverless cars that you would like to make comment on or ask questions about?

To keep the focus of an interview on the topic being researched, an interview guide is usually developed (see, for example, Textbox 4.2) and piloted. Inexperienced interviewers will benefit from interview training and observing an interview conducted by a more experienced interviewer before conducting interviews on their own. The emphasis in a qualitative descriptive interview is on the quality of the data that is yielded from the interview rather than consistency, as in essence the interview is a co-construction between the older person and the interviewer. The richness of qualitative data, and I argue the key contribution, lies in that co-construction. As Mishler (1986) contended, the research interview is a joint construction of meaning between the interviewer and the respondent. The setting of an appointment to be interviewed about their views on a particular topic will bring a person to thinking about that topic which they may not have done without being involved in the research study.

The way the questions are phrased and then re-formulated to elicit conversation with the participants, and the responses that are forthcoming, are shaped by the discourses between the interviewer and the participant. People being interviewed often ask if what they are saying is what the researcher is after, implying that researchers have an idea of a correct response. However, it is important to remember that the position of the researcher needs to be one of openness to whatever the participant is prepared to share. Their responses are shaped by the rapport built with the interviewer and by the reactions to what they were saying. Researchers may like to consider planning for a second interview to explore threads within the first interview that were not explored at the time, or to capture any thoughts that the interviewee had after the first interview had been concluded.

Questions for the focus groups are included in Textbox 4.2. The questions for the interview guide drew on the literature and the guide was constructed from my experience as a qualitative researcher to answer our research question. Relevant demographic information are collected at the time such as age, living situation, and self-reported health status to be able to describe the sample in a subsequent report or publication. On conclusion of the focus group or interview, it is good practice to write a reflection about the interview including contextual notes and impressions. When conducting large studies, I use data sheets in either Word documents or Excel spreadsheets to assist in keeping track of a large number of participants that include participant details, the date of the interview, the demographic information, and my reflections.

Each focus group was run by two members of the team with one facilitating and the other observing and making notes. We also had the support of staff from our industry partner. I always have at least one or two people assisting to run a focus group so that someone else is available to support participants in finding the venue (particularly for late comers) and with refreshments.

All focus groups were digitally recorded and transcribed verbatim by professional transcriptionists. There are pros and cons to using a professional to transcribe rather than transcribing data oneself. If researchers do their own transcription the familiarity with the data is greatly increased; however, it can be time-consuming depending on their speed and ability to touch type and having access to technology such as a transcribing kit with a foot pedal or learning to use keyboard shortcuts. For every one hour of recorded interview, it can take three to four hours to transcribe or longer depending on the quality of the recording. The time spent has to be weighed up against the costs of having transcription done professionally as it can be expensive. Davidson (2009) argued that transcription is theoretical and part of the analysis process and identified several issues with utilizing professional transcriptionists, including omission or alteration of words, but also offered suggestions for working with professionals. We ensured that the professional transcriptionists signed a confidentiality agreement and transcribed verbatim, including all the umms, ahs, and laughter, and note where they could not distinguish the text due to more than one person talking at a time or being inaudible. It is tempting to use voice to text apps that are readily available; however, it is important that researchers do due diligence and know the privacy arrangements of the app provider and where data are stored. The quality of the voice transcription is also variable and it may take just as long to correct errors as it does to fully transcribe the interview.

Data Analysis

Analysis is not a straight linear process as might be indicated by the presentation of steps of analysis in reports or publications. Rather, it is an iterative recursive process as will be evident in most of the chapters in this book. Analysis in qualitative descriptive studies draws on generic approaches, and methods for analysis are not as well articulated as analysis approaches for other methodologies. That said, researchers still need to be able to clearly articulate their analytic pathway, including keeping an audit trail of decisions made. There are a range of approaches to analysis which can be placed on a continuum in terms of levels of induction and interpretation. The decision about the choice of analysis approach needs to be in keeping with the overall epistemological and ontological approach taken with the study. At one end of the continuum there is content analysis, through to framework analysis; and at the other end of the continuum a more inductive interpretive approach of reflexive thematic analysis. All approaches involve some process of transcription; familiarization with the data; coding, grouping of like codes, and then collapsing those grouped codes into themes. I will expand on the three common approaches below.

Content Analysis

Content analysis involves examining the data for patterns and trends. Liamputtong (2013) suggested that codes for content analysis are pre-determined which means that the researchers already anticipate what they will find in the data. Content analysis is a pragmatic approach to analyzing text which requires little induction and interpretation. It is more akin to counting or looking at the frequency of certain words and phrases occurring in the data. In my opinion, content analysis is a useful analytical approach for short sections of text; for example, responses to open ended questions on a questionnaire (c.f. Strecker & Hitch, 2021). Having said that, there is not a shared understanding of what content analysis is and some authors will use the term content analysis to describe what I would term thematic analysis. Novice researchers need to be aware of the conflation of terms and to be a critical reader of the published literature.

Framework Analysis

The framework method was developed in the United Kingdom by social researchers in the 1980s (Ritchie & Spencer, 1994). In common with the other approaches to analysis described here, the analysis begins with familiarization and coding (Gale et al., 2013; Goldsmith, 2021). The departure comes at the stage of categorizing codes where the researcher develops an analytical framework which is applied to the data and the data charted into the framework matrix to enable interpretation of the data. The matrix consists of rows which contain the interviewee data (one row per interviewee) and columns for the codes and the cells include the quotes and summarized data. See Goldsmith (2021) for a worked example. The proponents of framework analysis argue that it is a more transparent approach to analysis and that the structure enables the researcher to easily compare data to identify similarities and differences while keeping the data in context.

Some studies will use the literature to generate a list of start codes for analysis but still remain open to the possibility of the data not fitting theses codes and being able to generate new ones. For example, Kosma et al. (2013) examined 37 publications and conducted an analysis using a framework they had constructed from textual analysis of Wilcock's seminal work to ascertain the impact that Wilcock's theoretical work has had within occupational therapy research and practice.

Thematic Analysis

My preference for analyzing data from descriptive qualitative studies obtained through interviews or focus groups is thematic analysis. I believe that it is a missed opportunity to collect rich data to then lose the richness in analysis by using content analysis or even framework analysis. The thematic analysis needs to be inductive moving through a process of coding in layers of abstraction and interpretation. For example, if the outcome of analysis of a study of barriers and facilitators to maintaining physical exercise following a stroke results in a theme called 'barriers' and another theme called 'facilitators,' it is evident that there is very little interpretation and abstraction during analysis.

In recent years, the approach to thematic analysis, first proposed by Braun and Clarke (2006), has been used extensively. There are six clearly articulated steps which offer an appealing structure to the novice or experienced researcher (see Textbox 4.3). In updates of their work, Braun and Clarke (2022) have argued for a more reflexive approach to thematic analysis which reflects developments in their thinking and approach that have occurred over time. Researchers who choose a thematic analysis approach following Braun and Clarke need to be aware of developments and changes and seek later publications. The authors are extremely generous and offer published worked examples that are helpful to people learning the approach as well as teaching materials (refer to extra readings and resources at the end of this chapter).

Textbox 4.3   Six Steps of Analysis

1 Familiarization with the data
2 Generating initial codes
3 Generating themes
4 Reviewing potential themes
5 Defining and naming themes
6 Producing the report

Drawing on my experience as a researcher and a research supervisor, I have identified three key junctures in the analysis process which can pose difficulty for those new to analysis. The first one is when a researcher starts coding and must make decisions about the unit of analysis and what code to assign. The unit for analysis can vary from a few words to a line, to a whole sentence or a whole paragraph. It is whatever makes sense and is covered by the code assigned. There is a temptation when one first starts coding to use abstract conceptual labels. My advice at this first open coding stage is to stay quite close to the participant's words at low levels of abstraction and to not move to a conceptual level too early. For example, the segment of text might say something like "I like to go to coffee with friends, and parties and visiting others," which could be coded with a single word 'social,' which is more like categorizing than coding as 'meeting others for social connection' which still captures some life and richness (refer to Table 4.3).

Table 4.3 Example of open coding of the transcript

Verbatim text	*Open coding*
I've got reservations	*Cautious concern*
because cars regardless of whether they computers and if they can make them hack proof,	*Computers can be hacked*
but the problem is they're programmed by humans.	*Room for human error*
And I don't think any human that I've ever heard of, can consider all the potential circumstances that can arise. And a car may be confronted by a decision that it has to make, for instance, a kid jumps in front of the car, does it stop or does is swerve and hit the oncoming traffic?	*Car has to decide between hitting a child or hitting oncoming traffic*

Author created

The most difficult point in the analysis is the bringing of categories and collapsing into a smaller number of themes. Which brings me to the second common issue of dimensionalizing of themes. Often analysis will reveal that the same phenomenon impacts data or participant experience in quite opposite ways; for example, in the driverless car study safety was identified as a concern and an inhibitor to using a driverless car and, paradoxically, others highlighted that safety would be enhanced by having less cars on the road. There might be the temptation to have separate themes where safety is identified as a barrier to uptake and a benefit from adoption of driverless cars. The opposites can be incorporated together in a theme about safety and trust with the contrasting views dimensionalizing the theme, but essentially still about safety and trust.

The third issue relates to having themes that move beyond simple description to a more conceptual theme. The researcher has to keep working at the analysis to 'lift' it to a more conceptual level without losing the richness of the data to what Thorne and Derbyshire (2005) called "bloodless findings" (p. 1109). One strategy to keep the richness is to draw on participants' words for theme names as Appleby et al. (2022) have demonstrated with one of the themes about parents' perspectives on owning an autism assistance dog being named "At the end of the day they're dogs". This theme describes views that there were logistics around owning a dog which required grooming, feeding, and an ongoing commitment to training. In the first edition, I wrote that the researcher should aim for a maximum of three to five themes, as too many themes or too few themes might indicate that analysis is not complete or that not enough data has been gathered. While I stand by my original statement, I have seen that idea cited as a definitive instruction where I offer it more as a guide. The reader may also enjoy reading Dickie's (2003) description of her approach to analysis and the process of being 'in' the data and distancing herself, then returning to the data.

The analysis of the driverless car data began by reading the interview through in its entirety, then open coding line by line. At this stage the coding stayed fairly close to the participants' words and made use of 'in vivo' codes, that is, the language of the participants. There are semantic codes which capture the surface meanings of the data and latent coding which capture the underlying meaning of the data (Byrne, 2022). Using latent codes enables the analysis to move from description to interpretation. Following open coding, similar codes were brought together to form categories. Iterative analysis continued until there was a smaller number of categories, then like categories were grouped and collapsed into three themes.

My personal preference is to use a manual process for analysis which includes printing transcripts single sided with double spacing and the transcript text only on half of the page leaving lots of room for writing. I then hand write the code into the space next to the segment of text. Then I literally cut the transcripts so that each segment and text is attached to its code. Each transcript is color coded so that I can track codes back to the interview for context. I painstakingly go through a process of sorting codes into piles on the table with other like codes and attach a category label to the group of codes. These category labels are tentative and can be changed as I keep working until all codes are sorted, and then categories are reviewed, and codes or categories moved around as I work through our iterative process. If the analysis has to be moved from the space I am working in I pack it away into plastic bags and attach the category label. I may well have a bag of codes that do not quite fit anywhere at the moment, but I will keep working on it until all data are accounted for. Gradually, the categories are reduced to a smaller number and themes developed. See Table 4.4 where I list early themes from our analysis and link them to the five dimensions that we derived at the end of analysis. With the driverless car study at this point, I shared the analysis with a co-author who worked on refining the categories into themes. At this stage, analysis was done by sharing Word documents and Excel spreadsheets.

Data analysis should yield a rich description of participants' views on the topic being explored, allowing the reader a better understanding of another's perspective. Once I have arrived at what I think are the themes, I begin writing 'the story of the theme' and slotting in direct quotes from the data which capture the idea I am trying to write about. In the writing process I may still identify where ideas and data need to be moved around as the data analysis is not finished until writing the account of the data is complete. I usually start the writing with one theme that for some reason 'jumps' out at me, and I think, yes I can

Table 4.4 Contrasting descriptive themes from early analysis with conceptual dimensions

Early theme	Final theme
Science fiction Technology Fear	A brave new world
Loss of control Danger Safety	Relinquishing control
Enjoyment Rite of passage	Driving is part of being Australian

Author created

write about that one and gradually work through each one. Once they are written I will review the order of presentation of themes and see if there is a more logical order or if I leave the themes in the order in which they were written. With the driverless car study, I decided to put the theme about 'Driving being part of being an Australian' first as it appeared to set the context for the rest of the themes.

Frequently, authors can be seen to report the themes that have 'emerged' from their thematic analysis, indeed I may well have been guilty of this myself in early work. That statement conjures up an image of themes emerging miraculously from the word swamp of analysis. Braun and Clarke (2022) argued that themes do not just 'emerge'; rather, it is a process of theme generation and development that involves the researcher(s)' interpretation of the data in the analysis process.

My manual process of analysis is not very practical when it comes to working in teams or for studies where this is a large amount of data. Most qualitative researchers will use software such as NVivo to help with data management. As I learnt data analysis before the widespread use of software, working manually is still my preference; however, I also know that it suits the way my brain works in that I need to literally handle my data and move it around. I do not have the same sense of knowing my data when it is within a software program. Even when using software during analysis I still find it useful to move away when it comes to finalizing themes to other ways of thinking about analysis such as drawing mind maps or moving sticky notes around on a table or vertical surface such as a wall. The writing of the story of the theme is still part of the analytical process as one does not really consolidate the themes until writing about them.

Rigor and Ethics

Given the broad nature of the qualitative descriptive approach, the researcher has a wide range of rigor strategies available to them to ensure trustworthiness. These strategies include journaling to provide a clear audit trail of methodological decisions made during the research process, member checking, peer debriefing including supervision or discussion with a more experienced qualitative researcher, as well as presentations to a range of audiences including colleagues and research stakeholders. With a large variety of strategies available, it is advisable for the researcher to be selective and choose strategies that best demonstrate the rigor of the study, rather than employing a multitude of strategies that only superficially address the issue of rigor.

Some of the strategies to ensure rigor in the driverless car study have already been described as I have laid out the data collection and analysis process that we undertook, for example the peer debriefing. We kept an audit trail of the project through team meeting minutes, in addition to keeping different versions of the analysis as it progressed to document the methodological and analytical decisions made along the way.

Member checking is a common rigor strategy for descriptive qualitative studies where the researcher returns to the participants at various points to check the accuracy of interpretations of the data. One often reads of researchers taking transcripts back to participants for checking the accuracy of the transcription. In my opinion, there are more useful times to use member checking if the interview has been digitally recorded, transcribed verbatim, and the accuracy of the transcription checked against the digital recording. The transcript is what the person said and there is no interpretation at this point, so I would argue that it is not the best use of the participant's goodwill or the researcher's time to be returning transcripts to participants at this stage in the process. I believe it is far more useful to return later in the analysis to check the interpretation of the data to see whether the findings resonate with the person's perspective. Usually, I send a short summary of each theme (no more than two to three pages in total) back to participants and invite feedback, and/or I publish a lay summary in an organizational newsletter.

Having an advisory panel or reference group comprising major stakeholders is a useful strategy for rigor, as well as for guidance regarding broader issues in relation to the topic, networking, and ideas for dissemination strategies. An advisory group can assist with recruitment and provide access to industry publications and presentations to disseminate findings. Members of such a group are generally made up of representatives of key stakeholders and/or end-users and those with lived experience.

Ethical approval for the driverless study was obtained from the university ethics committee. The study was not high in terms of risk so the ethical approval was straight forward; however, ethics committees often take a very conservative approach to research with older people as there is an assumption that older people are a vulnerable group. In studies drawing on samples from a clinical population, particular attention needs to be paid to the issue of participants being free to make up their own minds about volunteering to participate and not feeling obliged given the pre-existing and ongoing nature of the relationship between residents or service users and the organization or workers and their employer. Further, if collecting data in participants' homes and in rural locations, attention must be paid to researcher safety. Data collectors need to follow safety protocols including wearing name badges identifying them as coming from a university, carrying a mobile phone, and having someone know where they are going and when they are expected to return who can raise an alarm if required, as well as always having an exit strategy.

Gathering perspectives on driverless cars is not a particularly sensitive topic but often occupational scientists or occupational therapists are interested in exploring phenomena which can raise feelings of discomfort or even distress. Researchers need to have a protocol in place for managing that. For discomfort, the interviewer can offer to pause the interview to allow the participant to collect themselves or the interview can be stopped altogether. It is also important to provide information about community resources, remembering that the researcher role is different from the therapist role. Any topic that might result in participants experiencing distress will be highly scrutinized by any ethics committee or institutional review board, but sensitive topics cannot be avoided completely or there will be significant gaps in the research evidence for practice. The protocols for managing distress need careful thinking through and planning depending on the topic.

Application to Occupational Science

Findings from the driverless car study provide insight into the perspectives that older people have about changes to the way that people may be able to move about the community. They highlight that the occupation of driving has a range of meanings beyond the utilitarian function of being able to get oneself to the shops, attend appointments, and visit family and friends; and that for some people, the occupation of driving itself has significant meaning and connection with their identity. Even if the act of driving was not the main occupation, thinking about driverless cars made older people think about other occupations that could potentially be disrupted such as fishing or horse riding.

In addition, the findings from the driverless car study include consideration of the occupational disruption that arises from technological advancement. The recognition of occupational disruption can be unsettling and anxiety provoking; however, the older people could see that there were also potential positive outcomes and affording of possibilities for those who are unable to drive.

Application to Occupational Therapy

Qualitative descriptive studies offer great potential for occupational therapy research without the need to understand an underlying theoretical orientation. They are particularly useful for evaluating clients' and stakeholders' views on a program or service or a topic; and the findings can be used to inform quality improvements, more client focused services, and better targeted services. The findings from qualitative descriptive studies are also readily conveyed by occupational therapists to clients or other team members without them having to understand a theoretical orientation in order to comprehend the findings.

The findings from the driverless car study highlighted the need for therapists in the future to consider the use of driverless cars as another option for clients to be able to access the community for participation. Being able to participate despite poor mobility has the potential to prevent mental health issues arising from social isolation and loneliness, and enable older people to maintain an independent life if they desire. New competencies such as being able to use a mobile phone application to book a driverless car may need to be included in occupational therapy interventions in the future.

Critiquing Qualitative Descriptive Studies

While a generic approach to qualitative research with no alignment to a particular theoretical orientation is useful and appealing, it does pose some challenges for developing guidelines for critiquing qualitative descriptive studies. The questions I have developed (refer to Textbox 4.4) relate to qualitative descriptive studies that use a thematic analysis rather than a content or framework analysis.

Personal Reflections

A descriptive qualitative approach was a good fit for a driverless car study and is my 'go to' or 'default' approach for funded research and the work that I do now which is heavily influenced by co-design. I have conducted many other studies using a descriptive qualitative approach and supervised numerous student projects. Having used grounded theory for my PhD, and in my professional life having a strong attraction to processes, I would say that I

Textbox 4.4   Critiquing Qualitative Descriptive Studies – Questions to Ask

1 Has the *design* been chosen for an *exploratory, descriptive* study?
2 Does the research question fit with a *generic approach* that is not aligned to a particular theoretical orientation?
3 Are *methodological decisions* around sampling, recruitment, data collection, and rigor described in detail?
4 Are the steps used in *analysis described in detail?*
5 Do the findings presented show *interpretation and abstraction* without losing sight of the data?
6 Does the author make explicit how the *findings contribute to knowledge?*

---

approach a descriptive qualitative design from a grounded, emergent, and social constructivist perspective. So, while I might claim no particular alignment with a theoretical orientation for descriptive qualitative, I think that my view of reality as socially constructed influences my teaching and my research without me being consciously aware of that. My preference in data analysis is always, 'let's see what is in the data'; what emerges from analysis, rather than imposing a coding framework which could be an appropriate way to do the analysis. The key difference here is that the aim is to build a rich description rather than a theory.

I like the open generic nature of this approach. It lends itself to many of the research questions that I am interested in which are about gaining the perspective of various groups of people with lived experience as their view is often absent from the research literature but perhaps, more importantly, provides a unique perspective to knowledge and evidence for therapy. The outcome is a rich description of another's perspective. There is an appeal in revealing findings that might have been anticipated and that confirm what is already 'known' but for which there is scant evidence. More importantly, I love how qualitative descriptive studies, when done well, can reveal the 'taken for granted' or the unknown, as that is where the very special contribution to knowledge or practice lies. The theme in the driverless car study which captured the importance of driving as a meaningful occupation and being a driver for older Australians is a very good example of revealing the unknown or 'taken for granted' and I contend makes an important contribution to knowledge.

Summary

In this chapter I have described the most generic methodology within qualitative research designs. I have taken examples from a study of older people's perceptions of driverless cars to show how a qualitative descriptive methodology can be utilized. In drawing on that experience, one of the features of this chapter has been to show how the methodology can be applied in a large project which attracted nationally competitive funding with attention paid to rigor. Just because the methodology is generic and not aligned to any particular theoretical orientation, it does not follow that it is second rate or less serious than other methodologies. Indeed, as was the case with the driverless car study, seeking the perspective of the participants reveals the 'taken for granted.' Therein lies a great beauty.

In the title of this chapter, I called on a line from a song from a well-known musical, *The Sound of Music*, "Let's start at the very beginning, a very good place to start." So many of the considerations that researchers need to learn about and make for a descriptive qualitative study can be taken and applied to other approaches, which is why I argue that when it comes to considering qualitative research methodologies it is, indeed, a very good place to start.

References

Appleby, R., Wright, S., Williams, L., & Stanley, M. (2022). Australian parents' experiences of owning an autism assistance dog. *Health and Social Care in the Community, 30*(6), e4113–e4121. https://doi.org/10.1111/hsc.13805

Braun, V., & Clarke, V. (2006). Using thematic analysis in psychology. *Qualitative Research in Psychology, 3*(2), 77–101. https://doi.org/10.1191/1478088706qp063oa

Braun, V., & Clarke, V. (2021a). One size fits all? What counts as quality practice in (reflexive) thematic analysis? *Qualitative Research in Psychology, 18*(3), 328–352. https://doi.org/10.1080/14 780887.2020.1769238

Braun, V., & Clarke, V. (2021b). To saturate or not to saturate? Questioning data saturation as a useful concept for thematic analysis and sample-size rationales. *Qualitative Research in Sport, Exercise and Health, 13*(2), 201–216. https://doi.org/10.1080/2159676X.2019.1704846

Braun, V., & Clarke, V. (2022). *Thematic analysis: A practical guide.* SAGE.

Byrne, D. (2022). A worked example of Braun and Clarke's approach to reflexive thematic analysis. *Quality & Quantity, 56*(3), 1391–1412. https://doi.org/10.1007/s11135-021-01182-y

Council of the Aging South Australia. (2020). *Country listening posts.* COTA.

Creswell, J. (2007). *Qualitative inquiry and research design. Choosing among five approaches* (2nd ed.). SAGE.

Davidson, C. (2009). Transcription: Imperatives for qualitative research. *International Journal of Qualitative Methods, 8*(2), 1–52. https://ejournals.library.ualberta.ca/index.php/IJQM/article/viewFile/4205/5401

Denzin, N. K., & Lincoln, Y. S. (2005). Introduction: The discipline and practice of qualitative research. In N. K. Denzin & Y. S. Lincoln (Eds.), *The SAGE handbook of qualitative research* (3rd ed., pp. 1–32). SAGE.

Dickie, V. A. (2003). Data analysis in qualitative research: A plea for sharing the magic and the effort. *American Journal of Occupational Therapy, 57*, 49–56. https://doi.org/10.5014/ajot.57.1.49

Gale, N. K., Heath, G., Cameron, E., Rashid, S., & Redwood, S. (2013). Using the framework method for the analysis of qualitative data in multi-disciplinary health research. *BMC Medical Research Methodology, 13*(1), 117. https://doi.org/10.1186/1471-2288-13-117

Gillham, B. (2000). *The research interview.* Continuum.

Goldsmith, L. J. (2021). Using framework analysis in applied qualitative research. *The Qualitative Report, 26*(6), 2061–2076. https://doi.org/10.46743/2160-3715/2021.5011

Guba, E. G., & Lincoln, Y. S. (2005). Paradigmatic controversies, contradictions, and emerging confluences. In N. K. Denzin & Y. S. Lincoln (Eds.), *The SAGE handbook of qualitative research* (3rd ed., pp. 191–215). SAGE.

Hess-April, L., Dennis, L., Ganas, N., Phiri, L., & Phoshoko, P. (2017). Occupation-based practice in a tertiary hospital setting: occupational therapists' perceptions and experiences. *South African Journal of Occupational Therapy, 47*(3), 25–31. https://doi.org/10.17159/2310-3833/2017/v47n3a5

Kibele, A., & Llorens, L. A. (1989). Going to the source: The use of qualitative methodology in a study of the needs of adults with cerebral palsy. *Occupational Therapy in Health Care, 6*(2/3), 27–40. https://doi.org/10.1080/J003v06n02_04

Kosma, A., Bryant, W., & Wilson, L. (2013). Drawing on Wilcock: An investigation of the impact of her published work on occupational therapy practice and research. *British Journal of Occupational Therapy, 76*(4), 179–185. https://doi.org/10.4276/030802213X13651610908416

Liamputtong, P. (Ed.). (2013). *Research methods in health: Foundations for evidence-based practice* (2nd ed.). Oxford University Press.

McCarthy, K., Ballog, M., Carranza, M. M., & Lee, K. (2022). Doing nonbinary gender: The occupational experience of nonbinary persons in the environment. *Journal of Occupational Science, 29*(1), 36–51. https://doi.org/10.1080/14427591.2020.1804439

Merrill, S. C. (1985). Qualitatiave methods in occupational therapy research: An application. *Occupational Therapy Journal of Research, 5*(4), 209–222.

Mishler, E. G. (1986). *Research interviewing. Context and narrative.* Harvard University Press.

Murray, C., & Lawry, J. (2011). Maintenance of professional currency: Perceptions of occupational therapists. *Australian Occupational Therapy Journal, 58*(4), 261–269. https://doi.org/10.1080/14427591.2011.602628

Neergaard, M. A., Olesen, F., Andersen, R. S., & Sondergaard, J. (2009). Qualitative description: The poor cousin of health research? *BMC Medical Research Methodology, 9*(52), 1–5. https://doi.org/10.1186/1471-2288-9-52

Patton, M. Q. (2002). *Qualitative research and evaluation methods* (3rd ed.). SAGE.

Patton, M. Q. (2015). *Qualitative research & evaluation methods: Integrating theory and practice* (4th ed.). SAGE.

Peoples, H., Nissen, N., Brandt, Å., & la Cour, K. (2021). Perceptions of quality of life by people with advanced cancer who live at home. *British Journal of Occupational Therapy, 84*(11), 723–730. https://doi.org/10.1177/0308022620976839

Ritchie, J., & Spencer, L. (1994). Qualitative data analysis for applied policy research. In A. Bryman & R. Burgess (Eds.), *Analyzing qualitative data* (pp. 305–329). Routledge.

Sandelowski, M. (2000). Whatever happened to qualitative description? *Research in Nursing and Health, 23*, 334–340.

Sandelowski, M. (2010). What's in a name? Qualitative description revisited. *Research in Nursing and Health, 33*, 77–84. https://doi.org/10.10022/nur.20362

Strecker, C., & Hitch, D. (2021). Perceptions of current occupational therapy practice with older adults experiencing delirium. *Australasian Journal on Ageing, 40*(3), e190–e198. https://doi.org/10.1111/ajag.12882

Thorne, S. (2013). Interpretive description. In C. T. Beck (Ed.) *Routledge international handbook of qualitative nursing research* (pp. 295–306). Routledge.

Thorne, S., & Derbyshire, P. (2005). Land mines in the field: A modest proposal for improving the craft of qualitative research. *Qualitative Health Research, 15*(8), 1105–1113. https://doi.org/10.1177/1049732305278502

Werner, J. M., & Jozkowski, A. C. (2022). Comparing graduate occupational therapy students' perceived time use, temporality, and tempo of occupational participation before and during the COVID-19 pandemic. *Journal of Occupational Science, 29*(3), 295–305. https://doi.org/10.1080/14427591.2022.2061037

Additional Resources

Sage Publications. (2020). *Thematic analysis by Virginia Braun and Victoria Clarke.* https://study.sagepub.com/thematicanalysis

Sage Zoom. (2022). *Common challenges in thematic analysis and how to avoid them with Virginia Braun and Victoria Clarke.* www.youtube.com/live/tpWLsckpM78?feature=share

The University of Auckland. (2023). *Thematic analysis.* www.thematicanalysis.net/

5 Grounded Theory

Kate D'Cruz and Shoba Nayar

In a textbook written for occupational scientists and occupational therapists, it would be natural to argue that humans are inherently occupational beings; just as they are social beings. Combining these two aspects—the occupational and the social—offers a rich world for qualitative exploration. It can also be argued that using grounded theory methodology for any study is both a social and occupational journey that can reveal much about the field being studied, as well as about ourselves as researchers and humans. In this chapter we outline key considerations for the planning and implementation of grounded theory research, with a more focused consideration of best practice application. To illustrate, we draw on Kate's research, which used grounded theory to uncover the relational process of narrative storytelling in brain injury rehabilitation (D'Cruz, 2020). In doing so our aim is to make explicit the 'fit' between grounded theory methodology and occupationally focused inquiry.

Described as an "empirical approach to the study of social life through qualitative research and distinctive approaches to data analysis" (Clarke, 2005, p. xxi), grounded theory guides the exploration and understanding of social processes that occur within society. Indeed, it was through the collaboration of sociologists Barney Glaser and Anselm Strauss (1967) and their studies of the topic of dying in hospitals, that grounded theory first emerged. As an approach to analyzing qualitative data, it immediately resonated with social scientists who were interested in generating new theory as opposed to testing existing theory in what was otherwise a positivist environment (Birks & Mills, 2015). Together, Glaser and Strauss "joined epistemological critique with practical guidelines for action" (Charmaz, 2006, p. 5); and, although they later parted ways, their work transformed the world of qualitative research.

Over 50 years later, grounded theory methodology has evolved to encompass a range of nuances and approaches. These iterations have been led by many former students of Glaser and Strauss, from their time teaching at the University of California, San Francisco. For instance, Charmaz (2006, 2016), a former occupational therapist, has been one proponent advancing the development of grounded theory, along with contemporaries such as Birks and Mills (2015), Clarke (2005), Bowers (Bowers & Schatzman, 2009), and Corbin (2009), who, together, have become known as the second generation of grounded theorists (Morse et al., 2016). Despite the variations, grounded theory methodology has one goal—to uncover and explain the underlying social processes shaping interaction and human behavior. It is this aim that underpins the resonance between grounded theory and occupation focused research.

DOI: 10.4324/9781003456216-5

Grounded Theory and the Study of Occupation

In 2003, Stanley and Cheek (2003) advocated for grounded theory as a methodological approach to study the "use of occupations to enhance health and wellbeing" (p. 143); while Charmaz (2014c) has championed the use of a constructivist approach to grounded theory in exploring the social psychology of illness and disability. In the healthcare context, nursing scholars have embraced this methodology and, since the first edition of this book, there has been an increase in the use of grounded theory by occupational science and occupational therapy researchers. Some researchers have used grounded theory both as methodology and methods to explore topics such as the process of health in mothers during caregiving of children with cerebral palsy (Dehghan et al., 2022), the settlement experiences of immigrants (Kim et al., 2015; Nayar & Wright St. Clair, 2020), how early career occupational therapists learn once practicing (Murray et al., 2020), and the experiences of client-centered practice after stroke (Walder & Molineux, 2020). Other researchers have combined grounded theory methods with other methodologies, most commonly qualitative descriptive, for example, to better understand the interplay between being and belonging through meditation (Chisman & Brooks, 2018) and financial management among adults with acquired brain injury (Engel et al., 2019).

As evidenced, the scope for occupation focused grounded theory studies is considerable, reflecting that many social processes involve engagement in occupation. As a discipline, occupational science seeks to understand and influence societal practices, while keeping the notion of occupation central to understanding the everyday experiences of people's lives. Implicit in the *everyday experiences* is the notion of *process* or doing as it unfolds over time. From this perspective, grounded theory methodology has much to offer for extending understanding of people's occupational engagement (Nayar & Stanley, 2015).

The work that occupational therapists are engaged in is, primarily, process driven. Whether it is assisting clients in their recovery from mental illness or stroke, transitioning from unemployment to paid work, or encouraging children in play, all are examples of occupation rich processes. Furthermore, the work of occupational therapists shifts within and across time, similar to the practice of grounded theory methods which involves the interplay between data collection and data analysis (Charmaz, 2006). Concurrent data collection and analysis means that the researcher is constantly moving from the present to consider what has happened in the past and what may happen in the future. A social process is dynamic, much the same as engagement in occupation. Both contain movement and develop as new pieces of data/understanding become apparent or previously analyzed data takes on new meaning. The ultimate act of grounded theory is, therefore, to uncover the social processes individuals use in response to a particular phenomenon that includes elements of the past, present, and future.

One approach to grounded theory that has taken hold within social and healthcare research is constructivist grounded theory (Charmaz, 2014a). Central to constructivist grounded theory is the co-construction of data, recognizing and engaging with the participant–researcher relationship, as well as the broader relational context of the research enquiry. This co-construction approach is complementary to the theoretical underpinnings of occupational science and occupational therapy such as the person–occupation–environment relationship, as well as person-centered engagement, and supports a collaborative partnership approach to qualitative research. In this chapter, the discussion and examples are drawn from constructivist grounded theory.

Epistemology, Ontology, Axiology

The variations within grounded theory such as classic (Glaser, 1992), critical (Belfrage & Hauf, 2017), or constructivist (Charmaz, 2006) approaches makes defining the theoretical orientation challenging. Indeed, Charmaz (2006) has argued that grounded theory methods "need not be tied to a single epistemology" as the "research process is fluid, interactive, and open ended" (p. 178). That said, constructivist grounded theory is situated within the symbolic interactionist methodological framework which focuses on the ways by which individuals interact, interpret, and make meaning of their world (Blumer, 1969).

From a symbolic interactionist perspective, the social and political context within which a person operates is central in shaping personal beliefs, values, thoughts, and actions. It is the environment within which one resides that constructs the self and subsequent actions. The self in symbolic interactionism is a duality comprising both a *me* and an *I*. The thinking part of us is directed by the *I*. The *I* processes information and decides how the interaction will proceed. The actual act—or interaction—is led by the *me* aspect of self which is the interactor between the self and society. Thus, it is the *I* which interprets and contributes meaning to an event, and it is the *me* which subsequently acts (Bowers, 1988). The environment, with its variety of conditions and contexts, elicits change in people and shapes their actions to make sense of the world. Reality is, therefore, a social construct; hence the synergy between symbolic interactionism and grounded theory.

In considering one's methodological position, alongside epistemology, it is necessary for researchers to also consider notions of ontology and axiology. It is important to consider one's ontological position, or stance from which the world is understood (Birks & Mills, 2015). In the context of Kate's study, the ontological position was evidenced in the partnership approach to gathering and making sense of data with research participants. Reflecting Kate's background as an occupational therapist, the study embraced a co-constructive approach to research data collection, analysis, and generation.

With regards to axiology of the study, researchers are encouraged to identify the values that are central to the research process, ensuring they are integrated into the implementation of the study (Birks & Mills, 2015). For example, in Kate's study, central to the research question and implementation of the study was an underlying commitment to ensuring that the voice of people with cognitive and communication difficulties was captured through an inclusive approach to the design and implementation of the study.

In summary, one's methodological position should be congruent with the chosen research design and methodology, guiding the design and implementation of the study. Ultimately, though, no matter how the researcher positions themselves, clearly articulating the theoretical orientation is pivotal for laying the foundations of a rigorous study as it will guide data analysis and presentation of findings.

Topics and Questions Best Suited to Grounded Theory Studies

When considering the use of grounded theory methodology, a useful approach is to consider the following questions: (1) is this an area of practice or study in which little is known? (2) is the study seeking to explore an underlying social process? (3) is the aim of the study to generate new knowledge grounded theoretically? Grounded theory is particularly useful in areas where little is known about the phenomenon of interest or where there are few existing theories to explain an individual's or group's behavior. Furthermore, as outlined later in this chapter, the analytical process of grounded theory guides an in-depth exploration of the processes underpinning a phenomenon of interest, shifting the analysis from descriptive to theory generating. It is this generative nature of grounded theory research that is particularly complementary to occupation-focused research that is often grounded in a complex relational space between the person, the environment, and occupational participation.

Working as an occupational therapist in acquired brain injury rehabilitation, Kate became interested in better understanding humanizing partnership approaches such as person-centered practice to support community re-integration. Underpinning this interest was recognition of the impact of social isolation and loss of pre-injury identity for people with brain injuries and an emerging understanding of the potential of narrative storytelling to support meaningful social connection and identity re-construction. Kate sought to explore the use of narrative storytelling in brain injury to address the research evidence gap and to inform rehabilitation practice. Constructivist grounded theory was the chosen methodology given the emerging nature of the evidence base, as well as recognition of the socio-relational context of the processes of storytelling and identity construction (Gergen & Gergen, 2014; McAdams, 2001). By adopting constructivist grounded theory, the methodology also enabled recognition of the research participants as partners with the researcher in a collaborative sense, supporting the notion of shared wisdom between the participants and researcher.

In addition to researchers' personal interests, the literature can also be used to help define the topic. There is much debate about the place of a literature review in a grounded theory study. Glaser (1978) contended that the researcher should not look at the literature prior to undertaking the study as it may influence their assumptions and analysis of data. However, this stance is not reasonable in a world where funding bodies, ethics committees, and academic institutions often require some review of the literature when writing research proposals. Consistent with these expectations, more contemporary grounded theorists, such as Charmaz and Birks and Mills, suggest a review of the literature prior and during a grounded theory study. Indeed, a review of the literature can orient the researcher to the field of study and assist with ascertaining the gap to be studied, as well as contributing to theoretical sensitivity and incorporated as data are collected and analyzed (as discussed later in this chapter).

Having decided on a topic, the next step is to develop the research question. In a grounded theory study, the research question commonly starts with 'how'; for example, 'how do Indian immigrant women settle in New Zealand?' or 'how do occupational therapists use evidence to inform practice?' By posing the question in this way, the research inquiry is shaped for in-depth exploration of the underlying social processes impacting the experience of a phenomena or life situation, resisting a more superficial or surface level exploration of the experience. Further, structuring the question in this manner differentiates grounded theory from other qualitative methodologies. In some instances, questions may begin with 'what'; for example, 'what happens when occupational therapists undertake postgraduate study?' or, as in Kate's study, 'what is the experience and impact of narrative storytelling following acquired brain injury?' Key to constructing a grounded theory question is the focus on process; and, in the context of constructivist grounded theory, examination of process in a socio-relational context.

Lived Experience

Lived experience involvement in the design and implementation of research is increasingly an expectation of best practice research. Lived experience involvement in research is commonly described as co-design, co-production, or co-creation. Co-design supports collaboration between researchers and end-users who have lived experience wisdom or knowledge of the area of investigation. There is a range of levels of co-design involvement, from one-off consultation such as focus groups/workshops to more active engagement or partnering in the planning and implementation of research such as stakeholder reference groups (Lindblom et al., 2021). The underlying philosophy of co-design as a collaborative relationship is complementary to the symbolic interactionist foundations of constructivist grounded theory and is central to ensuring the development of a research topic that resonates with the lived experience of participants, contributing to impactful translation of research into practice.

Participants' lived experience, however, goes beyond that of the individual and the collaborative relationship of participant and researcher. Qualitative studies demand "researchers address in detail the complexity of the context within which the study is being undertaken" (Nayar & Wright St. Clair, 2020, p. 133). Historically, the cultural foundations of grounded theory have remained implicit (Charmaz, 2014a) wherein differences of race and ethnicity, and culture are erased in the generalizing of grounded theory methods of analysis (Clarke, 2008). However, Charmaz (2014a) has argued that methodologists have a responsibility to "explicate the national and cultural underpinnings of his or her method" (p. 1082). Therefore, articulating the researcher's lived experience, as well as the cultural context in which the research is undertaken, is a fundamental step in the process of a constructivist grounded theory study. For instance, in a recent constructivist grounded theory study of living with mental ill health undertaken in Singapore, the first author clearly noted his personal lived experience of being a Singaporean and the potential for his perspectives to impact the way data were collected and analyzed. To help mitigate this possibility, two Australian mental health scientists were included in the research team, thus bringing their professional lived experience to the research (Kuek et al., 2022).

Recruitment and Sampling

In a grounded theory study, recruitment follows techniques common to many qualitative studies; for example, the use of flyers or advertisements on notice boards or internet sites (e.g., Facebook groups), word of mouth, or intermediaries. A hallmark of grounded theory is the concurrent processes of data collection and analysis. Thus, in a grounded theory study, sampling occurs across two stages: (1) purposive and (2) theoretical.

Initially, a purposive sample of people who fit the inclusion criteria is sought. Purposive sampling is commonly used in qualitative research and involves the deliberate selection of research participants based upon their experience and the knowledge they can offer in addressing the research question (Liamputtong, 2012). In Kate's study, the selection criteria for storyteller participants were inclusive of (a) aged between 19 and 65 years, (b) severity of acquired brain injury, (c) living circumstances, and (d) time elapsed since injury. In this study, selection criteria were influenced by Kate's experience as an occupational therapist; for example, recognizing that time elapsed post-injury influenced people's experiences of their injury and recovery or re-integration into the community. It was, therefore, an explicit strategy to recruit participants with a range of time post-injury to better understand the relationship between storytelling, identity re-construction, and social connection as a complex evolving process, rather than a static experience at one time point. It was also important that participants with cognitive and communication difficulties were not excluded. Kate sought to reflect the broad acquired brain injury population in the sample of participants. Thus, strategies to effectively support the engagement of people with cognitive and communication difficulties were integrated into the study design.

During this phase, it may be possible to return to participants to ask further questions or clarify data. For example, in Kate's study, each of the storytellers were interviewed at least twice as a strategy to support the participation of participants with cognitive and communication difficulties. This enabled investing time in the first interview to build rapport with participants and to tailor the interview approach to maximize their participation. The follow-up interview (also a form of theoretical sampling wherein new or clarifying interview questions are asked to flesh out analysis; see below for a discussion of theoretical sampling) acted as an opportunity to 'check-in' with participants following the first interview, to clarify understanding of interview data and to probe further areas of inquiry.

In recruiting participants for a grounded theory study, purposive sampling for maximum variation is used to add depth to the evolving theory. In the context of Kate's research, participants were purposively recruited from an advocacy organization in Australia that facilitates storytelling workshops for adults with disability who have entered or are at risk of entering a nursing home. The workshops support story sharing between storytellers and facilitators, resulting in the production of personal narratives that are used, with the permission of storytellers, as part of the organization's advocacy strategy. The produced personal narratives are either in the format of a short co-constructed digital story narrated by the storytellers, or a profile in an electronic or paper document written in the third person with a photograph of the storyteller. Given the nuance of the storytelling focus, it was not feasible to recruit participants beyond the context of this specific organization; however, both formats of the produced narrative were included in the study. As analysis progresses, the researcher shifts to the second stage of theoretical sampling.

Theoretical Sampling

Concurrent with data collection and analysis, a core principle of any grounded theory study is theoretical sampling (Charmaz, 2014a; Corbin & Strauss, 2015; Glaser, 1992), which enables selection of participants in response to emerging theoretical understanding from the data analysis (Charmaz, 2014a). More simply put, theoretical sampling is used to seek participants who can best provide answers to enhance understandings of emerging concepts. Charmaz (2006) contended that theoretical sampling should be used to delineate and saturate the properties of a category, check hunches about categories, distinguish and clarify relationships between categories, and identify variation in a process.

As a decision-making tool, theoretical sampling guides the researcher to seek participants who can provide data; thus, participants are selected as research progresses, rather than being pre-determined. According to Strauss and Corbin (1998), theoretical sampling is key to grounded theory methodology as it enables the researcher to obtain a participant population that will maximize opportunities to compare events and "bring about greatest theoretical return" (p. 202). In the context of Kate's study, theoretical sampling guided recruitment of two participants who were living in a nursing home, in contrast to the earlier participants who had moved from a nursing home into more independent living. Theoretical sampling enabled an opportunity to further explore people's motivation for participating in storytelling, in response to an emerging understanding of the importance of advocacy impact for the storytellers. While the storytelling appeared to be a personally impactful experience for the storytellers, this seemed less important as a motivator for participation than the opportunity to contribute to the advocacy work of the organization. We were interested to see if this view held true for people who were living in a nursing home, as well as those who had moved to more independent living.

Ideally, through the process of theoretical sampling and collection of data, the researcher seeks to achieve theoretical saturation. It should be noted that saturation in this instance is not "seeing the same pattern over and over again" (Glaser, 2001, p. 191); which is how the term is commonly understood. Rather, theoretical saturation occurs when "gathering fresh data no longer sparks new theoretical insights, nor reveals new properties of core theoretical categories" (Charmaz, 2006, p. 113). Research experience suggests that data saturation can occur with as few as seven participants and is usually evident with 14 participants. However, it needs to be acknowledged that project constraints (e.g., time or financial limitations, sample size) may prevent this from happening. In studies that draw data from more than one group of participants (i.e., Kate's study of storytellers and story facilitators), data saturation is often achieved through the combined data, as opposed to a discrete number of participants in each group.

Data Collection

Consistent with other qualitative research methodologies, grounded theory research typically includes collection of participant data from interviews and/or focus groups. In this context, a range of data can be included such as interview transcripts, participant observation, analytical memos, the researcher's reflective journal, as well as other relevant documentation. In the context of Kate's study of narrative storytelling, sources of data included in-depth interviews conducted with the storyteller and facilitator participants, as well as the personal stories produced from the storytelling workshops.

Individual In-depth Interviews

Individual in-depth interviews enable a one-to-one discussion between the researcher and the participant and can be tailored to the needs of the individual participants. There are a range of factors that need to be considered when planning for interviews (see Textbox 5.1) such as whether interviews will be conducted in-person or online via a video conferencing platform such as Zoom or FaceTime (Topping et al., 2021).

It is important to invest time in the development and piloting of an interview guide. The interview guide is designed to support in-depth exploration of the participant's lived experience of the area under investigation. Therefore, the interview questions are often

---

Textbox 5.1   Factors to Consider When Planning Research Interviews

- Will the interview be conducted in-person or online?
- If in person, what is the participant's preferred location and is it private and free of distraction? Does the participant have access needs, such as wheelchair accessibility?
- Does the participant need a supporter/close other present at the interview?
- Could the interview be an emotional trigger? What strategies are in place to minimize risk?
- Does the interview guide include language that is easy to understand for the participant?
- Does the participant use a communication device?

open ended, with use of phrases such as, 'can you tell me about your experience?' or 'what was that experience like for you?' For example, in Kate's study of narrative storytelling, interview questions included: Can you tell me about the day that you shared your story with X? What did you expect or think the day would be like? Was the storytelling like you expected? How did you feel while you were telling your story? How did you feel after you told your story?

In grounded theory studies, the aim of the interview is to move from descriptive story sharing to further probe and understand the social processes underpinning the lived experience. Often this involves traversing the complex relational space between the person, the environment and occupational participation. For example, Kate used interview questions to further explore the experience of the storytellers in the context of relationships, such as family/friends and the storytelling facilitators, as well as the impact of the experience upon their sense of self, or identity. These questions included: Did you have family/friends at the storytelling workshop? Did you tell family/friends about the workshop? Has anything changed for you or your family after the storytelling? Was there anything the facilitator did that helped or hindered your storytelling? How do you see yourself now after the storytelling?

Consistent with the use of concurrent data collection and analysis in grounded theory studies, it is often helpful to adapt the interview guide in response to emerging understandings generated from the data analysis. Defined as theoretical sampling, this often includes the use of additional prompts within question areas to further probe and test out understanding. For example, in the context of Kate's study the following questions were developed: 'I am really interested in understanding more about your relationship with the storytelling facilitators. I would like to know from your perspective, what did [name of facilitator] do to help you share your story? To make you feel comfortable? How would you describe the role of the facilitator?

When conducting interviews, whether in-person or online, it is necessary to consider the structure of the interview and to invest time at the beginning of the interview to build rapport and at the end of the interview to provide closure. In the context of Kate's study, she took time to consider the use of strategies to maximize the engagement of participants with cognitive and communication difficulties. Most of the participants had slowed communication due to dysarthria or used a communication device, as well as having reduced concentration and attention and mild memory difficulties. Key strategies used in the data collection included the use of: (a) multiple short interviews of 45–60 minutes; (b) email, text, and social media posts to scaffold face-face discussion in the interview; (c) email questions (three maximum) in advance of interview; (d) reminder phone calls before and after the interview; and (e) use of storytelling technique to connect and build rapport (Paterson & Scott-Findlay, 2002).

Other Forms of Data

In addition to forms of verbal data (e.g., storytelling, individual interviews, focus groups), constructivist grounded theory can draw from multiple and diverse data sources to generate rich and sufficient data to gain a full picture of the topic (Birks & Mills, 2015; Charmaz, 2014b; Mills et al., 2006). One such form of data are observations, which, in grounded theory, can help explain what is happening in complex social situations and provide fresh theoretical insight and direction for theory construction (Charmaz, 2014b; Mulhall, 2003; Nilsson, 2012). Observations are particularly useful for providing additional information,

---

Textbox 5.2   Example of a Narrative Profile Written About a Storyteller Participant

Katherine is a mum and a stroke survivor who sustained her stroke 4 years ago. She is in her 40s and lives in a nursing home. Katherine described herself as 'sporty,' 'funny,' and 'sentimental.' She shared that she likes a "good comedy" and used to do gymnastics, diving, and running when she was younger. Katherine's use of the word 'sentimental' seemed a very apt choice for the person who I got to know in the interviews. She said, "I'm a sentimental person at heart … I take everything personally." Katherine spoke of acceptance, personal learning, and development, caring for other residents, and being hopeful and determined for a better future. She ended our interview saying, "… the longer term, I'll go home. I will go home."

---

such as context, regarding participants' actions and interactions which they may have been unaware of or unable to articulate (Corbin & Strauss, 2015). Additionally, observations can provide an opportunity to confirm whether participants' reports of experiences align with what is happening in action (Mulhall, 2003; Savin-Baden & Major, 2013), thus capturing information that may not have been possible to adequately capture through the spoken word alone (Mulhall, 2003; Nilsson, 2012).

Another form of data is that of texts (Charmaz, 2014a; Savin-Baden & Major, 2013). These may be in the form of field notes documented during interviews or observations that supplement and extend understandings of data derived first hand from the participant; or sociohistorical documents such as relevant policies that have a direct influence on the actions and interactions of participants in a particular setting. Considering the research site from multiple perspectives offers a comprehensive understanding of the field; while using a combination of methods adds robustness to the constructed theory through triangulation of sources (Flick, 2019; Glaser & Strauss, 1967).

In the context of Kate's study, the storyteller's produced stories (written profile or digital story) were re-visited with each of the storyteller participants in the interviews. Written transcripts of these stories were included as data for analysis, as well as written profiles of each of the storyteller participants. The profiles were written as a reflective exercise after each of the interviews, drawn from interview data, observations, and information shared in the produced stories (see Textbox 5.2). The produced stories and written profiles provided rich information about the lived experience of the participants that could not have been collected from the interviews due to time constraints, especially with those participants with cognitive and communication difficulties. Written profiles also encourage consideration of research participants as unique individuals, positioning their shared stories or experiences in their own unique context; for example, the complexities and richness of race, culture, ethnicity, and gender.

Memo Writing

Memo writing or 'memoing' is a technique used by researchers to record their thinking throughout the research process. Early memos might capture researcher thoughts regarding reflections on interviews and the type of data gathered. Theoretical memos may occur further along the study wherein memos capture the researcher's thoughts concerning the process of analysis or directions for further analysis (Richards, 2005). For the grounded theory researcher, memoing is a central process (Strauss, 1987). Glaser (1978) argued, "the

---

Textbox 5.3   Example of a Memo: Focused Coding of Storyteller Data

Sharing MY STORY to help other is emerging as central to the storyteller analysis. All of the participants were motivated to tell their story to help others. I have emphasized 'MY STORY' as, despite the overall altruistic aim to help others through storytelling, both the storytelling process and the end products are highly personal. There is strong identification by the storytellers with their profile or digital story because 'it is me.' There is perhaps a tension between the public purpose of the stories and their personal nature. I see this as the 'above the surface' intended impact of the storytelling (helping others) and the 'below the surface' unintended impact of the storytelling such as therapeutic reflection and self-learning.

---

bedrock of theory generation, its true product is the writing of theoretical memos. If the analyst skips this stage by going directly from coding to sorting or to writing – he is *not* doing grounded theory" (p. 83). Memos may involve drawing models and/or diagrams that designate relationships between categories to help progress theory or may be written reflections on the research process as it unfolds. In whatever manner memos are constructed, they are meant to be "analytical and conceptual rather than descriptive" (Strauss & Corbin, 1998, p. 217). In Textbox 5.3 we include an example of a memo written in Kate's study.

Researcher's Reflective Journal

In addition to memo writing, researchers are encouraged to write a reflective journal. Writing a reflective journal typically involves a systematic routine of thinking about the research process and the way in which 'you' as the researcher engage with the research. Journal writing is one strategy to ensure that grounded theorists are reflexive researchers (Birks & Mills, 2015; Charmaz, 2014a). Reflective journals work best when written throughout the research project; from planning the study to dissemination of the research findings. In our experience, reflective journaling is a particularly helpful practice to do before and after conducting research interviews. The act of writing about the interview experience, supports learning about interviewing technique, while also anchoring the data collection with the analysis. Furthermore, journaling promotes reflexive thinking about the co-constructed nature of the research. As described by Charmaz (2014a), researchers are "not passive receptacles into which data are poured" (p. 27). Reflexivity is a key strategy for researchers to recognize their own pre-existing assumptions about the world and how they might influence the research.

In Kate's study, reflective journal writing was an essential part of the research process and her experience as a grounded theory researcher. Influenced by her background as an occupational therapist in brain injury rehabilitation, Kate came to the study with an appreciation for the complexity of brain injury and an intent to acknowledge the personal impact of acquired brain injury with each of the participants. Through the processes of intentional listening and reflective journaling, Kate was challenged to identify and moderate preconceived ideas about survivors of acquired brain injury finding meaning in the injury experience through storytelling. Kate came to better appreciate the capacity and strengths of each of the storytellers, understanding storytelling as a way for acquired brain injury survivors to contribute to the lives of others. Journaling enabled Kate to recognize pre-conceived ideas, possibly grounded in her rehabilitation experience, and to challenge these by more deeply listening and engaging with the lived experience of the research participants.

Data Analysis

Data analysis follows the constant-comparative method of simultaneous data collection and analysis. This method is an active and iterative process of constructing understanding through seeking the perspective of research participants while critically questioning and exploring data and returning to the field for more data. Some novice researchers are drawn towards grounded theory as they perceive the process of grounded theory analysis as tending to be more structured than other qualitative approaches; however, this is not necessarily the case. Data are read and analyzed word by word, line by line, as part of a coding process. Charmaz (2014a) described grounded theory coding as involving two main phases: initial coding and focused coding, with axial and theoretical coding as secondary processes. As analysis progresses, the initial codes are grouped as 'categories' or 'concepts,' which refer to the context, strategies, and conditions under which the social process unfolds. Ultimately, each of these categories is linked to a central process or core category.

The Coding Process

Initial coding, sometimes described as open coding, is the first stage of coding in which segments of data are summarized, typically in a line-by-line process (Charmaz, 2014a). Where possible, *gerunds* (active words) are used to focus the coding on processes of action. For example, the gerund 'seeking to help others' was used to capture the storytellers' motivation for sharing their story. To help ensure that the analysis is grounded in the participant experience, it can also be useful to consider use of in-vivo coding in which codes are drawn from words or specific terms used by the research participants. An example of an in-vivo code from Kate's study is, 'being belittled in the nursing home' which aptly captured participant's experiences in language shared across participants.

The next stage of analysis is focused coding. Focused coding is an iterative process of refining the codes generated from initial coding. The most frequent codes are identified and systematically compared within and across transcripts resulting in the development of emergent categories and sub-categories. Memo writing and diagramming are useful strategies to support reflexive thinking about the properties of the coded data and the researcher's emergent theoretical understanding. For Kate, memo writing (see Textbox 5.4 for an example) included reflections about the similarities and differences in experiences both within and across the two groups of participants (storytellers & facilitators).

Textbox 5.4   Example of a Memo Written During Focused Coding

My understanding is that Felicity facilitates storytelling based on her observations and developing awareness of the needs of the storytellers, perhaps more than the intended message of the advocacy organization. This is quite different to Gideon and Jemima, who were very focused on the audience, but quite similar to Anna. Interesting, as Anna and Felicity seem to cope with the emotional demands of the job more comfortably than Jemima and Gideon. But then Gideon identifies as an emotional person. I am interested in enquiring more about this at the upcoming interviews.

Following focused coding, axial coding is described by Charmaz (2014) as a process of bringing the analyzed data back to a coherent whole. While the storyteller and facilitator data were analyzed separately, relationships between the data became increasingly evident, informing analytical thinking. At this stage of analysis, additional interviews were conducted to further explore the relational nature of storytelling. For example: *I am really interested in understanding more about your relationship with the storytelling facilitators. I would like to know from your perspective, what did [name of facilitator] do to help you share your story? How did they make you feel comfortable? How would you describe the role of the facilitator?*

Theoretical coding is the final stage of grounded theory data analysis and is a process of connecting all substantive codes or categories to the core category, thereby creating a relational model (Hernandez, 2009). There are different approaches to theoretical coding. Novice researchers might appreciate the structure of Strauss and Corbin's (1998) coding matrix consisting of three phases—open, axial, and selective coding, which are similar to Charmaz' steps of open, focused, and theoretical coding. Alternatively, some researchers may find the flexibility of Glaser's (1978) coding families—"sets of general sociological concepts organized into loosely connected frameworks" (p. 91)—more useful in supporting this phase of theory development.

In the context of Kate's study, theoretical coding involved a rigorous process of comparing and contrasting the analyzed data with core theories of occupation, identity formation, and narrative storytelling. Through this process, a theoretical understanding of storytelling was produced with the development of a model of narrative storytelling. While this model can be used to guide an understanding of the process of storytelling engagement, it is grounded in the participants' experiences and situated within the context of the advocacy storytelling program.

Constant Comparative Analysis

Data collected in a grounded theory study are analyzed using constant comparative analysis—a hallmark of grounded theory studies. This method requires the researcher to work through the interview transcripts comparing codes and looking for similarities and points of difference in the analysis. According to Hutchinson (1986), this type of interplay between the data allows for a proposed theory that is "molecular in structure rather than causal or linear" (p. 122). Constant comparative analysis is used within grounded theory studies to aid with theoretical decision-making and can be used to assist with preparing and asking questions in later interviews to deepen understanding of emerging concepts.

As data analysis proceeds, the use of constant comparative analysis both guides further interviews and what to look for in the data. It can also lead the researcher back to the literature. In grounded theory, literature becomes part of the method by which the theory is compared, contrasted, sorted, and expanded (Glaser, 1992). For example, in addition to going back to participants to test out emerging theoretical understanding, to further explore the relational nature of storytelling, literature on the topic was also sought. This initially involved re-visiting writing on storytelling as a relational experience (Gergen & Gergen, 2014) and expanded to an exploration of new areas of inquiry such as intersectionality (Gerlack, 2015; Gerlach et al., 2017; Thayer-Bacon, 2003) to better situate the emerging theoretical understanding of the research.

Developing the Theory

It is important to carefully consider which variant of grounded theory will be used for a grounded theory study. Indeed, as one strategy for rigor, researchers are advised to make explicit which version of grounded theory they are using and to describe and justify any deviation from the chosen approach (Cutliffe, 2000). Throughout this chapter, and in reference to Kate's study of narrative storytelling, we have profiled constructivist grounded theory methodology and the methods described by Charmaz (2014a).

While all approaches follow the methods of open coding and constant comparative analysis, the process of developing codes into abstract categories and eventually a theory to explain the social process can differ. For example, Glaser (1978) described a process of selective coding followed by theoretical coding. Strauss and Corbin (1998) developed a conditional matrix, a more structured approach for the novice grounded theorist, and Charmaz (2006) identified axial and theoretical coding as secondary process to initial (open) and focused coding.

Findings: Core Category

Traditionally, a fully developed grounded theory study must have a core category. The core category captures the social process and human interactions that occur in the phenomenon and has the explanatory power to pull together the theory (Glaser, 1978)—linking categories and explaining any variation in the process. More recent iterations of grounded theory (Charmaz, 2014b; Clarke, 2005) have lessened the emphasis upon a core category, focusing more on the development of an abstract grounded theory. Charmaz (2014a) argued, "A constructivist approach does not adhere to positivist notions of variable analysis or of finding a single basic process or core category in the studied phenomenon" (p. 132). Rather, Charmaz suggested the development of a theoretical understanding of the data as a social process, recognizing the evolving nature of the generated theory. In other words, the generated theory is contextualized within the focus area of research and may be presented as a framework or model of understanding. In the context of Kate's study, this approach to theory generation supported the development of a process model of narrative storytelling, grounded in the experiences of the research participants, and the advocacy context of the storytelling program.

Data Management

Qualitative studies can generate large amounts of data; therefore, before commencing analysis it is important to consider how data will be managed. Remote access to data is increasingly in demand as researchers increasingly work in virtual ways and as part of international collaborations. Traditionally, qualitative research was performed as a pen and paper exercise, and use of cards to sort and organize data. Qualitative data analysis computer software is an alternative tool that can store large amounts of data and ideas, which can then be retrieved quickly and efficiently (Richards, 2005). Furthermore, in response to our increasingly collaborative and virtual world of research, data analysis computer software offers a flexible space in which multiple researchers can analyze the same data. Examples of software include NVivo, ATLAS.ti, and MAXQDA to name a few. Each software offers different tools and options; for example, the ability to accommodate the upload of filmed observations for analysis, or the integration of multiple users collaborating in analysis of the same dataset.

While software tools are becoming increasingly intuitive and responsive, ultimately it is still the responsibility of the researcher to interpret and make meaning of the data.

Rigor and Ethics

Good grounded theory is not about imposing pre-existing theories; rather it is about generating theory that is grounded in the data. Yet, researchers are never completely impartial. As humans, researchers bring their past experiences, knowledge and values to the process. Indeed, Glaser (1992) suggested that it is the researcher's professional and personal experience together with their in-depth knowledge of the data that gives them the sensitivity to generate categories. Further, from a constructionist perspective, Charmaz (2006) has argued that the researcher is a co-participant in the study whose experiences contribute to the phenomenon being explored.

Charmaz (2006) identified four criteria for rigor in grounded theory studies—credibility, originality, resonance, and usefulness. Credibility involves making explicit the steps in the process of developing the theory, including the collection of appropriate data and evidence of procedures used in analysis. Researcher positionality and a thick description of the context are also necessary. A primary technique to assist with achieving credibility is memoing. As written records of analysis, memos make explicit the researcher's decisions and assist with exploring issues of concern throughout the data collection and analysis process. Originality pertains to "whether the study has helped develop new insights about the phenomena" (Priya, 2013, p. 4) and asks whether the findings "challenge, extend, or refine current ideas, concepts, and practices" (Charmaz, 2006, p. 182).

Additionally, appraisers of qualitative rigor often look for the use of member checking and triangulation; however, these are not mandatory in a grounded theory study. The researcher uses theoretical sampling to determine who to talk to next, or which interview questions to ask to expand on the emergent theory rather than using member checking. Thus, resonance is the degree to which the findings depict participants' lived experiences and whether participants are able to identify their journey in the grounded theory. From an ethical perspective, theoretical sampling may present challenges. For instance, a number of participants may volunteer; yet not all may be sampled to take part in the study due to the need to follow the research process and interview participants who can best speak to emerging theoretical concepts. If potential participants are recruited but not interviewed for the study, it is important, at a minimum, to offer them a summary of the research findings. We believe this to be an expression of respect in recognition of their willingness to be involved. Finally, usefulness requires researchers to explicate the contributions the study has made to their field and how the findings may be used by researchers and others impacted by the study (e.g., health services, health professionals, service user groups).

Critiquing Grounded Theory Studies

The findings in a grounded theory driven study must include four key elements: "(1) taking the word "grounded" seriously, (2) capturing and explaining context-related social processes, (3) pursuing theory through engagement with data, and (4) pursuing theory through theoretical sampling" (Timonen et al., 2018, p. 1). While many researchers who frame their studies with a qualitative descriptive methodology choose to use grounded theory methods, such as constant comparative method, to guide data analysis, there is a tendency to miss some or all of the aforementioned 'key elements.' For instance, the findings of many grounded theory studies are often presented as 'themes'; which, especially for novice researchers, can lead to confusion associating 'themes' with grounded theory studies. Thus, when reading articles that purport to be a grounded theory study, it is important to ask some critical questions (refer Textbox 5.5).

Textbox 5.5   Critiquing Grounded Theory Studies – Questions to Ask

1   Is the *epistemology* (constructivism, symbolic interactionism, or otherwise) clearly stated and justified?
2   Do the authors state what *version of grounded theory* is being used?
3   Does the research question start with a *how* or *what*?
4   Does the research question seek to uncover a *social process*?
5   Is there discussion of *theoretical sampling*?
6   Have the authors explained their method of *constant comparative analysis*?
7   Is there a *core category* presented?
8   Do the categories relate to each other and form a *coherent theory*?
9   Have the authors used *memos* as part of rigor?
10 Has the theory been *situated in current literature*?

Application to Occupational Science

Why do people choose to engage in certain occupations in a particular situation? How do they decide what occupation will be best for them or their community? What are the ways in which the same occupation is undertaken in multiple different cultures? These are just some questions that occupational scientists might be interested in answering when considering the relationship between people, occupation, and the environment. In Kate's study of narrative storytelling in brain injury rehabilitation, while not explicitly framed as an exploration of the occupation of storytelling, the occupational nature of storytelling was central to the research findings. Storyteller participants described their storytelling experience as occupationally meaningful. They were motivated to participate in the storytelling to help others and through the storytelling they experienced community connection.

Grounded theory methodology uncovered the relational process of storytelling underpinning these humanizing experiences of sharing and connection. Given Kate's background as an occupational therapist and the participants' occupational experience of storytelling, analysis inevitably became more closely situated to occupational science. Applying an occupational lens to the final stage of theoretical analysis generated a grounded theory of storytelling, depicted in a model of narrative storytelling. This model encapsulates the dynamic and multidimensional relationships between storytelling, occupational engagement, and identity construction. By 'playing' with analysis at the points of intersection between constructivist grounded theory and occupational science, the produced model enables a better understanding of how and why storytelling is an impactful experience.

Application to Occupational Therapy

Occupational therapy seeks to enable people to transform and transition through action (or the doing of occupation) for the betterment of their health and well-being. As a process, occupational therapy involves two or more people who influence the actions of each other (e.g., therapist and client); thus, the process can change, depending on those involved, while the intended outcome remains the same. Understanding the relational process of narrative storytelling in brain injury rehabilitation, as evidenced through Kate's research, has direct relevance to occupational therapy practice. Storytelling is framed as a series of humanizing relational experiences between the storyteller, the facilitator, and the advocacy context, that contribute to a transformative process of change for the storytellers. Through storytelling, the storyteller 'insider' or 'lived' experience of feeling heard and valued, releasing emotions and being occupationally productive, contribute to a developing sense of agency and connection with the wider community. The findings of this study have been translated into practice recommendations, organized around the constructs of (1) meaningful occupational engagement; (2) humanizing relational experience; and (3) personal reflection and self-learning (refer to Textbox 5.6). Resulting from the robust process of constructivist grounded theory, the practice recommendations are firmly grounded in the experiences of the research participants, while evolving from a co-constructed process of data analysis.

Textbox 5.6   Practice Recommendations

- Embed opportunities for sharing stories of lived experience into rehabilitation, for example initial assessment, goal planning, goal review, discharge planning and family meetings.
- Frame listening to stories as gathering information about the values, preferences, and needs of clients.
- Find strengths in stories that reinforce the message of lived experience as a recourse of knowledge and wisdom.
- Consider ways to share stories in the community to build community connections

---

Author Reflections

Qualitative research offers a rich experience of listening to the experiences of others, and actively engaging in analysis to seek a deeper understanding of a phenomenon of interest. As occupational scientists and occupational therapists inherently oriented to listening to and privileging the stories of lived experience of disability or migration, qualitative research is a gift. In doing qualitative research, we have been particularly drawn to constructivist grounded theory due to the co-constructed approach.

Kate: In my earlier work as a practicing occupational therapist in brain injury rehabilitation, years of experience taught me that I worked best when partnering with clients and their families. At times this work was harder, requiring flexible working hours to ensure I met with families when they were available and a readiness for emotional sharing. Partnering with clients and families taught me to be reflexive, flexible, and open to new ways of seeing, doing and being. At times, I had to abandon pre-conceived ideas, other times I was challenged to explain my views in pursuit of shared understanding, or a new path forward. At all times, I enjoyed the authenticity of this work. Similarly, in my research role, I value the challenge and opportunity to grapple with analysis in partnership with others, including research participants and colleagues.

Shoba: My interest in undertaking research in the field of migration and culture reflects my personal journey as an immigrant trying to find my way in a world that has involved straddling multiple cultures. Migration as an inherently social process is a field rich for grounded theory research. While initially I was drawn to grounded theory as it appeared to be one of the more 'structured' qualitative methodologies with regard to analytic methods; like Kate, the flexibility and rigor of the methodology has challenged me time and again to remain open to collaboration, learning about the processes of participants, communities, and society at large.

Constructivist grounded theory, with strong theoretical foundations and an evidence base, has a clearly defined framework from which to engage in a collaborative approach to qualitative research. And while the process is clearly defined, the process of concurrent data collection and analysis encourages reflexivity, creativity, and deep analytical thinking to generate a grounded theory of understanding. Constructivist grounded theory is now a familiar but ever challenging process of analytical thinking that is, at its heart, collaborative and centered around better understanding lived experience processes.

Summary

Throughout this chapter, we have sought to provide a comprehensive illustration of the process of constructivist grounded theory. As occupational scientists, occupational therapists, and qualitative researchers, we have drawn upon our shared experience, contextualizing with examples from Kate's research. Grounded theory is a recursive process that requires perseverance, patience, and partnership. Perseverance is needed to keep working with the data to develop a core category and a theory that coherently and robustly explains the social process. Patience is required for sitting in those times of 'not knowing'—where a potential theory lies but has not yet been generated. During these times, it is important to keep memoing every decision, question and plan. Finally, a grounded theory study requires passion, a desire to partner with others in building a co-constructed understanding of the research area. When approached with these three values, grounded theory, as a qualitative methodology, has much to offer researchers in occupational science and occupational therapy who are interested in uncovering a world of process within which people engage in occupation.

References

Belfrage, C., & Hauf, F. (2017). The gentle art of retroduction: Critical realism, cultural political economy and critical grounded theory. *Organization Studies*, 38, 251–271. https://doi.org/10.1177/0170840616663239

Birks, M., & Mills, J. (2015). *Grounded theory: A practical guide* (2nd ed.). SAGE.

Blumer, H. (1969). *Symbolic interactionsim: Perspective and method*. University of California Press.

Bowers, B. J. (1988). Grounded theory. In B. Sarter (Ed.), *Paths to knowledge: Innovative research methods for nursing* (pp. 33–59). National League for Nursing.

Bowers, B., & Schatzman, L. (2009). Dimensional analysis. In J. M. Morse, P. N. Stern, J. Corbin, B. Bowers, K. Charmaz, & A. E. Clarke (Eds.), *Developing grounded theory. The second generation* (pp. 90–132). Left Coast Press.

Charmaz, K. (2006). *Constructing grounded theory: A practical guide through qualitative analysis*. SAGE.

Charmaz, K. (2014a). *Constructing grounded theory* (2nd ed.). SAGE.

Charmaz, K. (2014b). Grounded theory in global perspective: Reviews by international researchers. *Qualitative Inquiry*, 20(9), 1074–1084. https://doi.org/10.1177/1077800414545235

Charmaz, K. (2014c). The power of constructivist grounded theory for critical inquiry. *Qualitative Inquiry*, *23*(1), 34–45. https://doi.org/10.1177/107780041665710

Charmaz, K. (2016). Shifting the grounds: Constructivist grounded theory methods. In J. M. Morse, P. N. Stern, J. Corbin, B. Bowers, K. Charmaz, & A. E. Clarke (Eds.), *Developing grounded theory. The second generation* (pp. 127–154). Routledge.

Chisman, E., & Brooks, R. (2018). The interplay between being and belonging through meditation: A grounded theory methods study. *Journal of Occupational Science*, *25*(4), 542–553. https://doi.org/10.1080/14427591.2018.1514320

Clarke, A. E. (2005). *Situational analysis: Grounded theory after the postmodern turn*. SAGE.

Clarke, A. E. (2008). Sex/gender and race/ethnicity in the legacy of Anselm Strauss. In N. K. Denzin (Ed.), *Studies in symbolic interaction* (pp.161–176). Emerald.

Corbin, J. (2009). Taking an analytic journey. In J. M. Morse, P. N. Stern, J. Corbin, B. Bowers, K. Charmaz, & A. E. Clarke (Eds.), *Developing grounded theory. The second generation* (pp. 35–54). Left Coast Press.

Corbin, J., & Strauss, A. (2015). *Basics of qualitative research*. SAGE.

Cutliffe, J. (2000). Methodological issues in grounded theory. *Journal of Advanced Nursing*, *31*(6), 1476–1484. https://doi.org/10.1046/j.1365-2648.2000.01430.x

D'Cruz, K. (2020). *Narrative storytelling following acquired brain injury: Creating connections and exchanging wisdom through sharing stories of lived experience* (Doctoral dissertation, LaTrobe University, Melbourne). http://hdl.handle.net/1959.9/570949

Dehghan, L., Dalvand, H., Hadian Rasanani, M. R., & Kelly, G. (2022). Exploring the process of health in mothers of children with cerebral palsy: Changing "clinical reasoning". *British Journal of Occupational Therapy*, *85*(4), 283–291. https://doi.org/10.1177/03080226211020659

Engel, L. L., Beaton, D. E., Green, R. E., & Dawson, D. R. (2019). Financial management activity process: Qualitative inquiry of adults with acquired brain injury. *Canadian Journal of Occupational Therapy*, *86*(3), 196–208. https://doi.org/10.1177/0008417419833839

Flick, U. (2019). From intuition to reflexive construction: Research design and triangulation in grounded theory research. In A. Bryant & K. Charmaz (Eds.), *The Sage handbook of current developments in grounded theory* (pp. 125–144). SAGE.

Gergen, M. M., & Gergen, K. J. (2014). The social construction of narrative accounts. In K. J. Gergen & M. M. Gergen (Eds.), *Historical social psychology* (pp. 173–189). Psychology Press.

Gerlach, A. J. (2015). Sharpening our critical edge: Occupational therapy in the context of marginalized populations: Aiguiser notre sens critique: L'ergothérapie dans le contexte des populations marginalisées. *Canadian Journal of Occupational Therapy*, *82*(4), 245–253. https://doi.org/10.1177/0008417415571730

Gerlach, A. J., Browne, A. J., & Greenwood, M. (2017). Engaging Indigenous families in a community-based Indigenous early childhood programme in British Columbia, Canada: A cultural safety perspective. *Health & Social Care in the Community*, *25*(6), 1763–1773. https://doi.org/10.1111/hsc.12450

Glaser, B. G. (1978). *Theoretical sensitivity: Advances in the methodology of grounded theory*. Sociology Press.

Glaser, B. G. (1992). *Basics of grounded theory analysis*. Sociology Press.

Glaser, B. G. (2001). *The grounded theory perspective: Conceptualization contrasted with description*. The Sociology Press.

Glaser, B. G., & Strauss, A. L. (1967). *The discovery of grounded theory: Strategies for qualitative research*. Adeline De Gruyter.

Hernandez, C. A. (2009). Theoretical coding in grounded theory methodology. *Grounded Theory Review: An International Journal*, *8*(3). https://groundedtheoryreview.com/2009/11/30/theoretical-coding-in-grounded-theory-methodology/

Hutchinson, S. (1986). Grounded theory: The method. In P. Munhall & C. Oiler (Eds.), *Nursing research: A qualitative perspective* (pp. 11–130). Appleton-Century-Crofts.

Kim, H., Hocking, C., McKenzie-Green, B., & Nayar, S. (2015). Occupational experiences of Korean immigrants settling in New Zealand. *Journal of Occupational Science*, *23*(2), 181–195. https://doi.org/10.1080/14427591.2015.1126531

Kuek, J. H. L., Raeburn, T., Chow, M. Y. Z., & Wand, T. (2022). Lived experiences of mental health conditions in Singapore: A constructivist grounded theory study. *International Journal of Social Psychiatry*. https://doi.org/10.1177/00207640221135111

Liamputtong, P. (2012). *Qualitative research methods* (4th ed.). Oxford University Press.

Lindblom, S., Flink, M., Elf, M., Laska, A. C., von Koch, L., & Ytterberg, C. (2021). The manifestation of participation within a co-design process involving patients, significant others and healthcare professionals. *Health Expectations*, 24, 905–916. https://doi.org/10.1111/hex.13233

Mills, J., Bonner, A., & Francis, K. (2006). Adopting a constructivist approach to grounded theory: Implications for research design. *International Journal of Nursing Practice*, *12*(1), 8–13. https://doi.org/10.1111/j.1440-172X.2006.00543.x

McAdams, D. P. (2001). The psychology of life stories. *Review of General Psychology*, 5(2), 100–122. https://doi.org/10.1037/1089-2680.5.2.100

Morse, J. M., Stern, P. N., Corbin, J., Bowers, B., Charmaz, K., & Clarke, A. E. (Eds.). (2016). *Developing grounded theory: The second generation*. Routledge.

Mulhall, A. (2003). In the field: Notes on observation in qualitative research. *Journal of Advanced Nursing*, *41*(3), 306–313. https://doi.org/10.1046/j.1365-2648.2003.02514.x

Murray, C. M., Edwards, I., Jones, M., & Turpin, M. (2020). Learning thresholds for early career occupational therapists: A grounded theory of learning-to-practise. *British Journal of Occupational Therapy*, *83*(7), 469–482. https://doi.org/10.1177/0308022619876842

Nayar, S., & Stanley, M. (2015). Occupational adaptation as a social process in everyday life. *Journal of Occupational Science*, *22*(1), 26–38. https://doi.org/10.1080/14427591.2014.882251

Nayar, S., & Wright St. Clair, V. (2020). Multiple cultures – one process: Undertaking a cross cultural grounded theory study. *American Journal of Qualitative Research*, *4*(3), 131–145. https://doi.org/10.29333/ajqr/9310

Nilsson, L. (2012). Using video methods in grounded theory research. In V. B. Martin & A. Gynnild (Eds.), *Grounded theory: The philosophy, method, and work of Barney Glaser* (pp. 103–116). Brown Walker Press.

Paterson, B., & Scott-Findlay, S. (2002). Critical issues in interviewing people with traumatic brain injury. *Qualitative Health Research*, *12*(3), 399–409.

Priya, K. R. (2013). Grounded theory methodology. In K. D. Keith (Ed.), *The encyclopedia of cross-cultural psychology* (1st ed.). John Wiley & Sons.

Richards, L. (2005). *Handling qualitative data: A practical guide*. SAGE.

Savin-Baden, M., & Major, C. H. (2013). *Qualitative research: The essential guide to theory and practice*. Routledge.

Stanley, M., & Cheek, J. (2003). Grounded theory: Exploiting the potential for occupational therapy. *British Journal of Occupational Therapy*, *66*(4), 143–150. https://doi.org/10.1177/030802260306600403

Strauss, A., & Corbin, J. (1998). *Basics of qualitative research: Techniques and procedures for developing grounded theory* (2nd ed.). SAGE.

Thayer-Bacon, B. (2003). *Relational "(e)pistemologies"*. Peter Lang.

Timonen, V., Foley, G., & Conlon, C. (2018). Challenges when using grounded theory: A pragmatic introduction to doing GT research. *International Journal of Qualitative Methods*, *17*, 1–10. https://doi.org/10.1177/1609406918758086

Topping, M., Douglas, J., & Winkler, D. (2021). General considerations for conducting online qualitative research and practice implications for interviewing people with acquired brain injury. *International Journal of Qualitative Methods*, *20*, 1–15. https://doi.org/10.1177/1609406921101961

Walder, K., & Molineux, M. (2020). Listening to the client voice: A constructivist grounded theory study of the experiences of client-centred practice after stroke. *Australian Occupational Therapy Journal*, *67*(2), 100–109 https://doi.org/10.1111/1440-1630.12627

Additional Resources

Bryant, A., & Charmaz, K. (Eds.). (2019). *The SAGE handbook of current developments in grounded theory*. SAGE.

Charmaz, K. (2017). An introduction to grounded theory [*Video*]. SAGE Research Methods. https://dx.doi.org/10.4135/9781473991798

Chun Tie, Y., Birks, M., & Francis, K. (2019). Grounded theory research: A design framework for novice researchers. *SAGE Open Medicine*, *7*. https://doi.org/10.1177/2050312118822927

Deakin University. (2022). *Grounded theory*. https://groundedtheory.weebly.com/

Grounded Theory Institute. (2008). *The official site of Dr. Barney Glaser and Classic Grounded Theory*. www.groundedtheory.com/

6 Phenomenology

Kirk Reed

Phenomenology holds as a central value the premise that most human truths are accessible through deep understanding of human subjective experiences, and the phenomenologist strives to "work through and around the filter of human thinking in order to obtain knowledge of the deeper essential structure of what it means to be human" (Thorne, 2016, p. 32). The scope of phenomenology offers an approach to the study of human occupation that goes beyond merely describing a person's lived experience. Literally, phenomenology is the study of 'phenomena,' the appearances of things, or things as they appear in our experience, or the ways we experience things—thus, the meanings things have in our experience. In essence, phenomenology is a Western Euro-centric philosophical tradition rather than a research methodology; therefore, it is important for a phenomenological researcher to at least have a beginning understanding of the underpinning philosophy when designing, developing, and conducting research. More generally, phenomenology is a way of investigation (Dreyfus, 1991); and a way of thinking, questioning, writing, and of being a researcher.

The tradition of phenomenology emerged in the first half of the 20th century influenced by Edmund Husserl, Martin Heidegger, Maurice Merleau-Ponty, Jean-Paul Sartre, and others. Edmund Husserl (1859–1939) is considered to be the founder and central figure of the phenomenological movement (Willis et al., 2016). Husserl criticized the positivist sciences and proposed an alternative to try and re-integrate the world of science with the 'lifeworld.' Husserl (1913/1962) described phenomenology as the science of the essence of consciousness, centered on the defining trait of intentionality, approached explicitly 'in the first person.' In this spirit, it might be said that phenomenology is the study of conscious experience of various types—as experienced from the first-person point of view. Thus, humans characterize experiences of seeing, hearing, imagining, thinking, feeling, wishing, desiring, willing, and also acting, that are embodied willful activities such as walking, talking, cooking, etc. However, phenomenological analysis of a given type of experience will feature the ways in which the researcher would also experience that form of conscious activity. How I see or conceptualize or understand the object I am dealing with defines the meaning of that object in my current experience. Thus, phenomenology features a study of meaning in a broad sense that includes more than what is expressed in the language used to describe the experience.

Over time, the contributions of key philosophers—Husserl, Heidegger, Merlau-Ponty, Schutz, and Derrida (see Table 6.1)—have generated important dimensions that are central to the philosophy and have potential implications for the study of human occupation. Indeed, the work of Lala and Kinsella (2011) identified that phenomenology could be useful for occupational science in terms of knowledge generation, intentionality, *Being*, and the lived body experience.

DOI: 10.4324/9781003456216-6

Table 6.1 Key phenomenologists over time

Philosopher	Research paradigm	Key contributions
Edmund Husserl	Positivist	Considered to be the founder of phenomenology which he developed as the rigorous "scientific study of things as they appear to be" (Pernecky & Jamal, 2010, p. 1063). Interested in essential experiences of things and consciousness, and analyzing intentionality. Proposed the method of 'bracketing' where judgment of the world is suspended to focus on the experience.
Maurice Merleau-Ponty	Post-positivist	Focused on perceptions and embodiment and the role of the body in human experience and resisted the separation of mind and body.
Martin Heidegger	Interpretivist	A student of Husserl, credited with the philosophical turn toward 'existential phenomenology.' Interested in understanding humans as Being-in-the-World and the contextual relationship to things. Focused on uncovering and interpreting people's situated experiences.
Alfred Schutz		A social phenomenologist, interested in how people create and construct social reality influenced by historical social and cultural structures.
Jacques Derrida	Deconstructivist	Developed the philosophical approach known as 'deconstruction.' Interested in dismantling traditional constructs as a means of providing alternative interpretations and meanings.
Max van Manen	Hermeneutic phenomenology	Specializes in phenomenological research methods, the meaning of the pedagogical relation, pedagogical tact, the pedagogy of self-identity in interpersonal relations, the pedagogy of recognition, and the meaning of writing in qualitative research.

Author created

As outlined in Table 6.1, there are a range of key philosophers that have contributed to the tradition of phenomenology. This chapter, however, will focus on interpretative phenomenology and the work of Heidegger based upon my own experiences of using Heidegger's work to explore the meaning of occupation (Reed et al., 2010). As the chapter progresses, I will strive to show how the philosophy guided the research question, methodology, and methods. Interpretive phenomenology sits within the philosophical scope of hermeneutics, of which Hans-Georg Gadamer (a student of Heidegger) was a key proponent. Gadamer's work extends that of Heidegger's by asking 'how is understanding possible?' and placing a strong emphasis on language and the importance of dialogue, especially in being open to discovering something new and letting new understandings emerge.

As a means of inquiry, interpretative phenomenology can be complex as it requires moving on from phenomenology as a philosophy to thinking about it as a guiding research methodology. Unfortunately, there is no recipe to guide the application of the philosophy to the research process. As a field of inquiry, interpretive phenomenology is the study of a phenomena as it appears in the world. Finding a way of uncovering and discovering phenomena is the challenge of phenomenology, where a phenomenon is any observable fact or occurrence of something. Heidegger (1927/1962) described phenomena as "that which shows itself in itself" (p. 52) and is a distinctive way in which something can be encountered. The phenomenon may, at some point, be uncovered (or obvious) and at other times remain hidden.

Interpretative phenomenology may be seen as a process of capturing the meaning of phenomena, unpacking the often "seen but unnoticed" (Hasselkus, 2006, p. 628) first-hand experience of engagement in occupation. It involves a refined and thoughtful exploration, an uncovering of what is taken for granted in relation to occupational engagement situated in the world, of going beyond physical engagement to consider the meaning of the experience and the social, cultural, and historical factors that have contributed to this meaning. Considering a person's occupations in the context of meaning provides the occupational therapy practitioner with an opportunity to understand occupation beyond the confinement of self-care, leisure, and productivity. Doing so, has the potential to develop a more significant relationship with the client; to explore outcomes beyond function and performance, often expected within the confines of the medical model and neo-capitalist health and social service provision; and to work with a person to build and maintain a sense of identity and meaning in contexts that are important to them.

Epistemology, Ontology, Axiology

Interpretative phenomenology is not so much interested in how people come to know things; rather, it seeks to interpret and understand the ontology or the meaning of everyday human existence (Inwood, 1999). The ontology of phenomenology is not about what and how certain things exist or figuring out categories and how things are related, it is much more about coming to understand the authentic meaning of being human. Heidegger challenges phenomenologists to discover the meaning of being, where being is not a substance or process or an event; rather, a central aspect of what a person is. He contended that Being is a phenomenon that conceals and hides itself and as such resists every attempt at "definition" (Heidegger, 1927/1962, p. 21). Being is familiar, natural, and so close to us that it is not actually recognized and, as such, it is a struggle to know what it is. Heidegger considers that one of the unique characteristics of human beings is the capacity to wonder about and reflect on our existence—he used the term 'Dasein' to describe this characteristic. Dasein has the ability to understand its being in terms of its existence in the world with others, but it is with relative ease that "Daseins fundamental tendency is to turn away from himself [sic] to a self-forgetful absorption in his occupations in company with other people" (as cited in King, 2001, p. 41). From an ontological perspective interpretative phenomenological research draws on philosophical assumptions that contend there are multiple and unique constructions of reality depending on context and how a person engages with the world. Heidegger's notion of Dasein calls on the researcher to 'tap into' the participants' experiences, to share their understandings of themselves and their connection to the world in relation to the phenomena of interest.

In attempting to find meaning, Heidegger's notion of 'horizons' is also important; this is explained by King (2001) who contended that "the world of our own existence is the horizon in which our everyday understanding moves" (p. 6). This is taken to mean that a person, including the researcher, interprets their everyday experiences through the eye of background meaning, which includes past knowledge, attitudes, values and experiences which are passed down through the language and culture a person is born into. These pre-understandings are always in motion as knowledge and experiences change, this is connected to the epistemology of the method. The data gathered are based on the interaction between the researcher and the participants, particularly from the participants' subjective reality of the experience. The researcher should create opportunities for research participants to share what they deem relevant in terms of their own experiences and to bring to the fore their horizon. In addition, the data are analyzed through the researcher's interpretations based on their own understanding of the phenomena.

For the interpretative phenomenology researcher, the notions of Dasein and horizons contribute to articulating the axiological nature of the study. This involves the researcher making explicit their own horizons (e.g., their professional knowledge and experiences, and personal values and beliefs) and how these values and prior understandings influence the aim, purpose, and design of the study, as well as their understanding of the phenomena. In my study, I sought to understand the meaning of occupation. From my own horizon and understandings, I assumed that meaning is likely to be hidden in the doing of an occupation, because occupation is people's everyday doing and happens with little consideration, unless they are no longer able to do that occupation.

Topics and Questions Best Suited for Phenomenological Studies

Research questions in interpretative phenomenology will be recognizable by naming the phenomena of interest and in defining the identified gap in knowledge. For Heidegger, people and their activities are always 'in the world'; our being is Being-in-the-world, so phenomenologists do not study activities by bracketing the world. Rather, activities are interpreted in terms of the meaning things have for a person by looking to the contextual relations between things in the world. Interpretative phenomenology is a suitable mode of inquiry when little is known about the hidden phenomenon of interest. Research questions are often 'what' questions, and are framed around the phenomenon of interest using the research question stem: what is the experience of X? Examples include 'what are health professionals' experiences of working with people from other disciplines?' (Flood et al., 2019); 'what is the experience and meaning of doing for people who are recovering from mental illness?' (Sutton et al., 2012); and 'what is the lived experience of professional musicians with playing-related injuries?' (Guptill, 2012).

Knowing what draws one to a topic of interest is a task for the phenomenological researcher. It is acknowledged with this type of research that the researcher comes to their inquiry with prior understandings and from a place from which the word is viewed. These pre-understandings are an accumulation of culturally held beliefs, ideas, historical events, or practices (Gadamer, 1960/2004; Heidegger, 1927/1962). Having someone interview the researcher about their 'pre-understandings' on the topic of interest, makes explicit how the research was conducted from the researcher's own experiences, and is useful to complete prior to fully reviewing the literature and gathering any data. Instead of bracketing off the researcher's subjective perspective, interpretive phenomenology recognizes that the researcher, like the research subject, cannot be rid of their *lifeworld*. Instead, the researcher's past experiences and knowledge are valuable guides to the inquiry.

When I was interviewed by my research supervisor, I talked about growing up in my family, family values, my work history prior to and as an occupational therapist, engaging in further study, and the transition to working in a university. Because I was interested in the meaning of occupation, I was asked to talk about an everyday occupation. I chose preparing a meal and thought about it in two different contexts. Textbox 6.1 is an extract from my 90-minute pre-understandings interview.

Textbox 6.1   Example from a Pre-understandings Interview

My experience of cooking a meal only ever happens once and it is my experience! I had never thought of occupation in this way until today. Occupation is a clearly identified individual experience that only the person experiencing the occupation can really understand what it means to them. I recall what it is like when I am at home at Christmas time with my family and the coming together of the family in the cooking of the meal, we all do our little bit to contribute, but Mum always has oversight of the whole meal; when the meat be cooked, when the vegetables need to go on, who will set the table, who will be in charge of the music. This is completely different of my experience of coming home after work and having to decide what to cook for myself and eat alone in front of the television. It is such a vastly different experience!

Through transcribing and reflecting on my stories, I came to understand more about the meaning of occupation related to my own experience. Until the point of undertaking the interview, the differences between a meal at Christmas and a meal after work was not something I had thought about—the phenomena had remained hidden. There was a connection to people (or lack of connection) in the different experiences; there was a sense of excitement, anticipation, and of the meal being orchestrated at Christmas as opposed to the mundaneness of a meal after work. I realized that how I experienced the Christmas meal was my own and might have been different for other family members (like my mother who was 'in charge'). I still did not fully understand the meaning of occupation, but now I had asked the question I wanted to know more. The pre-understandings interview is something I went back to, it enabled me to step back, to open up new questions, and let knew understandings show. For the interpretative phenomenological researcher, reflecting on how pre-understandings influence thinking and taking these into account when gathering and analyzing data is part of methodological trustworthiness. In seeking a person to conduct a pre-understandings interview, the interviewer should be familiar with the phenomenological philosophy and research approach. They should encourage the researcher to articulate their own perspectives; philosophical positions; theoretical and disciplinary assumptions; knowledge, political, and cultural views; ideas about the topic, and how these will inform and shape the research.

In an interpretive phenomenological study, the review of the literature also plays a key part in coming to understand the topic or question. The review might be done in two phases: an initial search to scope the field and identify the knowledge gap/s, and then a second search that aligns with the philosophical intent of the study. The second review is underpinned by Gadamer's (1960/2004) notion that "language is the universal medium in which understanding occurs" (p. 390). In hermeneutical interpretation, language is much more than mere words, it is bound up with traditions, with the present, and in negotiating and making sense of the world. Philosophical integrity guides the phenomenological researcher to uncover the meanings that already exist in the literature regarding the phenomenon of interest. These meanings may exist in the scientific literature but may also be found in novels, journals, songs, and poetry.

In my literature review I first reviewed the professional literature of occupational science and occupational therapy to understand how these disciplines understood the meaning of occupation and to identify what the gaps were in the current knowledge base. In the second part of the literature review I focused on how the meaning of occupation had appeared in Western history through time and some of the key historical influences on people's doing (Reed et al., 2013). This involved turning to some of the classic texts such as the Bible, those from the Ancient Greeks and Romans, and then through to the Middle Ages, the Renaissance and Reformation, and the Industrial Revolution periods. I also explored the etymology of the word occupation to uncover the development of the word and how it has been used over time. Once the question and topic of inquiry is defined, the next key decision is to determine from whom to gather the 'lived experience' stories.

Recruitment and Sampling

In a phenomenological study, recruitment is almost always a purposive sampling approach, as the aim is to identify potential participants with the experiences of the phenomenon of interest, and who can offer insightful reflections and share their stories in a way that gives the full sense of their experience. When recruiting and selecting participants it may be useful to recruit some participants who have enough and others who have a lot of experience of the thing of interest to enable diversity of experience both in terms of range and depth. The range of experiences, in turn, contributes to deep thinking about the phenomena. The means for locating potential participants will vary; but the aim is always to locate people with a rich experience of the phenomenon.

In this kind of research, it is important that the researcher and the participant can communicate in the same language, so nuances in language, tone, and meaning can be gained. Determining choice of language should be established early on in the study proposal and set as an inclusion criterion for potential participants. Other inclusion criteria to consider for a study might include: culture, ethnicity gender, an age range, or a specific health condition. For example, in Flood et al.'s (2019) study, they decided participants needed to have been working with healthcare professionals within the last five years, with a minimum of one year's practice experience within an Aotearoa New Zealand health care context. Sutton et al. (2012) were much more specific in that participants should be diagnosed with a serious and enduring mental illness, who saw themselves as making significant progress in their recovery from their illness, were able to give informed consent, were able to communicate in English, and were free of acute symptoms. Conversely, Guptill (2012) decided that professional musicians who had self-identified as experiencing a playing-related injury was sufficient.

In my study, I sought adults who had experienced some kind of disruption to their usual occupations, such as a change in job, retirement, or the way occupations were usually carried out due to a health issue. The disruption was a 'a way in' to enable participants to reflect on how their occupations had changed. Participants also needed to be able to communicate in English (my first and only language) and be available for a face-to-face interview. The size of the sample should be based on the nature of the question, up to eight will likely be adequate for a small study, while up to 20 would ensure the range of experiences. In my study, I recruited 12 participants, aged between 27 and 67 years, with an assortment of occupational disruptions (e.g., one participant had had a head injury, another had retired, and another had ruptured their Achilles tendon). Initially I interviewed three participants. Following these interviews, data were collected in groups of three participants at a time over a 12-month period, giving me time to collect, transcribe, and interpret each person's data.

Phenomenology suits common methods of recruitment in qualitative research such as advertising on social media, or more direct methods such as inviting professional networks, health practitioners, or key individuals to pass on information about the study. Snowball sampling can also be a useful strategy once recruitment has started, particularly if participants are hard to locate. I used informal professional and personal networks to enlist intermediaries who were supplied with information sheets about the study. The involvement of an intermediary was to ensure that there was no coercion from myself as the researcher toward potential participants. Unlike other research methods, recruiting all the participants and collecting and analyzing all the data does not have to happen all at once. To allow thinking along the way, a rolling recruitment method can be implemented, one or a few participants can be recruited at a time so each participant's data can be interpreted before interviewing the next. This strategy allows the researcher to refine interview questions, seek further participants with new and different experiences, and to enable rich and deep experiences to be gathered. Ideally, recruitment continues until no new notions emerge which will mean that the number of participants might vary.

Data Collection

An individual interview is likely to be the data gathering method of choice because the researcher needs to get as close as possible to the individual participant's experience of the phenomena and descriptions from the participants need to be rich, deep, and thick (van Manen, 1997). The interview itself will likely be guided by pre-set questions, but will largely be an unstructured conversation, to allow the space to be opened up for participants to tell their stories. There is often a fine balance between allowing the conversation to flow and interrupting to seek more detail or clarify a point. Taking a semi-structured interview approach, using a guideline of topics and/or questions, allows for new questions and notions to emerge within and across the interviews; and asking open ended questions allows participants to say things that could not be anticipated.

As noted above, philosophically it is assumed that being or ontology is hidden. Gadamer placed a strong emphasis on language and the importance of dialogue. He highlighted the significance of the movement between question and answer, which is relevant for the researcher to consider in terms of developing understanding. Hence, in the collection of the data it is not just about hearing the stories from the participants, but for the researcher to "remain open to the meaning of the other person or text" (Gadamer, 1960/2004, p. 271). This openness means that as a researcher you do not go in search of agreement with your understandings; rather, you are prepared to let the stories tell you something new. It is in this way that new understandings emerge.

The practicalities of collecting data from a one-to-one interview means consideration needs to be given to where the interview occurs, ideally somewhere private of the participant's choice, free from interruption, and where the tone can be set for a relaxed informal conversation. Usually an interview of between 60 to 90 minutes is sufficient, but in some instances a further interview may be required to seek additional information or ask clarifying questions. The interview/s need to be digitally audio recorded so they can be transcribed verbatim as it is the text from the interview that will be used in the data analysis process. While some online platforms provide a transcription function these are not always accurate. Furthermore, for the researcher to listen and re-listen to the recording while typing the transcript is a way of dwelling with the data, picking up on changes in tone, and becoming familiar with the text.

In my study, I invited each participant to share the kinds of things that they had been doing over the last seven to ten days. I did not seek specific information on the disruption that occurred. I sought stories about the everyday occupations in which the participant had engaged. As the conversation unfolded, so did the details of the disruption. I asked the participants to tell me if and how the disruption impacted on engaging in their occupations in any way, ensuring the conversation remained focused on their occupations. I was able to follow the lead of the participants; only occasionally did I have to prompt them to uncover stories of their everyday occupations. Several participants shared that they had not revealed to anyone the impact the disruption had on their everyday occupations; and on more than one occasion participants became visibly upset as they told their stories. This highlighted to me how personal these stories were and that together the individual participant and I had created a place that was 'safe' enough for them to share their experiences. Creating a 'safe' space requires connecting with a participant on a personal level, finding a point of connection with the person, inviting the conversation, being an open an authentic listener, and going at their pace. Inviting a person to share their often-personal stories can be best achieved in a place that is familiar and comfortable to them (e.g., their own home), which may be a useful strategy to put the person at ease.

Textbox 6.2 provides an example of a story from a participant who retired at the age of 40 years and now spends much of her week days alone in a rural setting tending to her garden. I asked her to tell me about her usual day.

Textbox 6.2   Excerpt from Participant One Transcribed Story

I'm one of those people that doesn't finish a job, I wander through the garden and notice what needs to be done. I will go out there with a list of about ten things that I have noted in my mind from the previous day, and I try and get through my list, but I never do, so the list carries on. I might start something and get distracted by something else that needs to be done, so I will go and do that and then come back to what I originally started, but that might not be until the next day. Really, I have created this garden so that I won't ever get bored. Now that I don't have to go to work, I can do the housework when I like and go out into the garden when I like. I don't have a rigid structure, but I keep to the habit of going out into the garden every day. The garden is my passion and my project, and I like it looking nice and I get a certain enjoyment from the plants. At the weekends, my partner is here during the day so there is another person around and we will go out and do a couple of things or just communicate because we haven't seen each other all week. The weekends are a lot more relaxed and my partner will have a sleep-in and then we will have coffee together and decide what it is we are going to do.

Beyond gathering stories of particular moments and events, interpretative phenomenology gives scope for eliciting participants' reflections and interpretations of things. Textbox 6.3 refers to a participant's reflection on the impact a head injury had on her day to day and how she sees the future.

As well as collecting data from participants, keeping a reflective journal is congruent with this methodology. A journal is a way of recording events and observations and emerging thoughts. I often wrote in my journal the things I noticed after each interview and the

---

Textbox 6.3   Excerpt from Participant Two Transcribed Story

I remember thinking at one stage, it was about eight months after I hit my head, what more can be taken away from me? Physically I was so incapable. I could hardly do anything visual like read or drive or watch television. All you are left with is your thoughts and emotions and if you haven't got good thoughts then you are in trouble. I knew the most important thing for me was getting myself together for myself and for my daughters and husband. I wanted to get my thoughts in a good place, because that is what it says in the Bible, and then everything else would come together. Now I feel like I'm in a good place in myself and I am actually choosing to occupy myself with the things that I like doing, things that I am passionate about, like floristry. It feels like a step in the right direction.

---

ideas that came to mind as the participants told me about their experiences. I used journal entries to re-orientate me to the interviews during the data analysis process.

Data Analysis

Interpretative phenomenological analysis is an inductive, iterative process. There is no one-way of doing the interpretation, the researcher needs to 'find their own way' in the interpretation, but certain features should be evident. Importantly, analysis begins with and continues alongside data collection: one informs the other. When engaging in data analysis there is often a dynamic interplay between activities, as identified by van Manen (1997), which include: turning to the phenomenon, investigating the experiences as it is lived, reflecting on essential themes, interpreting, and writing a description of the phenomenon.

The analysis progresses with drawing out stories, or anecdotes, from the data that say something about experiencing the phenomenon of interest from the multiple interview transcripts. Because interview transcripts are an accurate record of what was said, they are often jumbled and untidy, as is the nature of a person recalling their experience—one story might start, then lead to another, before being revisited somewhere else in the flow of the interview. Sentences may be incomplete which may make them clumsy to read and the messiness of the transcribed conversational text can act to conceal its meaning (Caeli, 2001). In my study, all the transcripts contained several stories of participants' occupations. To identify what the stories were about I gave each a title which named the occupation. These stories were then crafted into more refined stories using the participant's own words verbatim, but removing duplications and tidying up grammar, in order to reconstruct the story into a logical order. The refined stories, along with the pieces of the transcript, were returned to the participants for clarification, addition, or deletion of words, and for verification. Full transcripts were also provided to participants for their information. It is up to the researcher to work through the text to identify and extract the stories. There is no 'ideal' number, but once there is a sense of 'knowing' that all the stories say something of the phenomenon of interest have been captured, it is then time to move on to interpreting the stories. There is no one right way of doing the analysis; however, the essential feature of the analysis of the stories is that it is interpretative. The process of analysis is one of thinking engagement (Harman, 2007). It is not a thematic analysis of the content; rather, a way of thinking about the meanings within the text.

The next phase of analyzing the data is to investigate experience as it is lived, rather than as it is conceptualized, and reflect on the essential [phenomenological] themes that characterize the participant's experience with the phenomenon. There is no rule for how many themes you should end up with, between three and four is common. Having too many themes is a sign of superficial engagement with the data; and, at some point, adding an extra theme no longer provides useful information and it is likely that some themes will be merged. The ideas that are presented in a theme should convey the essence and intent of theme, each theme must make sense to a range of people. Working with an experienced interpretative phenomenological researcher who may ask critical questions and get you to consider new possibilities can help with determining the themes. Simultaneously, the researcher needs to reflect on their own experiences and pre-understandings to ensure these standpoints or experiences are not limiting or confining how they engage with the data. Researchers capture their reflections in writing and then reflect and write again, creating continuous, iterative cycles to develop increasingly robust and nuanced analysis through the creation of themes and sub-themes that bring to the fore the phenomenon of interest.

Throughout the analysis, the researcher must maintain a strong orientation to the phenomenon under study and attend to the interactions between the parts and the whole. This last step, also described as the hermeneutic circle, which was first identified by Schleiermacher (1768–1834) evokes a sense of constant movement that is influenced by prior understandings and a quest for, and a move toward, new understandings. Schleiermacher (1998) identified the importance of "understanding the unity of the whole via the individual parts and the value of the individual parts in the unity of the whole" (p. 109). According to Gadamer, "all understanding emerges with the aim and in a context of meaning of which the circle invites us to take note" (Grondin, 1999/2003, p. 84). The hermeneutic circle emphasizes the practice of deliberately considering how the data (the parts) contribute to the evolving understanding of the phenomena (the whole) and how each enhances the meaning of the other.

In my study, once I had the refined stories, I read and re-read each one, each time asking questions of the stories to gain greater understanding. These questions included: why does this occupation have meaning for the person? What was the experience like? What did or not did happen as part of engaging in the occupation? What was not said? I then took a blank piece of papers and noted down what 'seemed to matter' in relation to participants' occupations. At regular intervals I discussed these ideas with my research supervisors who shared their responses and questions which helped me to see things I had missed. This in turn lead me back to the data with fresh eyes.

Gradually I moved from description to interpretation. As themes began to emerge, I used 'mind mapping' to visually represent each of the emerging themes and the elements that were connected to a particular theme which helped to clarify the essence of each theme and to give it a name. This was an iterative and creative process where components were moved between themes and themes were clarified and refined. As clarity was gained and I began to write about each theme, I went back to the work of Heidegger and Gadamer, delving into their philosophical writings to bring new understandings to the data. During the process of interpretation, it was important to share emerging themes and notions with research and professional colleagues and with friends and family to ensure my interpretations were clear and justified. The critique, discussion, and the affirming nods suggested that the themes I had arrived at were supported.

You will recall the story from Participant One above, who talked about her day-to-day experience of gardening. In Textbox 6.4 below, the outcome of the analysis of this story is outlined which highlights the theme that was named 'The Call' in particular the sub-theme 'The Call as Passion.'

Textbox 6.4   Analysis of Participant One's Story

For Participant One there is a sense that her occupations are different at the weekend because there is someone else there. Her passion shows itself in two ways, the first is her garden and the second is her relationship. She is able to structure her week as she sees fit. Not having the restrictions of going to work means that she can spread the household and other tasks through her week. She is in the position of being able to choose how to spend her time. Because her partner is at home at the weekends she dedicates that time to being with her. She is her prime concern. Typically, she spends her week days alone, working on her garden attending to the wide range of tasks that are necessary to maintain a large garden. It is in her concern for her garden, for it to look nice, that 'calls' her to the garden. The call comes from what she notices needs to be done, which plant needs to be trimmed or which weed needs to be pulled out. The call is also from within, her garden is her 'passion and her project.' During the week there is little that distracts her from her project, it is the focus of her attention. We each in our own way have something that is our project, something that keeps us grounded and focused. The way in which Participant One carries out the occupation of gardening shows others something about herself. She moves from task to task and there is little pressure on completing what needs to be done, if a task is not completed it rolls over to the jobs to be done the next day. She sees the garden as a work in progress, it does not have an end point, and it continues to evolve.

In contrast, at the weekend Participant One has a fixed amount of time to spend with her partner. There is an impression that she wants to make the most of this time together, that in her solicitude for her partner she wants to create a relaxing atmosphere which allows her and her partner to come together. The occupations she engages in at the weekend are done in negotiation and partnership with the other. They are not things done for the sake of doing something. They are done for the sake of being-with her partner. There is a sense that for her she worries about her relationship and, in doing so, carefully selects what she and her partner do together to allow a re-kindling and a re-connection to maintain the being together. The worry keeps her in touch with the one for whom she cares and prompts her to create an atmosphere where they can be together side-by-side as they make their way forward.

In our dealings with the world, concern shows itself as "producing something, attending to something and looking after it, making use of something, giving something up and letting it go, undertaking, accomplishing, evincing, interrogating, considering, discussing, determining … All these ways of Being-in have concern as their kind of Being" (Heidegger, 1927/1962, p. 83). The occupations that we engage in have care at the heart of them, yet it is in our actions or activities that concern becomes an outward showing of that care. The things that matter to us show up through care. It allows us to see the world and others around us. Participant One's story shows that she is responding to things in the world, she is tending to and looking after her garden just as she is tending to and looking after her relationship. The meaning of occupation shows itself in what a person cares about and what calls them to action. Care calls for engaged action and attentiveness. Her occupations show others what is at the forefront in terms of her care, thus revealing something about herself.

Textbox 6.5   Analysis of Participant Two's Story

Not being able to engage in her usual occupations leaves Participant Two to dwell on the hopeless, helpless side of herself to the point where she can no longer see a future for herself. The focus of the other is still present and she is left to worry about what she is no longer able to do. It is in the not being able to do that she worries and the worry is from the solicitude she has towards her husband and daughters. She is focused on getting herself 'together' to be mother and wife to her husband and daughters. In her solicitude she is apprehensive about what the future will hold. It is not until the Bible 'leaps-in' that she has a sense of direction and she is able to stop dwelling on herself. The non-doing has given her the opportunity to find something she would like to do and that can show her family that she has the capacity to do things. For Participant Two, the worry prompts her to engage in the occupation of floristry. This gives her a sense of hope for the future. It is through occupation she is able to show both herself and her family that she is improving and her family has the opportunity to 'leap ahead' and let her stand on her own two feet. This small step gives her some hope that she will be able to take on some of the tasks she and her family associate with being mother and wife. Being able to engage in an occupation has significance for her because it shifts the anxiety from not being able to do anything to worrying about how she can return to be as mother or wife. Being 'able' to do matters more than what the actual doing is.

Participant Two, who had experienced a head injury, talked about returning to occupational engagement. The analysis of her story follows (Textbox 6.5); this also highlights the theme of 'The Call' but a different sub-theme which was named 'The Call Getting Myself Together.'

Rigor and Ethics

One of the tensions of interpretive phenomenological research is ensuring that the research stands up to the scrutiny of others and is trustworthy. The nature of the methodology requires meanings to 'emerge' from the data in the form of themes or categories whose origins often remain unclear (Nowell et al., 2017). The challenge for the interpretative phenomenological researcher is to establish a framework that makes explicit how decisions were made and how themes or categories were arrived at. Clearly articulating your judgement as a researcher is critical in order to determine which themes are important for your research question and how many themes should be generated.

The four criteria proposed by Annells (1999), while quite old, are a relatively straightforward and concise framework for determining trustworthiness. First, it involves evaluating whether the study is understandable and appreciable, this includes findings being presented in a way that is interesting, comprehendible, and appreciated by the audience; clear simple language that fits with the methodology should be used. Second, is whether the process of inquiry is understandable, where there is a description of a clear trail of philosophically and methodologically sound decisions. Third, Annells proposed that the research should be a useful product, the study must show that it has potential to impact either theoretically or practically. The final criterion is evaluating the appropriateness of the inquiry approach. In essence this involves naming the phenomenological approach used, describing how the approach is compatible and suitable for the research question, and that there is congruency between the method and the underlying philosophical notions that guide the study. To ensure the methodology is robust the researcher should make sure that the research question is aimed at exploring lived experience or meaning of the phenomenon and that philosophical assumptions underpinning the study are clearly articulated and inform the study design.

In terms of ethical considerations for this type of research, gaining informed consent from participants is key. Participants should be fully informed about what the study will involve. This will include that they will be asked to share personal experiences that for some may have an element of risk in terms of sharing events or experiences that may cause discomfort; in such instances information on appropriate supports should be provided. Participants may be provided with the choice to be named within the study or that their details will be altered to protect their privacy, in either instance this needs to be made explicit in the informed consent process. Participants also need to be assured that their data will be stored safely and kept confidential. In addition, partnership and/or consultation with Indigenous Peoples experts should take place to ensure that cultural factors and culturally appropriate data collection and analysis are built-in to the study design. In some jurisdictions, recruitment of participants from Indigenous populations or those considered to be vulnerable (i.e., a person who experiences mental health issues or young people) may elevate the ethical review process from low- to high-risk.

Application to Occupational Science

Given that the aim of occupational science is understanding the occupational essence of 'being' human (Wilcock, 2006), there is a philosophical coherence between occupational science and interpretive phenomenology. Phenomenology offers a unique perspective of the study of human occupation which both captures the meaning of phenomena (occupation) through firsthand accounts and involves a refined and attentive perspective that seeks to unpack the complex realm of ordinary everyday doing in context. For occupational scientists, understanding culturally embedded meanings of occupation is important, along with defending, challenging, describing, and transmitting thinking about the meaning of occupation in order to uncover the complexity of what it truly means to be human. A phenomenological perspective is seen by Lala and Kinsella (2011) as offering occupational scientists five interwoven dimensions to inform current understandings of human occupation. These five dimensions are

> (a) a unique vision of what knowledge generation entails, (b) reveals human intentionality and lifeworld perspectives as significant, (c) views *Being* as of central concern, (d) attends to the lived body as a means of experiencing and knowing the world, and (e) brings the potential for critique of taken for granted interpretations of meaning.
> (Lala & Kinsella, 2011, p. 206)

More recently, Larivière and Quintin (2021) have proposed that occupational scientists need to establish a dialogue with philosophy and, more specifically, that Heidegger's ideas can "inspire occupational scientists to view meaningful occupations as a way of reflecting on one's world or to embrace an occupational disruption as a journey to making consciously explicit our 'Being-in-the-world'" (p. 1).

The interpretive findings from my study (Reed et al., 2010) contribute to occupational science by illuminating the interconnected meanings of occupation. The study highlighted that even occupations that might be considered mundane have complex layers of meaning. The meaning is shaped by a "dynamic interplay between the call, Being-with and possibilities" (Reed et al., 2010, p. 146), where 'the call' is what matters most; it is what a person cares about and what concerns them and reveals itself in the occupations a person chooses (or avoids) to engage in. The notion of 'Being – with,' which revealed itself as a significant dimension, is related to with whom we do an occupation, in that each time a person engages in an occupation the nature of who is present (or who is absent) will impact on the meaning of occupation. It is in the coming together that meaning shows itself. The final theme was that of 'possibilities.' The participants' stories suggested that occupation has meaning because it is through occupation that people become aware of their own capacities and the opportunities that open up (or close down) as they continue on the journey of who they are becoming. Each of these facets of meaning work in unison, showing that complex, yet usually hidden, layers of meaning exist in the context of the world.

Application to Occupational Therapy

Phenomenological research may be useful to complement or deepen quantitative empirical research data about what is clinically effective for occupational therapy practice. The findings from phenomenological research have the potential to contribute to stronger evidence informed practice by providing data of what matters to people as they go about their occupationally contextualized lives. The value of lived experience data can, as Wright St Clair et al. (2011) highlighted, "reveal deeper understanding of peoples engagement in everyday occupations" (p. 26) and get closer to understanding the meaning of things for them. If, as Hamell (2009a, 2009b) and Crabtree (1998) claimed, occupational therapy practice needs to focus on the client's sense of identity in context and on quality-of-life issues, then a shift in the profession's preoccupation with function and performance needs to take place. Phenomenology provides a means to think about engaging in dialogue with the people occupational therapists work with, inviting stories about what contributes to well-being and personal development and what hinders or contributes to occupational engagement. Narrative is one tool to get a sense of an individual's experience, allowing a person to reflect on their capacities and possibilities and their dreams and aspirations for the future.

While such a way of practice will reap benefits for recipients of occupational therapy, occupational therapists themselves can also explore their practice and uncover what being effective means for them. For example, Flood et al. (2019) found that interprofessional practice was seen as "a way of being that extends beyond known and measurable skills and knowledge, to dispositions and qualities. Dispositional qualities come from within a person and what they care about, and from experiences that shape their understandings" (p. 744). The study by Sutton et al. (2012) challenged assumptions about occupational engagement in recovery from mental health issues and found that "All forms of occupational engagement, including disengagement, can be meaningful in the recovery process. Increased understanding of different modes of occupational engagement will assist therapists to support recovery more effectively" (p. 142).

Critiquing Phenomenological Studies

When critiquing phenomenological studies, it is important that the philosophical underpinnings of the study are made explicit (van Manen, 2017), along with the how the researcher positions themselves and their pre-understandings in the context of the study.

Ensuring that there is congruence between the interview questions and phenomena that draw out participant experiences of the phenomena of interest, rather than generalized experiences and 'perceptions,' are important to look out for. In terms of data analysis, looking for a depth of analysis based on each participant's experience is crucial. The analysis should bring to the fore the interaction between the parts and the whole, rather than a thematic coding of narrative content. The writing up of the research should seek to make explicit the meaning of the phenomena which moves beyond a superficial description to one that is rich and deep. When critiquing phenomenological studies there are some critical questions (Textbox 6.6) than can be asked of the study.

Textbox 6.6   Critiquing Phenomenological Studies – Questions to Ask

1 Is the *ontological nature* of the methodology clearly stated and justified?
2 Do the authors indicate which *specific type of phenomenology* is being used?
3 Have the authors articulated how the *principles of the phenomenological approach* have been implemented in the study?
4 Is the research question aimed at exploring *lived experience or meaning* of the phenomenon?
5 Do the *authors state their pre-understandings* in relation to the phenomena?
6 Does participant inclusion criteria specifically seek *participants with lived experience* of the phenomenon?
7 Have the authors described a *transparent decision-making process* throughout the study (e.g., how each participant's stories were analyzed)?
8 Have *philosophical underpinnings* been used to deepen interpretation?
9 Have the authors described how they analyzed *both the parts of the text and the text as a whole*?
10 Is it clear how rigor was ensured as part of the study (e.g., reflective journaling and how preliminary findings were confirmed)?
11 Is the meaning of the phenomena interpreted and described in a way that is comprehendible?

Author Reflection

The doing of interpretive phenomenology is as much to do with becoming a phenomenologist as it is with doing the actual research; it is a transformative process in terms of thinking and seeing the world differently. It means reading philosophical texts, in this case the works of Heidegger and Gadamer, the complexity of some their notions and the constant questioning of what I already knew created a depth of thinking I had not experienced before. I often felt like my brain might explode! Nonetheless, I was always wondering what the meaning of occupation was.

I naively thought that understanding the meaning of occupation would come together easily. I recall the conversations I had with the participants and how openly they shared their stories with me and how powerful talking about occupation was to them. Often, they were moved to tears as they shared how the change in being able (or not able) to do their occupations impacted on the others around them. What surprised me was their willingness to share aspects about their lives with a stranger that turned up on their doorstep with little introduction and a recording device. The conversations made me aware of how much people told me when the focus was on occupation; and as I contrast this to the types of interviews I did as an occupational therapy practitioner, I realize how much I did not gain in the past about a person and their occupations. I was not there to be an occupational therapist, I did not have to solve a problem or report back to my multidisciplinary colleague. I was there as a researcher, there to listen and let people tell their stories—this, in and of itself, is an important learning about how I would work with people in the future.

My study confirmed for me how complex occupation is, much more so than I ever realized. I feel that I just touched the surface of uncovering the meaning of occupation and hope that others will build on this work.

Conclusion

Interpretative phenomenology, and phenomenology in general, offers a unique perspective for the study of human occupation. Attending to phenomenological understandings of the lived experience of occupation through first person accounts involves a refined an attentive perspective; however, a caveat is that this research method draws on Euro-centric philosophical underpinnings. The challenge for the phenomenological researcher is to bring together the philosophical underpinnings and rigorous and robust research design to generate new insights. The doing of phenomenological research means coming to terms with the slowness of thinking and writing until understanding emerges, it is as much about the researcher coming to understand themselves as it is about the depth of the lived experience of the participants. Interpretative phenomenology offers occupational science a means to gain insights into human occupation and for occupational therapy a way to generate evidence to contribute to and inform theory development and support authentic practice.

References

Annells, M. (1999). Evaluating phenomenology: Usefulness, quality, and philosophical foundations. *Nurse Researcher, 6*(3), 5–19.

Caelli, K. (2001). Engaging with phenomenology: Is it more of a challenge than it needs to be? *Qualitative Health Research, 11*(2), 273–281. https://doi.org/10.1177/104973201129118993

Crabtree, J. L. (1998). Occupational therapy: Building skills or transforming selves? *British Journal of Occupational Therapy, 61*(11), 504–508. https://doi.org/10.1177/030802269806101105

Dreyfus, H. L. (1991). *Being-in-the-world: A commentary on Heidegger's Being and time, Division I.* The MIT Press.

Flood, B., Hocking, C., Smythe, E., & Jones, M. (2019). Working in a spirit of interprofessional practice: A hermeneutic phenomenological study. *Journal of Interprofessional Care, 33*(6), 744–752. https://doi.org/10.1080/13561820.2019.1577810

Gadamer, H. G. (2004). *Truth and method* (J. Weinsheimer & D. G. Marshall, Trans.; 2nd, rev ed.). Continuum. (Original work published 1960)

Grondin, J. (2003). *The philosophy of Gadamer* (K. Plant, Trans.). Acumen Publishing Limited. (Original work published 1999)

Guptill, C. (2012). Injured professional musicians and the complex relationship between occupation and health. *Journal of Occupational Science, 19*(3), 258–270. https://doi.org/10.1080/14427591.2012.670901

Hamell, K. W. (2009a). Sacred texts: A sceptical exploration of the assumptions underpinning the theories of occupation. *Canadian Journal of Occupational Therapy, 76*(1), 6–13. https://doi.org/10.1177/000841740907600105

Hamell, K. W. (2009b). Self-care, productivity, and leisure, or dimensions of occupational experience? Rethinking occupational 'categories.' *Canadian Journal of Occupational Therapy, 76*(2), 107–114. https://doi.org/10.1177/000841740907600208

Harman, G. (2007). *Heidegger explained: From phenomenon to thing.* Open Court.

Hasselkus, B. (2006). The world of everyday occupation: Real people, real lives. *American Journal of Occupational Therapy, 60*(6), 627–640. https://doi.org/10.5014/ajot.60.6.627

Heidegger, M. (1962). *Being and time* (J. Macquarrie & E. Robinson, Trans.). Blackwell. (Original work published 1927)

Husserl, E. (1962). *Ideas: General introduction to pure phenomenology* (Gibson, W. R. B., Trans.). Collier-Macmillan. (Original work published 1913)

Inwood, M. (1999). *A Heidegger dictionary.* Blackwell.

King, M. (2001). *A guide to Heidegger's Being and Time* (J. Llewelyn Ed.). State University of New York Press.

Lala, A. P., & Kinsella, E. A. (2011). Phenomenology and the study of human occupation. *Journal of Occupational Science, 18*(3), 195–209. https://doi.org/10.1080/14427591.2011.581629

Larivière, N., & Quintin, J. (2021). Heidegger and human occupation: An existential perspective. *Journal of Occupational Science.* https://doi.org/10.1080/14427591.2020.1858941

Nowell, L. S., Norris, J. M., White, D. E., & Moules, N. J. (2017). Thematic analysis: Striving to meet the trustworthiness criteria. *International Journal of Qualitative Methods, 16*(1). https://doi.org/10.1177/1609406917733847

Pernecky, T., & Jamal, T. (2010). (Hermeneutic) Phenomenology in tourism studies. *Annals of Tourism Research, 37*(4), 1055–1075. https://doi.org/10.1016/j.annals.2010.04.002

Reed, K. (2008). Resituating the meaning of occupation in the context of living. [Doctoral thesis, Auckland University of Technology]. Tuwhera. http://hdl.handle.net/10292/398

Reed, K., Hocking, C., & Smythe, L. (2010). The interconnected meanings of occupation: The call, being-with, possibilities. *Journal of Occupational Science, 17*(3), 140–149. https://doi.org/10.1080/14427591.2010.9686688

Reed, K., Hocking, C., & Smythe, L. (2013). The meaning of occupation: A hermeneutic (Re)view of historical understandings. *Journal of Occupational Science, 20*(3), 253–261. https://doi.org/10.1080/14427591.2012.729487

Schleiermacher, F. (1998). *Hermeneutics and criticism and other writings.* (A. Bowie, Trans.). Cambridge University Press.

Sutton, D., Hocking, C., & Smythe, E. (2012). A phenomenological study of occupational engagement in recovery from mental illness. *Canadian Journal of Occupational Therapy, 79*(3), 142–150. https://doi.org/10.2182/cjot.2012.79.3.3

Thorne, S. (2016). *Interpretive description: Qualitative research for applied practice* (2nd ed.). Routledge.

van Manen, M. (1997). *Researching lived experience: Human science for an action sensitive pedagogy* (2nd ed.). Routledge.

van Manen, M. (2017). But is it phenomenology? *Qualitative Health Research, 27*(6),775–779. https://doi.org/10.1177/1049732317699570

Wilcock, A. A. (2006). *An occupational perspective of health* (2nd ed.). Slack.

Willis, D. G., Sullivan-Bolyai, S., Knafl, K., & Cohen, M. Z. (2016). Distinguishing features and similarities between descriptive phenomenological and qualitative description research. *Western Journal of Nursing Research, 38*(9), 1185–1204. https://doi.org/10.1177/0193945916645499

Wright St. Clair, V. A., Kerse, N., & Smythe, E. (2011). Doing everyday occupations both conceals and reveals the phenomenon of being aged. *Australian Occupational Therapy Journal, 58*(2), 88. https://doi.org/10.1111/j.1440-1630.2010.00885.x

Additional Resources

The BBC. (2023). *In our time. Phenomenology.* www.bbc.co.uk/sounds/play/b04ykk4m

Vagle, M. D. (2018). *Crafting phenomenological research* (2nd ed). Routledge.

Wisnewski, J. (2013). *Heidegger: An introduction.* Rowman & Littlefield.

7 Case Study Methodology

Simon Leadley, Margaret Jones and Clare Hocking

Textbox 7.1 Coco

Coco values "having family time. Like having a Christmas Eve movie fiesta and just sleeping out in the lounge … [or] a fish and chip picnic lunch in the lounge." Spending time with her parents and siblings provides emotional nourishment, a sense of security and happiness, helping her cope with the material hardship her family experiences. However, that can't undo poverty's impact on opportunities for recreational and social activities, the predominance of sedentary activities in her day-to-day life, or restricted family time due to her father's erratic, long hours as a shift worker.

Our case study of Coco, a pre-teen child, highlights the ways people and their occupations are intertwined with their environments. Case study provided the means of exploring the intricacies of Coco's occupations, all the while keeping to a view of these as they were interconnected with context.

Case study research commonly refers to the detailed examination of a specific situation or phenomenon in context. A range of different data sources are used, and there is careful attention to the particularities and complexities associated with each case and its natural situation (Simons, 2009). The 'case' in case study research is a natural, functioning, material phenomenon. It has defined boundaries, and is situated in a particular place and time; a thing that can be experienced. The case may center on an individual person, a group or community, an organization or political entity, or multiple groups that share a common feature, such as experience of a certain event. Because cases are intricately interwoven with their contexts, even a single-person case is regarded as a system (Stake, 1995; Yin, 2018).

It is important to differentiate case study research from the use of the term 'cases' in relation to medical records, the reporting of a typical or notable 'case' as an illustrative example or to raise awareness, or cases that are provided to support study and learning (Yin, 2018). We also note that literature variously refers to case study as a research methodology, an approach, a strategy, or a method (Simons, 2009), perhaps reflecting its application across time in diverse fields of practice and authors' terminological preferences. In this chapter, we refer to case study research as a methodology, which denotes that despite some variation in research applications and perspectives, case studies have commonality in their intentions, strategies, and processes, and ways of communicating (Jónasdóttir et al.,

DOI: 10.4324/9781003456216-7

2018; Mills, 2014), as illustrated in Figure 7.1. Although quantitative case studies are also conducted (Boyer, 2010), here we use the term 'case study' to refer to qualitative case study research. Unless otherwise stated, all information about the case is drawn from Simon's thesis (Leadley, 2019), presenting key terms bilingually (i.e., Māori/English), given that te reo Māori is the first language of Aotearoa New Zealand.

Case study research is thought to have its beginnings in the 19th and early 20th centuries through the work of Frederic LePlay, a founder of French sociological studies; in the Western Pacific studies of Bronislaw Malinowski, an Austrian-born pioneer of social anthropology; and in America, in social workers' case notes and in the field work of Robert Parks, William Thomas, and Florian Znaniecki in the Department of Sociology at Chicago University. Whilst the first case study researchers were internationally diverse, there were common concerns with the everyday activities and interactions of individuals within specific sociocultural groups, and the meanings group members attributed to those activities in their contexts. Correspondingly, these early case study researchers drew from a range of field data, including observations, interviews, and documents to give detailed, situated, and holistic accounts of the groups under focus (Hamel et al., 1993).

The early case study work in Chicago exploring the experiences and social challenges faced by immigrant workers shares historical linkages with the professional evolution of occupational therapy. Two of the earliest occupational therapists, Jessie Luther and Eleanor Clarke Slagle, spent time in Chicago early in the 20th century and worked from Hull House, a settlement house established to support new immigrants (O'Neill, 2022; Reed, 2018). Pragmatist philosopher John Dewey, who was based at the University of Chicago over this time, had an acknowledged influence on case study research (Hamel et al., 1993). Dewey also had close connections with programs offered at Hull House (Fischer, 2009) and with Adolf Meyer (Ghaemi, 2007), who played a key role in the early development of

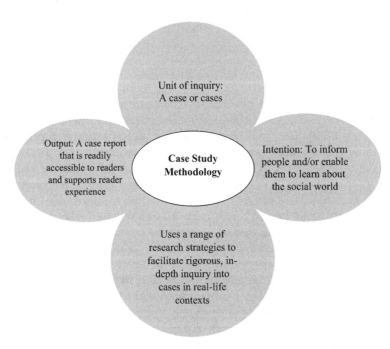

Figure 7.1 Case study methodology. Author created.

the occupational therapy profession (Loomis, 1992). Pragmatist influences on both case study and occupational therapy are reflected in a shared appreciation of common-sense ways of knowing, as they are directly derived through habits, action, and experience in context (Hamel et al., 1993; Reed, 2018).

The prominence of case study research waned in the mid-1930s, with a drive for quantitative research to inform social inquiry. Case study came to be seen as merely exploratory, paving the way for what were perceived as more robust studies that used statistical methods to validate theory (Hamel et al., 1993; Platt, 1996). Similar shifts began in occupational therapy in the 1940s and 1950s, when the profession moved away from a holistic view of people and their occupations to a reductionistic focus on body structures and functions, supported by research that could provide a 'scientific' rationale for addressing impairments in these elements (Kielhofner, 1992). However, in the 1960s and 1970s, there was a resurgence of interest in qualitative case study research in the social sciences. This was later paralleled by emerging recognition in the occupational therapy profession of the importance of a holistic focus in understanding and addressing people's occupational needs (Hamel et al., 1993; Kielhofner, 1992). Since these early beginnings, the use of case study research has extended, with widespread application in fields such as education, economics, urban planning, organizational and political studies, and health sciences (Flyvbjerg, 2011).

As a result of its evolution and diverse fields of application, there is variation in the way case study research is conducted. Its pluralistic approach has been critiqued, with the wide range of philosophical approaches, research designs, methods, and data analysis techniques seen as disadvantageous. Further points of critique include that it is an approach to research not a methodology; its lack of comparative analysis and generalizability (especially single case study designs); and that it is too onerous, not suited to developing theory; lacks rigor; and tends to confirm researchers' biases (Creswell & Poth, 2018; Schwandt & Gates, 2018; Yin, 2018). Nonetheless, a number of case study theorists have identified this research approach as a methodology (Jónasdóttir et al., 2018; Mills, 2014), and defend the rigorous processes involved (e.g., triangulation) (Simons, 2009; Stake, 2006; Yin, 2018). Furthermore, it has been argued that case study methodology creates no greater researcher bias than other forms of inquiry (Flyvbjerg, 2011) and that case study methodology's ability to accommodate pluralism is an advantage (Mills et al., 2010). Additionally, while the concept of statistical generalizability is not relevant to qualitative case study, analytical generalizations or inferences from cases are; thus, case study methodology can highlight a 'typical' case that offers insights about a broader set of cases. Further, case study methodology contributes to both empirical and normative (standards or values) theory development and testing, causal explanations, and insights into how and why interventions or processes work (Schwandt & Gates, 2018; Yin, 2018).

Epistemology, Ontology, Axiology

Qualitative case study research can accommodate different epistemological understandings, including critical, critical realist, relativist, post-positivist, pragmatist, or constructivist epistemologies (Crowe et al., 2011; Paparini et al., 2021; Yin, 2018). However, epistemological understandings can make a significant difference to the aim and questions asked, decisions about the design and methods employed, and the type of findings produced. Clarifying the epistemological standpoint of a case study is, therefore, important as a basis to support internal coherence and rigor (Stewart, 2014). Such concerns are addressed by seminal methodological authors including Gerring (2007), George and Bennett (2005), Yin (2018), Merriam (1998), Stake (1995), and Simons (2009), who have discussed ways case study research can be approached epistemologically, and proposed a range of research methods including some that are relevant across epistemological perspectives. Authors such as Gerring, George, Bennett, and Yin convey a post-positivist approach, with a realist epistemological position that assumes there is a single reality that can be discovered, which is independent of those who seek to know it (Harrison et al., 2017). The associated methods emphasize design based on a priori knowledge and theory, elimination of bias, and analytic strategies geared towards explanation, theory building, proof (or disproof), and generalization.

In contrast, authors such as Merriam (1998), Stake (1995), and Simons (2009) embody a constructivist approach to case study (Harrison et al., 2017). Drawing from the authors' backgrounds in educational research, their texts reflect a relativist epistemology that acknowledges multiple ways of knowing. These texts highlight the way knowledge is constructed by those who experience a phenomenon and who seek to know. From this perspective, meaning and understandings are of central importance when deciding on the methods used, and the ways the researcher's values and perspectives shape the research are made transparent. Findings are conveyed heuristically to support readers' vicarious experience of the phenomenon, enabling them to transfer their own constructed understandings within their own worlds (Merriam, 1998).

The epistemological positioning shapes the research aims and question, and the type of case study conducted. As case study methodology researchers, we adhere to a constructivism paradigm through which we seek to better understand the socially constructed world in which we live (Creswell & Poth, 2018; Schwandt & Gates, 2018). Our ontological position is that truth is relative, thus acknowledging multiple realities; and our epistemological stance is that knowledge is co-constructed through lived experiences and transactions, both individually and socially (Creswell & Poth, 2018; Lincoln et al., 2018). Axiology underpinning the study used to illustrate case study methodology in this chapter includes a belief in the right of all people to participate in meaningful occupations and that poverty is unjust. The study was informed by key theoretical perspectives of Dewey's pragmatism and transactionalism (Creswell & Poth, 2018; Cutchin & Dickie, 2012), occupational science (Wright-St Clair & Hocking, 2019), and a life course theory of human development (Humphry & Womack, 2019). Thus, we took a constructivist, qualitative approach to understand the phenomenon of interest—child poverty and its influence on patterns of occupation—that is based on multiple perspectives and situated in real life contexts.

Approaching the Research Topic

The desire to better understand the effects of poverty on tamariki/children's patterns of occupation was supported by a review of the literature identifying harmful impacts of poverty in children's development, physical and mental health, and educational and vocational outcomes; and our conviction that those impacts directly relate to restricted opportunities for regular participation in diverse occupations (Leadley & Hocking, 2017). We reasoned that if participation in a diverse range of occupations (i.e., personal cares, leisure, school/work) supports children's development, health, and well-being, then constrained patterns of occupation (i.e., habits, routines, roles, rituals) would have deleterious effects, despite tamariki/children and their whānau/families' best efforts to cope with this adversity. Our assumption was that child poverty is an occupational injustice, depriving children of the right to participate in socially valued occupations. We also believed the study could inform policy and practice that would contribute to addressing the issue of child poverty.

Considering our constructivist perspective and the exploratory nature of the research, qualitative case study methodology suited this enquiry because it can be used to examine issues from the differing perspectives of those who experience it (i.e., children, their families, community members) and is conducted in naturally occurring contexts (i.e., the child's home and neighborhood). Case study methodology also enables the complexity and transactional nature of phenomena to be examined; for example, the ways children cope, the supports available to them, and wider sociopolitical influences.

Types of Case Study

Depending on their purpose as exploratory, descriptive, explanatory, or evaluative, case studies have design variations (Merriam, 1998; Stake, 1995, 2006; Yin, 2018). Stake (1995, 2006) also discriminated between intrinsic, instrumental, and multiple case studies (Figure 7.2). Determining the best type to use for our study required deliberation about how the case could inform the research question and was informed by the theories

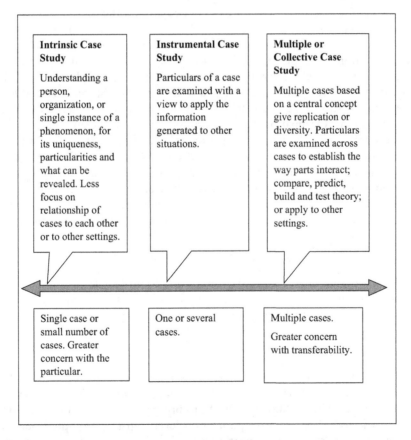

Figure 7.2 Continuum of case study designs. (Adapted from Stake, 1995, 2006). Author created.

underpinning the study (occupational science, transactionalism), a constructivist paradigm, and our goal of finding pragmatic ways to remediate the problem. Although we acknowledged this single case would be unique, we believed it would provide useful insights into the situation of other children and their families living in poverty in Aotearoa New Zealand. As the intent was to use in-depth understanding from this case to inform knowledge about the wider issue, an instrumental case study was proposed.

Dewey's (1925/1981) pragmatist philosophy also directed our understandings about our roles as researchers. Because people and their environments are seen as connected, taking part in research generates change in both the person and the environment. Therefore, when Simon was gathering data, rather than setting himself apart he interacted in a natural manner, taking account of his interpretation and influences on the data gathering process in his written reflections. Thus, data were seen as co-constructed by Simon and the participants.

Developing the Research Questions

Within case study methodology, research questions perform an important role in organizing the study. Case studies are well suited for answering 'how' or 'why' questions but are also useful for 'what' questions, where the study is exploratory (Yin, 2018). In situations where researchers are exploring or evaluating an organization against specified criteria, the case is already decided and research questions are developed around the case. As shown in Figure 7.2, this situation is characteristic of intrinsic studies, the focus being on a particular case or cases. Researchers responding to uncertainty over a more general situation would identify the research questions first, perhaps guided by theory. Cases are subsequently selected. These questions are more characteristic of an instrumental or multiple case study because cases are selected to provide understanding of a wider situation (Stake, 1995, 2006).

Our research question reflected our desire to understand the effect poverty has on children's occupations. Occupational science and occupational therapy theory (our theoretical perspectives) helped us define occupation as occurring in transaction with the person and their environment (Cutchin & Dickie, 2012; Nyman et al., 2014). Thus, a child's participation in occupations is a dynamic interaction of their abilities and skills, their whānau/family's material and personal resources, the features of their community, and the wider social context (e.g., policy that addresses child poverty). Accordingly, our research question was: How does material poverty affect a child's patterns of occupation?

Developing the Conceptual Framework

The next step is working out a conceptual framework, to provide foundations and boundaries for the study, and to bridge from existing knowledge to subsequent stages of the study. Developing a conceptual framework involves three stages, outlined below.

Issue Statements and Definitions

Conceptual issue statements (sometimes called issue questions or propositions) build on the research questions, drawing on researcher experience and theoretical understandings (Simons, 2009; Stake, 1995, 2006; Yin, 2018) to bring prior assumptions and likely areas of concern to the fore. For example, population level statistics prompted our concerns about children's time-use and participation in sports, leisure, and employment. Issue statements provide a conceptual base upon which the next stages of the study can be built. For example, guided by the child poverty literature and occupational therapy theory, one of our issue statements/assumptions was '*Children's occupations are patterned into habits, routines, and rituals that are responsive to their roles, their physical environment, societal patterns of time use (e.g., school hours), and people in their environment.*' Another issue statement described how environmental influences (e.g., available resources and material poverty) shape (afford/constrain) children's occupational patterns. Important terms, such as participation and poverty were also defined. While issue statements are proposed in the initial, conceptual stages of a study, they may undergo revisions in response to findings as the study progresses (Stake, 1995).

Delineating the Case

Case study methodology texts highlight the importance of defining the case or "unit of analysis" (Yin, 2018, p. 101) so that its components and boundaries are clear and there is control over the scope of the project. The case in our study was delineated as a child and their whānau/family living at or below the income-based poverty line, the low socioeconomic neighborhood in which they live, other adults who support the child's occupation, and also included relevant legislation and policy.

Different design features are considered at this point. Options include the number of cases and whether cases have embedded units of analysis (i.e., sub-cases contained within them). When conducting a multiple/collective case study, the number of cases is guided by the degree to which they provide diversity or similarity. Depth of understanding about the phenomenon and its interactions with the context is also sought. In our study, a single case study approach was chosen in order to learn as much about the case as possible, and consequently how this informed the research question (Stake, 1995, 2006). This decision was also influenced by time and resource restraints.

Developing Topical Questions

Topical questions focus in from the initial issue statements, specifying the information to be sought. For example, the issue statement "*Material poverty impacts a child's pattern of occupation*" led to the following topical question that was integral to all participant interviews, observations, and other data gathering methods: '*How does a lack of income in/directly impact a child's participation in and patterns of occupations?*' The issue statements and topical questions point to the types of data needed and data sources, and help frame inclusion and exclusion criteria. To keep track of the multiple components we needed to consider, we developed a table detailing the issue statements, related topical questions, methods to gather relevant data, and where or from whom the data would be gathered from (Stake, 1995; Yin, 2018). Arranging this information in a table helps pinpoint where information will be triangulated and highlights any gaps. The topical questions then inform development of interview and observation guidelines.

Project Management

Before commencing data collection, a project management plan is developed to ensure data are gathered systematically and that the overall project runs smoothly. This includes planning detailed information such as the conceptual structure and ethical approval/s.

Considerations include recruitment processes, securing participant contact details, safety procedures, equipment, and sequencing the data gathering. Strategies for data analysis and a proposed outline for the case study report assist focus and preparedness for subsequent phases of the project (Stake, 1995, 2006; Yin, 2018).

Recruitment: Case Selection

As discussed earlier, although a case may have already been identified, on other occasions cases are selected purposively, meaning the case and associated data sources are selected to best inform the research question. Selection of participants within a case needs to ensure that they meet the inclusion criteria, will generate answers to the topical questions, and provide adequate diversity or similarity between cases. People's availability and the location of the case also influence selection, given that data collection may extend over weeks or months.

Recruitment to our study began with building relationships with community organizations that support whānau/families who experience poverty. Representatives of these organizations put up recruitment posters and approached families they thought matched the study's inclusion criteria: A family living at or below the Aotearoa New Zealand income poverty line with a 10–13-year-old child who attended a school in a low socioeconomic area. The family then nominated a school teacher/sports coach and a youth group leader, who supported the child's occupations, to participate in the study.

Data Collection

Case studies are characterized by using multiple data sources, which supports trustworthiness and gives breadth of information. That is particularly useful if the study is exploratory and seeks new understandings. We employed multiple data sources, as detailed below.

Interviews

After an initial visit to complete consent forms and build connections with the family (whanaungatanga) (Egan-Birtan, 2010; Health Research Council of New Zealand [HRC], 2010), semi-structured interviews were conducted with Coco (the child's chosen pseudonym) and her mother, in the relaxed atmosphere of the family home (Creswell & Poth, 2018). Coco's interview was completed in two parts (approximately 50 minutes each), using age-appropriate language, and a friendly and relaxed approach. The interview with her mother included completing the NZiDep (a questionnaire about financial/household need over the last 12 months) (Salmond et al., 2014) and canvassing Coco's parents' views on the impacts of their poverty on her occupational patterns and their support of her participation.

The interviews with Coco's teacher and youth group leader focused on their perspectives about the family's financial situation, its effect on Coco's occupations, and the support they and the community provided for Coco and other tamariki/children in her socioeconomic position. Interview guidelines were used to ensure information gleaned aligned with the topical questions, whilst remaining open to new insights, such as the extent to which people in the community supported the occupations of children in the neighborhood and the importance Coco placed on time spent with her family.

A Daily Occupation Diary

Time-based data gathering methods are considered useful in revealing habits and routines, and their relevance in people's lives (Erlandsson, 2013; Hunt & McKay, 2015; Koome et al., 2012). For our study, a daily occupations diary using age-appropriate language and colorful graphic designs was created to capture Coco's pattern of occupation over a typical week. It had one page per day, with space allocated to describe each activity, its location and duration, and who was involved. This data supported information gleaned from interviews and other data gathering methods, revealing what proportion of Coco's occupations were passive or active, or occurred in or away from home.

Photo-elicitation

Photo-elicitation methods do not require advanced literacy or verbal skills, and can be a meaningful, creative, and fun data gathering strategy for children participating in research (Jorgenson & Sullivan, 2010). Child participants are provided with a camera and asked to take photos of places, situations, items, or occupations of importance to them and then discuss their photos. Coco's photos included the orchids she helped grow in their backyard, the Christmas pageant she performed in, and toys she played with in her room, which was the only private space she had to engage in restorative self-care occupations.

Mapping Activity

Mapping activities have been successfully employed in research, in particular with children, to capture the geographical spread and frequency of participants' occupations (Darbyshire et al., 2005; Huot & Rudman, 2015). The mapping method we devised used a hard copy map of the city and involved Coco and her mother drawing onto the map the locations of her occupations, access routes, and frequency of travelling those routes. Sticky notes with a brief description of modes of transport used and people supporting participation were attached. This data highlighted Coco's limited geographical range, the frequency of walking as a mode of transport (related to the cost of buses and the family owning only one car), and the number of people outside the family supporting various occupations by providing transport.

Observations

Observations can begin at the start of case study research, with diary entries about observations in the field and reflections related to the research question/s (Stake, 1995). In our study, observations occurred throughout data gathering, with three formal participant-based observations (Guest et al., 2013). These were selected by Coco and her parents from suggestions we offered: getting ready for school, afterschool routines (homework, preparing and sharing a meal), and a Christmas pageant Coco and her siblings took part in, and were guided by the topical questions and observation protocols. Observations were initially recorded in diary format before being written in full for analysis, ultimately informing our understanding of the family's hectic morning routine, how limited resources hindered afterschool occupations (e.g., access to the family computer to do homework), and the highly valued time spent eating meals and watching television as a whānau/family.

Document Review

Documents reviewed for this study were selected based on information needs highlighted by the topical questions and included websites and documents related to extracurricular occupations provided by Coco's school, and recreational opportunities provided by the city council and other community organizations in her neighborhood. These provided insights into the limited recreational opportunities on offer to her that did not involve fees, transport costs, equipment purchases, or adult supervision. However, the community did provide opportunities and resources, such as her teacher supporting engagement in water polo and a community center giving children bicycles.

Data Analysis

Given the variety of data collected using case study methodology, data analysis requires careful decisions about which analytic approach to use. In general, the process involves systematically breaking the data down into parts, discovering the meaning of those parts, then piecing them back together in a way that makes sense of the whole phenomenon and its context, and which provides answers to the research question/s. Common aspects of data analysis include in-depth description of the case and its context, preliminary interpretation of the data and coding, identification of patterns and connections in the coding, and development of assertions or propositions. Where there are several cases, a cross-case analysis may be performed. Throughout the process, researchers must consider alternative interpretations while staying focused on the issues. However, approaches to analysis vary according to the theoretical perspectives guiding the study, the types of questions an approach is designed to answer, and the degree to which the analysis is directed by the issue statements. Maintaining congruence of the methods with the study's epistemology is paramount.

The intention of our research question was to better understand the phenomenon. Therefore, analysis was guided by Stake's (1995) approach, which sees the researcher moving intuitively between direct interpretation of single instances of phenomena, and aggregation of instances, weaving meaning both inductively and deductively to connect the parts with the whole (Dewey, 1910; Stake, 1995). Where there is repetition, patterns and relationships begin to suggest themselves. Data may be methodically searched for instances that either refute or confirm patterns and relationships.

There was a need in our case study to represent both the unique qualities of this case and, in a pragmatic sense (Morgan, 2014), gain insights into the ways poverty affects children's pattern of occupation and how this knowledge might be used to address the problem. This confirmed the need for balance between direct interpretation (i.e., describing unique features in the case) and categorical aggregation (i.e., generating themes or assumptions based on the data), as forms of data analysis that help in the search for patterns and correspondence in the data (Stake, 1995). Furthermore, ensuring the findings are understandable to readers brings greater relevancy. This can occur through readers identifying with the case, or what Stake (1995) termed "naturalistic generalization" (p. 85). Of note, the strength of the qualitative single case study research approach is in accentuating the contextuality and depth of knowledge that comes from examining a single case in detail, in its real world setting (Simons, 2009; Stake, 1995).

The analysis in our case study followed a four-stage process. First, analysis occurred throughout the study as we created impressions and gave meaning to data, through reflexive approaches to clarifying topics in interviews, constant memos, reflective diary entries, and continued exploration of literature. The second stage involved intensive analysis of the data (e.g., repeatedly listening to audio recordings, reading transcripts, reviewing other forms of data, making memos) and use of mind mapping techniques to create codes and themes (Merriam, 1998; Stake, 1995). For example, insights gained from Coco's data were displayed on sheets of paper according to a key topic such as 'Coco's Pattern of Occupation,' with emerging conclusions grouped under subheadings such as 'time by myself' or 'helping out.'

The third stage consisted of developing categories aligned to the research question and issues statements (e.g., the case, patterns of and participation in occupations). We started by grouping all initially analyzed data aligned to each issue statement, using different colored paper for each transcript and other forms of data. The categorized data were then entered into data tables based on each issue statement. For example, one data table related to the issue statement "Resources will influence a child's patterns of participation in occupations," with data drawn from child and adult interviews, observations, and other forms of data gathering (see Table 7.1). As key themes such as 'low cost occupations: making do' and 'missing out on occupations' emerged, further data tables were developed (see Table 7.2).

The fourth and final stage involved combining all data analysis, grouping findings into sections (e.g., Introducing the participants, the context of the case study, and Coco's pattern of occupation: The impact of poverty) and using a narrative style of writing with rich descriptions, participant quotations, and visual forms of data to support naturalistic generalization.

Developing Assertions

A further level of analysis may be undertaken in relation to the research question/s by developing concluding statements about the case or cases (Simons, 2009). Stake (1995) referred to these statements as "propositional generalizations" or "assertions" (p. 86).

Table 7.1 Data table relating to Key Assumption/Issue Statement #4

Key Assumption/Issue Statement: #4 *Resources (i.e., physical, social, geographic, cultural, institutional, and temporal) will influence (i.e., constrain/afford) a child's patterns of participation in occupations.*	
Topical information question	*Data and data source*
1 What are the resources available to the child participant that support their engagement in occupations?	*Physical resources: Transport* – car, bike, buses, walking (child interview #2 p. 20; Parent interview p. 32; Observation (pageant) p. 5); *Home/house* – Observation (morning routine), Activity diary; *School & community center* – classroom, sports ground, playgrounds, river; *Opportunity shop* – recycled goods for sale *Social resources: Parents* – activities diary, mapping activity; *Family friends* – parent interview p. 32; *School & teacher* – teacher interview pp. 1, 5, 14, child interview #1 p. 25, additional funding for socioeconomically deprived schools; *Local church* – financial support and food parcels

Author created

Table 7.2 Example of data analysis table showing data, source, and emerging themes

Occupational patterns: participation		
Theme	*Description*	*Quotations*
Restricted occupational choices	*Do what we can* – This phrase sums up the restrictions on Coco's participation in a range of occupations she would like to do, due to financial and resource constraints	*"There are a few that she would like to do. She would like to join netball, quite possibly she would have liked to have done gymnastics... I would have loved to have been able to send her, but finances again."* (Parent interview, p. 35) *"I have a bike but I don't use it because I don't have a chain for it ... otherwise it will get stolen."* (Child interview #2, p. 11) *"She was invited to under 12 squad training for water polo ... and then her mum had to pull her out because of the cost."* (Teacher interview, p. 10)

Author created

To develop assertions in our case study, we examined the findings alongside key occupational science concepts, such as occupational deprivation, as well as the child poverty literature and found they supported our initial assumptions. Some of our tentative assertions were:

1 Child poverty is occupationally unjust.
2 Children living in poverty on a sustained basis experience occupational deprivation, characterized as having a restricted range of occupations, narrow social horizons, and negative effects on their well-being.
3 There are bi-directional relationships between child poverty, health, and occupation.

In Coco's case, poverty restricted engagement in social and physically active occupations, and supported a sedentary lifestyle (see Figure 7.3). In combination, her pattern of occupation was affecting her psychological well-being and had potential long-term implications for her health (Leadley et al., 2020).

The findings have practical implications for occupational therapists working in collaboration with tamariki/children, their whānau/families, and community agencies in impoverished communities, informing targeted prevention services and individualized interventions that build on their strengths/assets to enhance participation and promote healthier occupational patterns. Additionally, the occupational therapy profession can use the findings to advocate for change at a broader social and population level through policy, population-level interventions that enable participation, and through research (Pizzi, 2016; Scaffa, 2019).

Case Study Report

Presenting case study findings is an important part of the methodology. A report may be informed by the original conceptual framework but will also reflect new discoveries and assertions that were developed. Reports can include any combination of narrative, direct

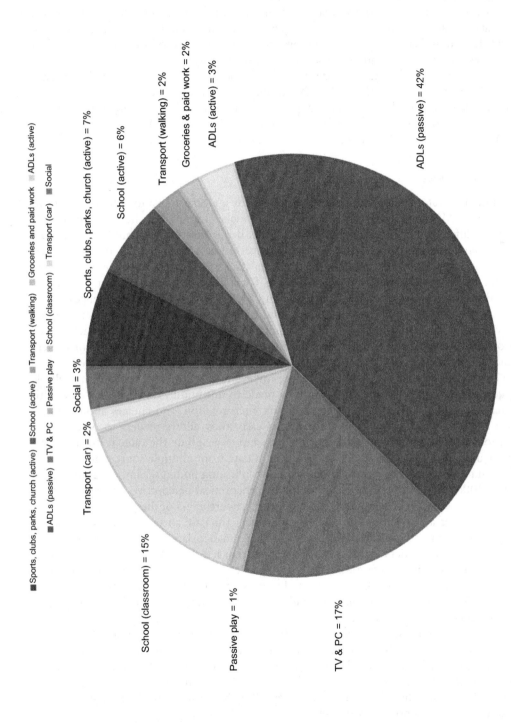

Figure 7.3 Analysis of Coco's occupations: active and passive. Author created.

quotations, diagrams, and quantitative data. They should provide vicarious experience of the case; therefore, the audience must be kept in mind when developing the format.

In writing the report for our case study, the need to convey meaning clearly and concisely was balanced against providing depth of experience and meaning for readers. It was anticipated that the audience may be occupational therapists, health professionals, child poverty advocates, or researchers and policy advisors. Consequently, the thesis was presented in an accessible format, including thick descriptions of the case, frequent use of participants' words, and visually displayed findings. Additionally, key findings were published in a peer reviewed journal (Leadley et al., 2020), presented at a national occupational therapy conference, and informed a submission made to the government's Child Poverty Unit on behalf of Occupational Therapy New Zealand Whakaora Ngangahau Aotearoa.

Rigor and Ethics

The primary strategy supporting rigor for a case study is clear articulation of the conceptual framework (Mitchell, 2000; Stake, 2006), which makes transparent the decisions undertaken at different stages in the research process. It demonstrates the connections between the research questions, the theoretical perspectives underlying the study, the issue statements, and the types of data sought from various data sources. In this way, readers can be assured of the logic underpinning the design. Their iterative design also supports rigor, with decisions and interpretations questioned in the light of new data, experiences, emergent understandings, and existing theory. Alternative interpretations are reflected upon. New avenues for data-collection may be sought. Researchers, therefore, look back as well as forward, changing and refining the conceptual framework, plan, or interpretations where indicated. Such changes are reasoned (Yin, 2018) and the rationale is documented.

Case study research necessitates the close involvement of the researcher with multiple aspects of the case. Although efforts may be made to not unduly influence the data, ultimately researchers shape the data gathered, its interpretation, and choices about what is most important to convey. A well-conducted case study allows readers to perceive the position of the researcher in relation to the data and to weigh up the value of the interpretation and assertions generated. Triangulation of data from multiple sources and via multiple data collection strategies is also a means of confirming findings (Simons, 2009; Stake, 1995, 2006; Yin, 2018). The use of alternative theoretical perspectives to explore study findings and member checking further support trustworthiness of the findings.

Most importantly, a rigorous case study conveys the case to readers in rich detail to support vicarious experience. Where assertions are made, data should be provided and explained so that readers can clearly see the path that led to those conclusions, and also consider different interpretations. These strategies enable readers to reflect on how that information relates to their experiences and understandings about phenomena, providing a foundation for learning and making a judgement about the degree to which information can be applied beyond reported cases.

In conducting a case study, researchers tread a fine line between accurately portraying the case and protecting participants' anonymity. Careful choices need to be made about obscuring identifying details without compromising the integrity of the findings. Dilemmas can be posed within a case if participants express views that may be hurtful or offensive to others. Researchers' first duty is to ensure the well-being of the participants, and data must be discarded if it cannot be used safely.

Careful attention was given to conducting our research as it involved tamariki/children under 18 years of age in the context of the sensitive issue of poverty (Graham et al., 2013; HRC, 2021). We designed the study to ensure both their protection and their participation. At a practical level, this meant parents' informed consent and the child's ongoing informed assent; child friendly data collection methods that, where possible, gave the child and her parents control; and maintaining a reflexive stance about the power imbalance between adult researchers and the participant/child.

Attention to specific cultural considerations highlights the cultural background/s of the researcher/s and the cultural context in which research took place. In Aotearoa New Zealand, all research occurs in the context of Māori as tangata whenua (Indigenous people) and Te Tiriti o Waitangi, a constitutional treaty (National Ethics Advisory Committee [NEAC], 2019). Acknowledgement of the negative impacts of colonization for Māori is required, along with respectful engagement with key principles: Tino rangatiratanga (sovereignty of Māori), Kawanatanga (governorship, authority for Māori), Ōritetanga (equitable access, treatment, and outcomes for Māori), and Wairuatanga (honoring Māori spiritual and health beliefs and practices) (Came et al., 2021; NEAC, 2019). In practice, this means working in partnership with and involving participation of Māori communities and protecting Māori rights and interests in relation to the issues of concern (HRC, 2010; NEAC, 2019).

In our study, we consulted with Auckland University of Technology's Mātauranga Māori Committee and engaged with a Māori cultural advisor throughout the study. All interactions with participants followed tikanga (correct Māori protocol) such as giving a mihimihi (Māori form of introduction), whanaungatanga (building connections), and manaakitanga (showing respect, kindness) (Moorfield, 2011).

Best Practice

Ensuring qualitative case study methodology is employed according to best practice is discussed broadly in a number of texts (Simons, 2009; Stake, 1995; Yin, 2018). Within occupational science and occupational therapy, case study research needs to accommodate the complexity of people's occupations including their experiences and perspectives, and contextual components (e.g., interactions with the environment, cultural values, and historical factors). Achieving that whilst adequately bounding the case study requires clearly stated research question/s, and a conceptual structure to guide the types and sources of information needed. To fully address concepts relating to people and their occupations in connection with context, a range of data collection methods such as interviews, participant observation, and document review (e.g., records, legislation or policy at individual, community, or population levels) should be considered for their ability to best provide detailed understandings relevant to the research question. Data collection should also be responsive to new ideas that are developed through interaction with the data, recognizing that new or different questions, strategies, and sources may become relevant as the study progresses. The analytical strategy chosen needs to enable interpretation of the multiple forms of data and also maintain a view of the transactional and contextual nature of occupations. Embedded in this process are carefully but pragmatically thought out ethical and cultural considerations, such as conducting research in people's homes/communities and where they are vulnerable, that both protects and enables their participation in the research.

Application to Occupational Science

The utility of case study methodology for studying phenomena in real-world contexts has a natural alignment with occupational science, specifically in exploring the transactions of people, occupations, and environments (Carey, 2020) and understanding the experience of occupation in context (Jónasdóttir et al., 2018). For instance, Murphy and Shiel (2018) used descriptive case study methodology to explore meaningful occupations within the restrictive institutional rules and practices of a community residential mental health facility, concluding that residents were subjected to occupational injustices. Conversely, case study methodology has been used to reveal how occupation affects people who engage in it, such as Phelan and Kinsella's (2014) exploration of occupations shaping the identity of children with disabilities, within their unique socio-cultural context. Case study methodology has also been used to uncover contextual factors shaping occupations, such as identifying skills family and community members use to enable children's participation after traumatic brain injury (Jones et al., 2017) or to depict how the continual presence of television in children's homes shapes their play activities, almost entirely displacing the traditional games their grandparents remember (Ramugondo, 2012). From our perspective, the uptake of case study methodology is making an invaluable contribution to understanding the complexity of occupation in context.

Application to Occupational Therapy

Endorsement of case study methodology to inform occupational therapy dates from at least 1996, when Colborn claimed its advantages for studying variables related to patient performance and intervention outcomes (Salminen et al., 2006). Over the following decade, its merits were further elaborated. Case study research designs, proponents argued, were well suited to developing new or validating existing theories about how and why things happen (Fisher & Ziviani, 2004) and for generating fresh insights into intervention processes, such as differences in therapist/client perspectives and the impact of specific contexts on therapy outcomes (Salminen et al., 2006). Arguments for the suitability of case study methodology for building the profession's evidence-base continue to be mounted (McQuaid et al., 2022).

Subsequent applications of case study methodology in occupational therapy fall into two categories: Studies to enhance understanding of complex occupational therapy processes and studies that elucidate practice in complex practice settings. Examples of the former include exploration of clinical reasoning processes, such as how therapists individualize interventions (Copley et al., 2008) and how to build therapeutic partnerships with a community (Hyett et al., 2019). Examples of the latter include analysis of practices and organizational systems across workplaces with effective retention and support strategies for people with mental illness (Gewurtz et al., 2021) and how adults with enduring mental illness participating in a group program, and its facilitators, perceived the change process. As befits case study methodology, such studies address entrenched, complex issues with intermeshed personal, organizational, structural, and environmental elements (Hercegovac et al., 2020).

Critiquing Case Studies

Given its diverse applications, case studies must be approached critically, recognizing a study's epistemology, ontology, axiology, and theoretical underpinnings, which influence the design and findings. Questions to guide a critical appraisal are listed in Textbox 7.2.

Textbox 7.2   Critiquing Case Studies – Questions to Ask

1 Are the *theoretical perspectives* clearly stated and justified?
2 Is the *role of the researcher* clearly articulated?
3 Does the *conceptual framework* clearly link to the question, theoretical perspectives, and types and sources of data sought?
4 Has the case been clearly defined?
5 Was the *safety and anonymity* of participants assured?
6 Were the data collection and analysis strategies systematic, clearly described, and justified?
7 Was the research process *responsive to unexpected events* or findings?
8 Were changes to the original protocol justified and reasonable?
9 Were *alternative explanations* for findings sought and discussed?
10 Is the *context* adequately described and integrated with the findings?
11 Is the case study report rich, engaging, and accessible?
12 Is the case cohesive, with *findings and assertions* considered in relation to the original questions and theoretical understandings?
13 Is it clear how the *assertions or issue statements* were derived? Do they make sense in relation to other information in the study?
14 Are *new insights* into the issue provided?

Author Reflections

Case study methodology initially appealed to Simon, as a novice researcher, because of the topic. Poverty is both personal and societal, meaning that a methodology that could encompass both was needed. An exploratory approach was also needed, as it has seldom been viewed from an occupational perspective. As Simon read and talked with others about case study methodology, he was drawn to its capacity to explore the phenomenon in a real-life setting (e.g., people's homes and community), drawing in diverse perspectives using data collection methods appropriate to the data sought. As a kaiwhakaora nganga-hau/ occupational therapist, he was comfortable with the narrative style of reporting Stake promoted.

Using case study methodology, however, has not been without its challenges. These have included: organizing the multiple types of data gathering (e.g., interviews, observations) in a variety of settings (i.e., home and community); negotiating sensitively the time spent with tamariki/children and whānau/family in their homes/communities; and managing and analyzing large amounts and varieties of data. These issues were managed using systematic data management strategies, by repeatedly consulting key texts, reflexive practices, and through the support of a supervisor experienced in case study methodology.

The most rewarding aspects of utilizing case study methodology were the rich insights generated about the phenomenon, which shaped the conclusions we reached. In collaboration with the participants, we shared a story about the ways a child, her whānau/family, other adults, and their community support children's participation in occupations while also elucidating how poverty constrains participation.

Conclusion

Our choice of case study methodology was justified as the complexity of Coco's pattern of occupation in the context of her whānau/family's material resources, their neighborhood and community, and the governmental assistance available for families living in poverty could be examined as an integrated whole. The range of data gathering methods, multiple participant perspectives, examination in a real-life context, along with strategies to ensure rigor, meant that this single case study succeeded in shedding light on the effects of material poverty on a child's pattern of occupation. The knowledge generated provides new insights that can inform practice, policy, and future research directions.

Acknowledgements

We thank Occupational Therapy New Zealand Whakaora Ngangahau Aotearoa and the Waikato–Waiariki Synod: The Methodist Church of New Zealand Te Haahi Weteriana o Aotearoa for funding support.

References

Boyer, W. (2010). Quantitative single-case research design. In A. Mills, G. Durepos, & E. Wiebe (Eds.), *Encyclopedia of case study research* (pp. 765–766). SAGE. https://doi.org/10.4135/9781412957397

Came, H., Kidd, J., McCreanor, T., Baker, M., & Simpson, T. (2021). The Simpson-led health sector review: A failure to uphold te Tiriti o Waitangi. *New Zealand Medical Journal, 134*(1532), 77–82.

Carey, H. (2020). An integrative review of case study methodologies in occupational therapy publications. *Cadernos Brasileiros de Terapia Ocupacional, 28*(4), 1284–1296. https://doi.org/10.4322/2526-8910.ctoAR2077

Copley, J., Turpin, M., Brosnan, J., & Nelson, A. (2008). Understanding and negotiating: Reasoning processes used by an occupational therapist to individualize intervention decisions for people with upper limb hypertonicity. *Disability and Rehabilitation, 30*(19), 1486–1498. https://doi.org/10.1080/09638280701654799

Creswell, J. W., & Poth, C. N. (2018). *Qualitative inquiry & research design: Choosing among five approaches* (4th ed.). SAGE.

Crowe, S., Cresswell, K., Robertson, A., Huby, G., Avery, A., & Sheikh, A. (2011). The case study approach. *BMC Medical Research Methodology, 11*(100), 1–9. https://doi.org/10.1186/1471-2288-11-100

Cutchin, M. P., & Dickie, V. A. (2012). Transactionalism: Occupational science and the pragmatic attitude. In G. Whiteford & C. Hocking (Eds.), *Occupational science: Society, inclusion, participation* (pp. 23–37). Wiley-Blackwell. https://doi.org/10.1002/9781118281581

Darbyshire, P., MacDougall, C., & Schiller, W. (2005). Multiple methods in qualitative research with children: More insight or just more? *Qualitative Research, 5*(4), 417–436. https://doi.org/10.1177/1468794105056921

Dewey, J. (1910). *How we think*. Retrieved from https://archive.org/details/howwethink000838mbp

Dewey, J. (1981). Experience and nature. In J. A. Boydston (Ed.), *John Dewey: The later works, 1925–1953* (Vol. 1). Southern Illinois University Press. (Original work published 1925)

Egan-Birtan, M. (2010). *'This is how I see it': Children, young people and young adults' views and experiences of poverty*. The Office of Children's Commissioner. www.occ.org.nz/assets/Uploads/Reports/Poverty/This-is-how-I-see-it.pdf

Erlandsson, L. (2013). Fresh perspectives on occupation: Creating health in everyday patterns of doing. *New Zealand Journal Of Occupational Therapy, 60*(1), 16–23.

Fischer, M. (2009). Addams and Dewey: Pragmatism, expression, and community. *Philosophy Faculty Publications, 155.* http://ecommons.udayton.edu/phl_fac_pub/155

Fisher, I., & Ziviani, J. (2004). Explanatory case studies: Implications and applications for clinical research. *Australian Occupational Therapy Journal, 51*(4), 185–191. https://doi.org/10.1111/j.1440-1630.2004.00446.x

Flyvbjerg, B. (2011). Case study. In N. K. Denzin & Y. S. Lincoln (Eds.), *The SAGE handbook of qualitative research* (4th ed., pp. 301–316). SAGE.

George, A. L., & Bennett, A. (2005). *Case studies and theory development in the social sciences.* Belfer Center for Science and International Affairs.

Gerring, J. (2007). *Case study research: Principles and practices.* Cambridge University Press.

Gewurtz, R. E., Harlos, K., Tompa, E., Oldfield, M., Lysaght, R., Moll, S., Kirsh, B., Sultan-Taïeb, H., Cook, K., & Rueda, S. (2021). Retaining and supporting employees with mental illness through inclusive organisations: Lessons from five Canadian case studies. *Equality, Diversity and Inclusion, 41*(3), 435–453. https://doi.org/10.1108/EDI-06-2020-0174

Ghaemi, S. N. (2007). Adolf Meyer: Psychiatric anarchist. *Philosophy, Psychiatry, & Psychology, 14*(4), 341–345. https://doi.org/10.1353/ppp.0.0141

Graham, A., Powell, M., Taylor, N., Anderson, D., & Fitzgerald, R. (2013). *Ethical research involving children. Florence: UNICEF Office of Research - Innocenti.* http://childethics.com/wp-content/uploads/2013/10/ERIC-compendium-approved-digital-web.pdf

Guest, G., Namey, E. E., & Mitchell, M. L. (2013). Participant observation. In G. Guest, E. E. Namey, & M. L. Mitchell (Eds.), *Collecting qualitative data: A field manual for applied research* (pp. 75–112). SAGE. https://doi.org/10.4135/9781506374680

Hamel, J., Dufour, S., & Fortin, D. (1993). *Case study methods.* SAGE. https://doi.org/10.4135/9781412983587

Harrison, H., Birks, M., Franklin, R., & Mills, J. (2017). Case study research: Foundations and methodological orientations. *Forum: Qualitative Social Research, 18*(1). https://doi.org/10.17169/fqs-18.1.2655

Health Research Council of New Zealand [HRC]. (2010). *Guidelines for researchers on health research involving Māori. Version 2.* www.hrc.govt.nz/sites/default/files/2019-06/Resource%20Library%20PDF%20-%20Guidelines%20for%20Reseasrchers%20on%20Health%20Research%20involving%20Maori%20.pdf

Health Research Council of New Zealand [HRC]. (2021). *HRC research ethics guidelines.* https://gateway.hrc.govt.nz/funding/downloads/HRC_research_ethics_guidelines.pdf

Hercegovac, S., Kernot, J., & Stanley, M. (2020). How qualitative case study methodology informs occupational therapy practice: A scoping review. *OTJR: Occupation, Participation and Health, 40*(1), 6–16. https://doi.org/10.1177/1539449219850123

Humphry, R., & Womack, J. (2019). Transformations of occupations: A life course perspective. In B. A. B. Schell & G. Gillen (Eds.), *Willard & Spackman's occupational therapy* (13th ed., pp. 100–112). Wolters Kluwer.

Hunt, E., & McKay, E. A. (2015). A scoping review of time-use research in occupational therapy and occupational science. *Scandinavian Journal of Occupational Therapy, 22*(1), 1–12. https://doi.org/10.3109/11038128.2014.934918

Huot, S., & Rudman, D. L. (2015). Extending beyond qualitative interviewing to illuminate the tacit nature of everyday occupation: Occupational mapping and participatory occupation methods. *OTJR: Occupation Participation and Health, 35*(3), 142–150. https://doi.org/10.1177/1539449215576488

Hyett, N., Kenny, A., & Dickson-Swift, V. (2019). Re-imagining occupational therapy clients as communities: Presenting the community-centred practice framework. *Scandinavian Journal of Occupational Therapy, 26*(4), 246–260. https://doi.org/10.1080/11038128.2017.1423374

Jónasdóttir, S. K., Hand, C., Misener, L., & Polgar, J. (2018). Applying case study methodology to occupational science research. *Journal of Occupational Science, 25*(3), 393–407. https://doi.org/10.1080/14427591.2018.1480409

Jones, M., Hocking, C., & McPherson, K. (2017). Communities with participation-enabling skills: A study of children with traumatic brain injury and their shared occupations. *Journal of Occupational Science, 24*(1), 88–104. https://doi.org/10.1080/14427591.2016.1224444

Jorgenson, J., & Sullivan, T. (2010). Accessing children's perspectives through participatory photo interviews. *Forum: Qualitative Social Research, 11*(1), 1–19. http://doi.org/10.17169/fqs-11.1.447

Kielhofner, G. (1992). *Conceptual foundations of occupational therapy*. F. A. Davis Company.

Koome, F., Hocking, C., & Sutton, D. (2012). Why routines matter: The nature and meaning of family routines in the context of adolescent mental illness. *Journal of Occupational Science, 19*(4), 312–325. https://doi.org/10.1080/14427591.2012.718245

Leadley, S. (2019). *Case study research exploring the impact of material poverty on a child's patterns of occupation* [Master's thesis, Auckland University of Technology]. Tuwhera. http://hdl.handle.net/10292/12215

Leadley, S., & Hocking, C. (2017). An occupational perspective of childhood poverty. *New Zealand Journal of Occupational Therapy, 64*(1), 23–31.

Leadley, S., Hocking, C., & Jones, M. (2020). The ways poverty influences a tamaiti/child's patterns of participation. *Journal of Occupational Science, 27*(3), 297–310. https://doi.org/10.1080/14427591.2020.1738263

Lincoln, Y. S., Lynham, S. A., & Guba, E. G. (2018). Paradigmatic controversies, contradictions, and emerging confluences, revisited. In N. K. Denzin & Y. S. Lincoln (Eds.), *The SAGE handbook of qualitative research* (pp. 108–150). SAGE.

Loomis, B. (1992). The Henry B. Favill school of occupations and Eleanor Clarke Slagle. *American Journal of Occupational Therapy, 46*(1), 34–37. https://doi.org/10.5014/ajot.46.1.34

McQuaid, L., Thomson, K., & Bannigan, K. (2022). Case study research: Building the occupational therapy evidence base one case at a time. *Scandinavian Journal of Occupational Therapy*. https://doi.org/10.1080/11038128.2022.2039758

Merriam, S. B. (1998). *Case study research in education: A qualitative approach* (6th ed.). Jossey-Bass.

Mills, A. J., Durepos, G., & Wiebe, E. (2010). Pluralism and case study. In *Encyclopedia of case study research*. SAGE. https://doi.org/10.4135/9781412957397

Mills, J. (2014). Methodology and methods. In J. Mills & M. Birks (Eds.), *Qualitative methodology: A practical guide* (pp. 31–47). SAGE. https://doi.org/10.4135/9781473920163

Mitchell, J. C. (2000). Case and situation analysis. In R. Gomm, M. Hammersley, & P. Foster (Eds.), *Case study method: Key issues, key texts* (pp. 165–186). SAGE. https://doi.org/10.4135/9780857024367

Moorfield, J. C. (2011). *Māori dictionary: Te Aka Māori-English, English-Māori dictionary*. Longman/Pearson Education New Zealand.

Morgan, D. L. (2014). Pragmatism as a paradigm for social research. *Qualitative Inquiry, 20*, 1045–1053. https://doi.org/10.1177/1077800413513733

Murphy, C. K., & Shiel, A. (2018). Institutional injustices? Exploring engagement in occupations in a residential mental health facility. *Journal of Occupational Science, 26*(1), 115–127. https://doi.org/10.1080/14427591.2018.1531780

National Ethics Advisory Committee [NEAC]. (2019). *National Ethical Standards for Health and Disability Research and Quality Improvement*. Ministry of Health. https://neac.health.govt.nz/publications-and-resources/neac-publications/national-ethical-standards-for-health-and-disability-research-and-quality-improvement/

Nyman, A., Josephsson, S., & Isaksson, G. (2014). A narrative of agency enacted within the everyday occupations of an older Swedish woman. *Journal of Occupational Science 21*(4), 459–472. https://doi.org/10.1080/14427591.2013.803433

O'Neill, J. (2022). *Jessie Luther: Artist, teacher, pioneer*. Westport Historical Society. https://wpthis tory.org/2022/02/jessie-luther-artist-teacher-pioneer/#:~:text=Jessie%20Luther%20(1860%20 %E2%80%93%201952)&text=She%20became%20steeped%20in%20the,important%20of%20 all%20settlement%20houses

Paparini, S., Papoutsi, C., Murdoch, J., Green, J., Petticrew, M., Greenhalgh, T., & Shaw, S. (2021). Evaluating complex interventions in context: Systematic, meta-narrative review of case study approaches. *BMC Medical Research Methodology, 21*(1), 1–22. https://doi.org/10.1186/ s12874-021-01418-3

Phelan, S. K., & Kinsella, E. A. (2014). Occupation and identity: Perspectives of children with disabilities and their parents. *Journal of Occupational Science, 21*(3), 334–356. https://doi.org/10.1 080/14427591.2012.755907

Pizzi, M. A. (2016). Promoting health, well-being, and quality of life for children who are overweight or obese and their families. *American Journal of Occupational Therapy, 70*(5), 1–6. https://doi.org/10.5014/ajot.2016.705001

Platt, J. (1996). *A history of sociological research methods in America: 1920–1960*. Cambridge University Press.

Ramugondo, E. L. (2012). Intergenerational play within family: The case for occupational consciousness. *Journal of Occupational Science, 19*(4), 326–340. https://doi.org/10.1080/144275 91.2012.710166

Reed, K. (2018). Henry B. Favill and the School of Occupations: Origins of occupational therapy practice and education. *Occupational Therapy in Health Care, 33*(2), 159–180. https://doi.org/ 10.1080/07380577.2018.1553087

Salminen, A.-L., Harra, T., & Lautamo, T. (2006). Conducting case study research in occupational therapy. *Australian Occupational Therapy Journal, 53*(1), 3–8. https://doi. org/10.1111/j.1440-1630.2006.00540.x

Salmond, C., Crampton, P., King, P., & Waldegrave, C. (2014). *NZiDep: An index of socioeconomic deprivation for individuals*. www.otago.ac.nz/wellington/otago020333.pdf

Scaffa, M. E. (2019). Occupational therapy interventions for groups, communities, and populations. In B. A. B. Schell & G. Gillen (Eds.), *Willard and Spackman's occupational therapy* (13th ed., pp. 436–447). Wolters Kluwer.

Schwandt, T. A., & Gates, E. F. (2018). Case study methodology. In N. K. Denzin & Y. S. Lincoln (Eds.), *The SAGE handbook of qualitative research* (5th ed., pp. 341–358). SAGE.

Simons, H. (2009). *Case study research in practice*. SAGE. https://doi.org/10.4135/9781446268322

Stake, R. E. (1995). *The art of case study research*. SAGE.

Stake, R. E. (2006). *Multiple case study analysis*. Guilford Press.

Stewart, A. (2014). Case study. In J. M. M. Birks (Ed.), *Qualitative methodology: A practical guide* (pp. 145–160). SAGE. https://doi.org/10.4135/9781473920163

Wright St. Clair, V. A., & Hocking, C. (2019). Occupational science: The study of occupation. In B. A. B. Schell & G. Gillen (Eds.), *Willard & Spackman's occupational therapy* (13th ed., pp. 124–140). Wolters Kluwer.

Yin, R. K. (2018). *Case study reseearch and applications: Design and methods* (6th ed.). SAGE.

Additional Resources

Baxter, P., & Jack, S. (2008). Qualitative case study methodology: Study design and implementation for novice researchers. *The Qualitative Report, 13*(4), 544–559. https://doi. org/10.46743/2160-3715/2008.1573

Haines, D. (2017). Ethical considerations in qualitative case study research: Recruiting participants with profound intellectual disabilities. *Research Ethics, 13*(3–4), 219–232. https://doi. org/10.1177/1747016117711971

Mason, W., Morris, K., Webb, C., Daniels, B., Featherstone, B., Bywaters, P., Nughmana, M., Hooper, J., Brady, G., Bunting, L., & Scourfield, J. (2020). Toward full integration of quantitative and qualitative methods in case study research: Insights from investigating child welfare inequalities. *Journal of Mixed Methods Research*. https://doi.org/10.1177/1558689819857972

Stake, R. E. (2010). *Qualitative research: Studying how things work*. The Guildford Press.

Swift, C., Hocking, C., & Jones, M. (2022). Exploring communication in families affected by chronic parental pain. *Scandinavian Journal of Occupational Therapy*. https://doi.org/10.1080/11038128.2022.2051601

8 Narrative Inquiry

Jens Schneider, Laetitia Zeeman, Natalie Edelman and Lee Price

Narrative inquiry has been used as a research design for many years by various scientific disciplines such as anthropology, health sciences, philosophy, psychology, and sociology (Bonsall, 2012). However, no single definition of narrative inquiry exists. Rather, there are multiple approaches to the application of narrative inquiry as a research design (Bonsall, 2012; Caine et al., 2013; Dwyer & Emerald, 2017; Josephsson & Alsaker, 2015; Riessman, 2013; Squire et al., 2013). Clandinin and Caine (2012) suggested that narrative inquiry is "first and foremost, a way of understanding experience" (p. 166), while Squire et al. (2013) outlined that "narratives carry traces of human lives that we want to understand" (p. 2). Humans live their lives and tell stories about their experiences. They assign meaning to their experiences and their environment and share their knowledge with other people with different intentions (Clandinin & Rosiek, 2007; Dwyer & Emerald, 2017). Clandinin and Rosiek (2007) further argued that narratives reflect a person's personality as well as the social influences they experience. For them, narrative inquiry seeks to understand how individuals' experiences are "constituted, shaped, expressed, and enacted" in transaction with their personal, social, and material environment (Clandinin & Rosiek, 2007, p. 42).

Taking the reasoning of Clandinin and Rosiek (2007), together with transactional perspectives on occupation (Cutchin & Dickie, 2013b), we further original understandings by arguing that narrative inquiry is a way of exploring "occupations as a ... response to situational elements" (Fisher & Marterella, 2019, p. 16). In addition, Clandinin and Rosiek (2007) considered narratives as a way of depicting the development of human experiences over the course of time. With this in mind, we regarded narratives as appropriate to represent experiences in a time-dependent manner that makes them particularly valuable for a study aiming to understand transgender men's meaningful occupations during their gender transition process over time and the "transformative capacity of [these] occupations" (Madsen & Josephsson, 2017, p. 417; Schneider, 2022). In this chapter, we draw on Jens' doctoral study (Schneider, 2022) as an example of how narrative inquiry can be applied in an occupation centered study.

Narrative inquiry is a research design frequently used to study human occupation (de Jong et al., 2021). Several authors have applied narrative inquiry to investigate occupations in different settings, or theorized about the suitability of narrative inquiry for research on occupation (e.g., Alsaker et al., 2013; Bonsall, 2012; Josephsson & Alsaker, 2015; Josephsson et al., 2006; Schneider, 2022; Schneider et al., 2019; Taylor & Kay, 2015). Josephsson et al. (2006) suggested that narratives are gates to capturing the meanings of human everyday occupations. Bonsall (2012) pointed out that narrative inquiry can be used to interpret occupations and their meanings for individuals, and proposed that describing narratives of occupations could help to increase interdisciplinary awareness of the meaning of occupation.

DOI: 10.4324/9781003456216-8

Considerations About the Narrative Inquiry Approach

Riessman (2013) considered narrative research as diverse and complex in its application. As a consequence, some authors have highlighted that there are no rules for performing narrative inquiry (Dwyer & Emerald, 2017; Squire et al., 2013). No clear recommendations exist as to which epistemology, ontology, and axiology are applicable; which data material are appropriate; how a study should be conducted; which media can be studied; how the interaction between the participant(s)and the researcher(s) should be structured; and whether stories should be analyzed in part or in full (cf. Squire et al., 2013). Caine et al. (2013) noted that narrative inquiry is often used as a research design in which stories are data, are analyzed in terms of content or structure, are studied as phenomenon themselves or serve as media to represent events (cf. Dwyer et al., 2017; Riessman, 2008; Squire et al., 2013). Dwyer and Emerald (2017) concluded that researchers have to choose the narrative inquiry approach that best fits their research aim(s). In order to cope with the dilemma of missing rules for conducting a narrative inquiry, we recommend looking for publications of studies that applied narrative inquiry and had a research focus similar to one's own (e.g., the exploration of experiences of occupations). By reading this literature and the references to further literature on narrative inquiry, one can successively develop and compile the approaches and methods suitable for their own research.

Philosophical Worldview

Dwyer and Emerald (2017) outlined that "narrative work is typically within a transactional frame – focused on the way knowledge is created in social settings" (p. 5). Clandinin and colleagues (e.g., Caine et al., 2013; Clandinin & Connelly, 2000; Clandinin & Rosiek, 2007) have drawn on Deweyan pragmatism to philosophically underpin narrative inquiry. In Jens' doctoral study, he applied Deweyan pragmatism as the philosophical worldview. This was done because Deweyan pragmatism also provides a foundation for the philosophical substantiation of elements such as occupations, experience, knowledge, and the research process (e.g., Biesta & Burbules, 2003; Cutchin & Dickie, 2013b; Dewey, 1938, 1938/1997; Madsen & Josephsson, 2017; Morgan, 2014). By taking the stance of a Deweyan pragmatist, we did not follow the traditional understanding of epistemology, ontology, and axiology. Instead, we considered "research as a human experience that is based on the beliefs and actions of actual researchers" (Morgan, 2014, p. 1051). This means that researchers draw on their beliefs, and thereby their values, to choose actions in their research which they consider as purposeful (Morgan, 2014).

A basic assumption of Deweyan pragmatism is that people and the world are intertwined – they are elements of a whole (Dewey, 1925/1929). Deweyan philosophy further considers these elements to be in constant interaction and mutual influence in what he termed 'transaction' (Biesta & Burbules, 2003; Dewey & Bentley, 1949). Biesta and Burbules (2003) argued that in Deweyan pragmatism knowledge of reality is constructed through the ongoing transaction between a person and the world. Actions and the conscious evaluation of the outcome of these actions construct knowledge (Biesta & Burbules, 2003; Morgan, 2014). In the context of knowledge construction, Dewey's (1925/1929, 1938, 1938/1997) understanding of 'experience' and 'inquiry' are of importance. 'Experience' can be regarded as an advancing everlasting circular process in which the elements of belief, action, and reflection are connected (Morgan, 2014). A person performs actions based on a reflection of their beliefs. The outcome of these actions is reflected and given meaning by the person in an interpretative process, shaping beliefs which in turn lay the foundation for subsequent actions (Morgan, 2014). The process of gaining experience can be unconscious. Dewey (1938) called the conscious experience process 'inquiry'.

In its final step of giving meaning to the outcome of an action, knowledge or, in the words of Dewey, "warranted assertions" (Dewey, 1938, p. 4; Dewey, 1941, p. 169) are created. It should be noted that warranted assertions derived from an inquiry do not reflect the reality of the world. Warranted assertions represent "relations ... between (our) actions and (their) consequences" (Biesta & Burbules, 2003, p. 45). Jens' study was specifically interested in revealing why and how the participants performed certain actions (occupations) during their gender transition process. In addition, he wanted to explore how the consequences of these occupations solved underlying "problematic situations" (Dewey, 1938, p. 35; Morgan, 2014, p. 1047); thereby, shaping the meaning attributed to the occupations by the participants. In other words, he aimed to understand which warranted assertions resulted from the participants' occupations and how these warranted assertions, in turn, shaped further occupations.

In the context of Deweyan pragmatism, experiences as they come to light during a narrative inquiry are not something that exist before the inquiry; rather, they emerge during the inquiry from pieces of experiences of both the participant(s) and the researcher(s) (Caine et al., 2013; Clandinin & Rosiek, 2007). Caine et al. (2013) referred to Dewey's (1938/1997) understanding of experience as changing in transaction with other people and the situation. According to Caine et al. (2013), narratives are thus based on the joint work of study participants and researchers. Hence, for researchers, it is necessary to be aware of all the elements which influence the narrative inquiry; among them the choice of recruitment process and the process itself, as well as the way in which the interviews are conducted, the narratives created, and the outcome presented. In addition, it is important not to neglect the "situational elements" (Fisher & Marterella, 2019, p. 23) with which participants and researchers transact and which may act as a frame for the narrative inquiry (cf. Caine et al., 2013; Clandinin & Caine, 2012).

Questions Best Suited for Narrative Inquiry

Clandinin and Connelly (2000) highlighted that the beginning of a narrative inquiry requires researchers who are interested in experiences. For scholars in the fields of occupational science and occupational therapy this means they need to be curious about how people experience occupation. The topics and questions that are best suited for narrative inquiry are therefore closely linked to a researcher's understanding of occupation. Acknowledging the transactional nature of occupation, Fisher and Marterella (2019) described occupation as "an ongoing response to the situational context" (p. 26); it is "what people do, what they experience in relation to that doing, and their experiencing personal value in that doing" (p. 28).

Guideline for Best Practice

General questions that researchers who aim to explore occupations using narrative inquiry should consider when designing a study can be:

- What occupation is performed?
- Why is it performed?
    - What is the problematic situation that caused a person to perform a particular occupation? What are the situational elements that frame or cause the problematic situation?

- How is the occupation performed?

    - How is the practical "doing"? How does the performance of the occupation change over time?

- What is experienced?

    - Has the problematic situation that caused the occupation been solved, or is another or additional occupation required to solve it? How are situational elements changed by an occupation?

- What meaning for their lives do the participants attach to the occupation?

Grounded in Dewey's understanding of experience and inquiry as ongoing processes, occupation needs to be explored in the context of participants' biographies and environments and the mutual ways they affect each other. Narrative inquiry as a research design enables the exploration of human experience of occupations in its contextual and temporal dimensions (cf. Caine et al., 2013). It is, consequently, a research design that allows researchers to gather deep insights into "how the relationship of occupation and situation unfolds" (Madsen & Josephsson, 2017, p. 413).

The aforementioned considerations and an identified knowledge gap in literature on the occupations of transgender men led Jens to the following general research question: "How do transmen experience the performance of meaningful occupations in their gender transition process?" (Schneider, 2022, p. 75).

Recruitment and Sampling

The description and understanding of human experiences by way of qualitative inquiry requires information-rich cases which can provide extensive descriptions of the topic in question (Patton, 2015; Polkinghorne, 2005). The recruitment of suitable participants is, therefore, of major importance. Patton (2015) has provided 40 purposeful sampling strategies that can be applied depending on the aim of a study. According to Patton, "there are no rules for sample size in qualitative inquiry" (p. 311), although he stated that it is more appropriate to recruit a small than a high number of people for studies that aim to gather detailed information from participants. Criteria such as topic of interest, research aim(s), resources, and available time are important guidelines to determine the sample size (Patton, 2015).

Taking into account that Jens conducted three interviews lasting 90 to 150 minutes, approximately one year apart, with each of the participants, he recruited eight participants in total, two of whom dropped out after the first interview round. Since Jens was interested in occupations of transgender and non-binary people in the German context, German speaking participants were recruited by applying "maximum variation (heterogeneity) sampling" to reveal "core experiences and central shared dimensions" of these people (Patton, 2015, p. 283). For this purpose, 93 specific forums for LGBTQIA+ people on internet platforms were approached by posting information about Jens' professional background and a call for research participants. As it was mainly transgender men who indicated their interest to participate, the focus of the study was subsequently narrowed to the gender transition process of transgender men (Schneider, 2022).

Data Collection

Narrative inquiry can include a variety of data sources such as transcribed interviews (e.g., Brinkmann & Kvale, 2015; Riessman, 2008; Squire et al., 2013); performed narrative-in-action (e.g., Josephsson & Alsaker, 2015); documents such as letters and diaries (e.g., Riessman, 2008); and visual art such as paintings, photographs, and videos (e.g., Lisahunter, 2017; O'Bryan, 2017; Riessman, 2008). Squire (2013) outlined that she and other authors have used further material such as field notes and external background material. Jens' study with transgender men used mainly transcribed interviews as data but also field notes recorded during the interviews.

Narrative Interviews

How narrative interviews are conducted and which questions are asked depend on the research question(s) and aim(s). As Jens conducted three in-depth narrative interviews with each participant over a period of two years, the aim of the first interview was to get to know the participants and their life situations, and to find out which occupations were meaningful to them in the context of their gender transition process. The second interview aimed to explore how the participants carried out up to three occupations of their own choice and which situational elements were involved. The purpose was to develop a deep understanding of the 'transactions' between the occupations of the participants and their environment (cf. Fisher & Marterella, 2019). Just before the start of the third interview, the participants were asked to select up to seven occupations that were most meaningful to them from all the occupations identified in the first two interview rounds. Seven occupations were chosen, together with the three occupations from the second interview round, with up to ten stories per participant that would represent a variety of occupations performed during gender transition processes. It appeared feasible in terms of time and resources to deal with up to ten stories per participant in Jens' thesis. The aim of the third interview was then to elaborate the meaning of these occupations in more detail than in the previous interviews and to supplement details not included in the first two interviews. The rationale for conducting three interviews at intervals of one year was to find out how the meaning of occupations changed over the course of the gender transition process.

The purpose of the interviews was to collect comprehensive and in-depth descriptions of the participants' occupational experiences, including the interpretations of the meaning of the occupations that participants described (cf. Brinkmann & Kvale, 2015; Clandinin & Caine, 2012; Clandinin & Connelly, 2000; Polkinghorne, 2005; Squire, 2013). For this reason, the interviews were unstructured, and interview guides with a few open-ended questions to start the interviews were used (cf. Brinkmann & Kvale, 2015; Clandinin & Connelly, 2000; Riessman, 2008). This gave the participants as much freedom as possible in the ways they wanted to narrate their stories.

Since both the study participants and Jens are native German speakers, the interviews were conducted in German. Given the research topic with potentially vulnerable participants, we considered it important to communicate in a language in which both parties were fluent. A rationale for our decision has been presented by van Nes et al. (2010) who stated "language … influences what can be expressed" and "metaphors [used to express the meaning of experiences] vary from culture to culture and are language-specific" (p. 314).

Textbox 8.1   Examples of Action Points to Structure an Interview Session

- Explain that you are interested in stories about the participants' lives and experiences in relation to the occupations which they chose and performed in order to cope with particular situations or during life events.
- Clarify that the focus is on the participants' performed occupations. Give a general example of an everyday occupation to illustrate that occupation meant something that is actively performed by oneself. To avoid influencing what the participants might relate, do not give any example of an occupation which is likely to be connected to your research topic.

Guideline for Best Practice

Prepare how to structure each interview session rather than the interviews themselves with an overall framework and several action points; for example, how to introduce the interviews. Some possible action points in addition to those outlined in handbooks on qualitative research interviews are presented in Textbox 8.1.

Photo elicitation (e.g., Harper, 2002), the creation of video diaries, and reflection on activity cards (cf. Baum & Edwards, 2008) can be included in narrative interviews. The aim of applying these methods in combination with interviews is to provide participants with direct and straightforward initial stimuli for reflection and discussion of different topics, and ultimately to inspire narratives and stories (cf. Asaba et al., 2015; Clark-Ibáñez, 2007; Lisahunter, 2017). Furthermore, the methods can be selected with the objective of facilitating exploration of the occupations in a targeted manner (cf. Hartman et al., 2011). These three methods are described in more detail below.

Photo Elicitation

The use of photo elicitation in the first interview round of Jens' study prompted the participants to describe occupations related to gender transition and to elaborate on the situational elements that affected these occupations.

Prior to the interview, invite participants to select personal photographs showing meaningful occupations. For the purpose of Jens' study, he asked the participants to select ten photographs that were related to their gender development and the occupations that reflected their gender transition process. Explain to the participants that they can use the photographs during the interview as a stimulus to tell their stories about special life events including meaningful occupations. Jens also indicated that the photographs would not be analyzed.

Video Diaries

Video diaries created by study participants allowed them to reflect in more detail on how they performed certain occupations. Joint viewing of the videos during the interviews leads to rich narratives, including accounts of occupational performance, occupational experiences, participation, and situational elements. In addition, it allows the interviewer to get a better understanding of the recorded occupation and the connected situational elements than a purely oral narrative would do. The creation of video diaries of meaningful occupations by research participants proved to be a particularly valuable tool to explore occupations in more detail (Schneider, 2022).

Several weeks before the interview date, ask participants to select meaningful occupations and to create a video diary. For instance, ask them to record three 20-minute video clips with a video camera or smartphone, each showing the selected, specific occupation(s). Inform the participants that they should be the only person recorded for reasons of privacy.

At the beginning of the interview review the occupation(s) that they have selected together with the participants. The following questions can be used to elicit further information afterwards:

- Why did you choose these occupations?
- How do or did these occupations facilitate you in [name the special life event under investigation]?
- How do you perform these occupations?
- How do or did these occupations facilitate you to live your life in the way you want?
- Have these occupations changed over the course of time and if so, how?

Activity Cards

Activity cards showing different occupations are used in occupational therapy as a means of exploring the occupations which need to be trained during interventions with clients; for example, the *Activity Card Sort* (2nd ed.; Baum & Edwards, 2008). They are also a useful tool to support participants in selecting occupations, and in reflecting on occupations that are meaningful for them. The cards may be self-developed and consist of a photograph that represents a particular occupation and the key terms or descriptions that label the occupation.

Create activity cards derived from the meaningful occupations identified in the transcripts of previous interview rounds of a study or in literature. The intention of using self-developed activity cards in Jens' study was to support the participants in the third interview round in selecting and reflecting on the occupations that were most meaningful to them during their gender transition process. The cards showed all the meaningful occupations that had been identified in the transcripts of the first and second interview rounds. The information shown on these cards enabled the participants to get a quick overview during the third interview of the meaningful occupations that all participants had mentioned. They could also check whether Jens had correctly identified and included the meaningful occupations they themselves had described in the previous interviews in the activity cards. Finally, the participants had the opportunity to reflect on all occupations which had come to light in the first two interview rounds. This enabled them to prioritize the importance of these occupations for their gender transition process. Activity cards used in the research interviews thus turned out to be a useful way of quickly identifying and presenting a large number of occupations as a basis for further actions. Participants prioritized the importance of the occupations in their own lives and discussed different aspects of occupations as well as situational elements.

To summarize, it can be said that the three research methods outlined in the current section – photo elicitation, creation of video diaries, reflection on activity cards – are excellent vehicles for facilitation of detailed narration in studies. During the interviews, participants elaborated on three elements of occupations – occupational performance, occupational experience, participation – and on the different situational elements which framed their narrated occupations (cf. Fisher & Marterella, 2019). The participants often did this spontaneously without being prompted. The methods used in Jens' study paved the way to obtain holistic pictures of meaningful occupations during research interviews.

Narrative Analysis

Since there are various ways to carry out a narrative inquiry, we draw on Jens' study as an example to illustrate the process of data analysis. Before commencing analysis of the interview data, transcribe the interviews. If the interviews were conducted in the researcher's mother tongue but the final results are to be published in another language, perform the steps to identify narratives about occupations in the original transcript. This procedure is in line with the recommendation by van Nes et al. (2010) to work "in the original language [for] as long and as much as possible" in order "to avoid limitations in the analysis" (p. 315). In his study, Jens, as a native German speaker, performed the analyses of the German transcripts and created the final narratives in German before he translated them into English. If researchers are doing cross-language research, which means that participants and researchers have different mother tongues, they should be aware that a foreign language may influence their data analysis differently compared to those analyzing in their mother tongue (cf. Jackendoff, 2009). In cross-language research, it is consequently advisable to involve research colleagues or professional translators who are native speakers of the participants' mother tongue in the analysis and creation of the narratives. These people can offer support in understanding cultural and language differences.

Guideline for Best Practice

For the narrative analysis, read each transcript closely to identify descriptions of occupations. When re-reading the text passages, identify whether accounts of occupations are accompanied by descriptions of elements of a Deweyan inquiry as listed in Table 8.1. This search can be supported by a search for structural elements of narratives as also outlined in Table 8.1. In addition, look for situational elements (cf. Fisher & Marterella, 2019) which can be relevant to understand possible accounts of occupations. The main purpose of this component of the analysis is to identify occupations which are connected to a participant's life event (e.g., a gender transition process). Furthermore, look for the participant's explanations of whether and how these occupations are meaningful during their life event.

When re-reading the identified text passages for particular occupations, apply the criteria given by Labov and Waletzky (1967) as well as Taylor (2008; Table 8.1) to investigate whether these passages are told as narratives. Although the criteria of Labov and Waletzky and Taylor used for the structural analysis of narratives may not fit the applied approach to narrative inquiry exactly, they can be helpful in identifying narratives in the transcripts. This approach is appropriate against the background of limited tools in narrative inquiry as raised by Patterson (2013), who subsequently recommended the use of the Labovian approach to match structures within transcripts. Moreover, as shown in Table 8.1, the criteria of Labov and Waletzky and Taylor fit comfortably with the components of a Deweyan inquiry. By applying the criteria outlined in Table 8.1, narratives of occupations can be identified in transcripts.

Table 8.1 Assigning elements of a Deweyan inquiry to parts of narratives

Parts of narratives (Labov & Waletzky, 1967; Taylor, 2008)	Assigned elements of Deweyan inquiry (Dewey, 1938; Miettinen, 2000; Morgan, 2014)
Abstract: A summary of the story, usually told at its beginning (not always available).	–
Orientation: An introduction which informs the audience about the "person, place, time and behavioral situation" of the narrator (Labov & Waletzky, 1967, p. 32).	This section of narratives includes reports of habitual actions that no longer lead to the desired result in a certain situation and represent "indeterminate situations" (Dewey, 1938, p. 105; Miettinen, 2000, p. 66). In addition, there are descriptions of the beliefs on the basis of which the narrator performs their habitual actions and the situational elements under which the habitual actions functioned but now no longer function.
Complication: A part which informs about an event; for example, in terms of "a problem, a crisis or a turning point" (Taylor, 2008, p. 82).	The problematic situation and probably the narrator's assumptions on the causes of this situation is told in this part of narratives.
Evaluation: A section which informs the audience about the meaning of the story.	In this section the narrator reflects on how they assess the importance of particular episodes in a story. This can mirror beliefs which are shaped by past experiences and situational elements, as well as by the meaning that the narrator assigned to an inquiry and its outcome.
Resolution: A description about the resolving action and outcome of it.	In this part, the performed action and its outcome is described. In addition, the meaning which the narrator assigns to the outcome of an action is presented here. This meaning can be understood as a description of warranted assertions gained or how an action changed the problematic situation.
Coda: A clause to connect the story to the present (not always available).	In this section the narrator reflects on their present beliefs as shaped by past experiences and situational elements as well as by the meaning that they assigned to an inquiry and its outcome.

Author created

Creating the Narratives

The narrative of each participant in Jens' study consisted of a curriculum vitae (CV) and several stories on meaningful occupations.

Curriculum Vitae

Clandinin and Caine (2012) emphasized the significant role of the environment in which participants are situated if narratives are to be understood. It is, therefore, important to consider how participants' experiences and warranted assertions were acquired through transaction with their situational elements. This is further underlined by scholars who have used transactional perspectives on occupation or have drawn on Dewey's theory of inquiry to understand occupations. They emphasized the need to understand the "situations in which occupation takes place" (Madsen & Josephsson, 2017, p. 412) when exploring occupations (e.g., Cutchin & Dickie, 2013a; Fisher & Marterella, 2019). Jens' solution to present situational elements was to write an informal CV from the participants' perspective. In addition, he considered this approach to give readers of the final narratives detailed impressions of the participants and set the scene against which background the participants narrated their experiences (cf. Schneider, 2022; Seal, 2014; Textbox 8.2). Depending on the research aim(s), it might be also useful to present occupational histories or profiles of participants as CVs as they might be revealed by 'occupational performance history interviews' (Hemmingsson et al., 2017) or comparable assessments.

Textbox 8.2 Excerpt from Nick's CV

Hey,

... When I was in kindergarten, I already felt like a boy. ... My boyish behavior and activities continued in primary school.

When I was 12, major changes occurred as a result of puberty. Due to all the physical changes, I tried to accept that I'd been born a girl. ...

At the age of 23, I started to think about what it would have been like to have been born a boy. I started to watch the gay series 'Queer as Folk' and knew straight away: 'Now something's got to change'. ... I disclosed as a transman to my partner and since that time I've been living as a man. ... I then made an appointment straight away with my psychologist and started with the therapy.

'You grow along with your tasks.' There are just certain things that change automatically. I copied from the men's world – how a man walks, for example. ...

At 25 I'd already completed my 'mandatory hours' of psychotherapy. ... The change in my civil status was carried out. ... A mastectomy, a hysterectomy, and an adnexectomy were also performed. ...

At this stage everyone considers me to be a man, because I definitely look like a man. I'm accepted everywhere – in the family, by friends, and at work – as a man.

Kind regards,
Nick

(Schneider, 2022, pp. 220–221)

Guideline for Best Practice: Extracting and Creating the CV

Extract the data for the CV from the narrated experiences on occupations; other speech elements, such as explanations and descriptions within the transcripts; and recorded field notes. Rearrange them in almost chronological order so that they take the form of a CV. Where required, add information from the interviewer's field notes. Information such as that already deemed necessary by Clandinin and Caine (2012) and regarding situational elements as described by Fisher and Marterella (2019) should be included in the CV. In the case of Jens' study, this comprised for example:

- Participant/personal elements (Fisher & Marterella, 2019): e.g., physical attributes; status and courses of hormonal treatment and gender-affirming surgeries; educational and professional background.

- "Geopolitical elements" (Fisher & Marterella, 2019, p. 17): e.g., areas where the participants had grown up and where they were living.
- "Temporal elements" (Fisher & Marterella, 2019, p. 17): e.g., the participant's occupational experiences and performances in childhood and youth.
- "Social environmental elements" (Fisher & Marterella, 2019, p. 17): e.g., statements about the beliefs and reactions of the environment to cisgender non-conforming behavior and other transgender related issues; how other people such as relatives, classmates, teachers, colleagues affected the lives of the participants.

Extracting the Stories

Extract the stories identified in the narrative analysis by copying the text blocks, including the elements of a narrative outlined in Table 8.1, that belong to a particular occupation into a new document. Jens looked for the stories of each participant in all three interviews of the occupations they had selected as particularly meaningful. The story of each occupation from the second and third interview transcript was used as the basic framework to create the final narratives. If this framework lacked important details and aspects which could be found in the first transcript, these were inserted to create a comprehensive story. Jens considered the extraction of a story as complete when he did not find any further information that contributed to this story (Schneider, 2022).

Creating the Final Narratives

Transcribed spoken language of interviews is often difficult to read. Consequently, clean-up of the extracted stories as suggested, for example, by Birch (2011), Riessman (2008), and Williams (1984), is often advisable. While doing clean-ups try to keep the stories as intact as possible (cf. Riessman, 2008). If it is required to make an extracted story comprehensive, rearrange parts of it. You may thereby order the story according to the structure provided in Table 8.1. Remove filler words, interruptions, and utterances as well as names of people, institutions, or locations which might allow the participant to be identified. Omit sentences or phrases, such as questions from the interviewer, digressions, discussions, and examples, which do not contradict the narratives but do not contribute to them. To shorten a story, remove repetitions if they were not told in order to put an emphasis on a particular aspect. Thereby, decide whether the first statement or the repetition fits the narrative better.

If, as in Jens' study, a translation needs to be performed, further preparation of the original narrative is required in order to achieve a comprehensible and meaningful translation. People do not always follow the grammatical rules of their language when talking. Moreover, they may use words, phrases, and grammatical structures of their local dialect. Where required, rearrange or replace words in sentences or add words to fulfil grammatical rules in order to prepare the sentences for translation. This measure changes the participant's quote, but that happens in any case by the translation. Be aware of the risk of misinterpreting statements during a clean-up and look at the transcripts for evidence to support your interpretations of the meaning narrators wanted to convey. When the clean-ups are completed, compare the drafted narratives with the original transcripts and re-work in cases where their content and meanings are found to diverge. Applying the 'four eyes principle' for this task by involving a member of your research team or by member checking can be of advantage.

Translating Narratives into Another Language

Van Nes et al. (2010) pointed out that translation from one language to another is an act of interpreting itself. They further contended that in qualitative research based on interviews, knowledge is acquired and transferred via texts and by interpreting texts, which means that much care needs to be taken in translating narratives. Riessman (2008) and van Nes et al. reported that many researchers from non-English speaking countries publish their research in English for various reasons without revealing how the translation was performed. Riessman suggested that authors neglect differences in languages by presuming an equality of meanings within different languages. Squires (2009) has recommended informing readers about the translation process and measures taken to avoid loss of meaning within the translation process.

As described above, from the start, consider the requirements for translation when writing the mother tongue narratives. Translate the narratives into the target language. Use the aid of a professional translator who is a native speaker of the target language (van Nes et al., 2010). Send the original narratives and your translations to the translator for review and possible correction. In cases of doubt, for example in cases where expressions originated from the original language's slang or dialects, the translator and the author should discuss and agree which phrasing in the target language best matches the content and meaning of the original statements for use in the related narrative.

Presenting the Narratives

It may be useful to present the stories based on a structure used by Birch (2011) and Seal (2014), consisting of a descriptive introduction or abstract of the story, the story itself, and a brief statement of the key message(s) conveyed in the story (Textbox 8.3). In some of the participants' stories, the structural elements "abstract" (Riessman, 2008, p. 92; Taylor, 2008, p. 82) and "orientation" (Labov & Waletzky, 1967, p. 32; Riessman, 2008, p. 92; Taylor, 2008, p. 82) may set the scene. This information is necessary to understand the "thematic thread" of the narrative (Polkinghorne, 1995, p. 5). In cases where the

---

Textbox 8.3   Example of Nick's Story

Singing as an emotional counterbalance and vocal training during the GTP [gender transition process]

An occupation which Nick performed almost daily and which helped him during the GTP was singing.

"I actually do it nearly every day. … It's really extremely important for me because it somehow simply acts as a counterbalance for me for bad times. … You don't always only have good times during this process. And it's also very good vocal training as well of course. When you sing along with the low parts of the male singers, it's also vocal training in order to make [your] voice a bit deeper."

[For] Nick, … singing [seemed to have two functions]: Firstly, it appeared to serve as emotional counterbalance to the difficulties of the GTP; and secondly, as vocal training during the process.

(Schneider, 2022, p. 227)

elements 'abstract' or 'orientation' are incomplete or missing, create these based on information from the transcripts to make the stories comprehensible to readers. The stories should be followed by a short summary. Drawing on the story's content, develop headings for the narrative of each participant, as well as subheadings for each story to guide the readers. These present the "contextual meaning" of the narratives and stories (Polkinghorne, 1995, p. 7).

Rigor

Dwyer and Emerald (2017) presented several ways of assessing qualitative studies for quality and rigor. They suggested the "twelve qualitative touchstones for narrative inquiry" developed by Clandinin and Caine (2012, p. 169) as a possible way of assessing rigor specifically tailored to narrative inquiry. Since the way that Jens understood and applied narrative inquiry in his study was significantly influenced by the work of Clandinin and colleagues (Caine et al., 2013; Clandinin & Caine, 2012; Clandinin & Rosiek, 2007), it was consistent to apply the quality criteria by Clandinin and Caine as guidelines for the narrative inquiry in Jens' study. In doing so, Jens aimed to ensure the quality of his study, to build trust in its findings, and, hence, to establish rigor. He thereby kept in mind "that there is no final telling, no final story, and no one singular story we can tell" (Clandinin & Caine, 2012, p. 176). This means that the findings of a narrative inquiry are only snapshots of the experiences of participants as experienced and recorded by researchers in the light of their own experiences. They are stories whose quality can hardly be judged by criteria such as "truth or accuracy and verifiability" (Clandinin & Caine, 2012, p. 176). However, that does not make them any less valuable. As highlighted by Clandinin and Rosiek (2007), "narrative inquirers study an individual's experience in the world and, through the study, seek ways of enriching and transforming that experience for themselves and others" (p. 42).

Guideline for best practice: Essentials of the qualitative touchstones (Clandinin & Caine, 2012)

1   Responsibilities in the research relations

- Your participants and you participate in each other's lives and shape the research process together.
- To ensure a trustful and fruitful relationship, comply with ethical principles.
- To ensure equality as well as social justice is important.
- Openness, mutuality, and caring but also awareness of each other's vulnerability are key aspects in the research relationship.

2   Awareness of situational elements of the participant(s) and the researcher(s)

- A narrative inquiry always begins in the midst of both the participants' and your lives.
- Become aware of how your situation is affected by your belonging to a research community, your social environment, your biography and experiences.
- Consider how your situational elements influence your view of the participants and the phenomena that may be revealed in the research process.
- Consider issues such as how potential participants are invited to take part in a study, the arrangement of joint communication and work in the research process.

3   Basis of relationships

- Negotiate with your participants the conditions under which collaboration will take place as well as the research aim(s) at the beginning of your collaboration.
- Discuss how you can assist the participants both during and after the research.

4   Start of the narrative inquiry

- Reflect on your own experiences and beliefs at the beginning and during a narrative inquiry.
- Present the results of your self-reflections in publications if these are necessary to understand the outcome of a narrative inquiry.

5   Awareness of the situation in which participants are embedded

- Pay attention to the "social, cultural, familial, linguistic, and institutional" (Clandinin & Caine, 2012, p. 171) backgrounds against which participants narrate their stories.
- Be aware of the potential complexity of the research associated with "ambiguities, … difficulties and uncertainties" (Clandinin & Caine, 2012, pp. 171–172).

6   Collecting data

- Be open to the many ways in which participants share their experiences; for example, interviews, photographs, diaries.

7   Transforming the data into the final narratives

- It is a complex process characterized by iterations.
- Negotiate the emerging texts with your participants.
- Produce preliminary texts that are guided by the research aim(s).
- Read the data several times with attention to the people, time, and places associated with the events described to capture the meaning of the experiences described.
- Create the final narratives from the preliminary texts.
- Align these narratives with the target audience, thereby paying attention not only to an academic audience, but also to the participants and the practical and social impacts this research can have.

8   Situational elements in narratives of experiences

- Include details of the time, place and social environment in which the experiences described took place. This enables readers to understand the complexity of the lives of participants with all their twists and turns.
- Narratives cannot provide definitive answers; rather, they are meant to make the reader think about the experiences described and how they can be related to other contexts.

9   Relational response communities

- Include people such as the research team, supervisors, and academic peers with whom you can regularly discuss your research approach and narratives at different stages of development.

10   Justifications for narrative inquiry

- Outline your personal interest in a research subject, your relationship to this subject and to the participants.

- Illustrate practical benefits of your research.
- Explain why narrative inquiry is used as the research design.
- Outline what kind of impact your study may have on society or politics.

11 "Attentive to audience" (Clandinin & Caine, 2012, p. 175)

- Address your participants as well as the scientific community with texts originating from narrative inquiries.
- The narratives shall be of such storytelling quality that they reflect the experiences of both the study participants and the researchers, and also the situations and environments in which they were experienced.
- The narratives shall also have scientific value by contributing to answering social and theoretical questions.
- Narrative research can have the character of an intervention because of the close relationship between participants and researchers. Through the telling of old experiences, new ones can be made. Be aware that the potential intervention character of narrative inquiry demands a high ethical responsibility that persists beyond the research end.

12 "Commitment to understanding lives in motion" (Clandinin & Caine, 2012, p. 175)

- Narratives of experiences are never finished.
- There is no such thing as 'one story.'
- Narratives are altered by telling or retelling.

Ethical Considerations

Within their 12 qualitative touchstones, Clandinin and Caine (2012) suggested that narrative inquirers comply with ethical standards. This is even more relevant for scholars conducting studies with members of vulnerable groups such as transgender people. Transgender people are considered as vulnerable because they belong to a minority group which is often confronted with discrimination, exclusion, or violence. Based on literature and experiences of former research, we assumed that sensitive topics such as sexual behavior and experience of discrimination and violence might arise within the data collection process (Beagan et al., 2012; Schneider et al., 2019). Jens, consequently, sought and obtained ethical approval from the research ethics committee of the University of Brighton (UK).

The ethical considerations resulted, among other things, in the setting up of a 'study advisory group' consisting of two transgender people who were involved in the development of the research plan and the application for ethical approval to ensure that the study focus met the needs of transgender people as well as ethical standards.

During the recruitment and before the first interview with each participant was started, the participants were reminded that their participation was voluntary and were informed about their rights to not answer a question and to interrupt or terminate the interview at any time without any negative consequences. Both written and oral informed consent were obtained before the interviews started.

Terminology is an important issue in research with transgender people. In line with recommendations by Adams et al. (2017) and Vincent (2018), Jens asked the participants which term and pronoun he should use to describe them. Furthermore, he requested that they should state on the participant consent form whether they would like to be described by a pseudonym or their original first name in the study. This was in accordance with a recommendation by the study advisory group and Vincent (2018) regarding the ethical principle of autonomy of the participants. Data protection in general was applied in line with the legal requirements in Germany and the European Union.

Application to Occupational Science and Occupational Therapy

We argue that the way narratives are told corresponds to the passage of everyday Deweyan inquiry processes (Dewey, 1938; Miettinen, 2000; Morgan, 2014). Narratives enable researchers and therapists to understand occupations and situational elements in which people find themselves and perform occupations. In addition, narratives may allow the identification of indeterminate situations in which therapy clients find themselves and of which they are unaware due to health, social, and occupational issues. The identification of indeterminate situations allows therapists to make clients aware of their problematic situations. Narratives can already contain descriptions of problematic situations in people's lives and how they try to find solutions while reflecting on these situations. During these reflections, people take their beliefs, emotions, and experiences into account and narrate them. This allows researchers and therapists to gain deeper insights into what enables or hinders individuals to perform occupations to cope with problematic situations.

Descriptions of occupations that research participants and clients performed to achieve certain goals, how these occupations changed the problematic situation and framing situational elements, and how participants and clients evaluate the achievement of the goals are essential for the body of knowledge in occupational science and occupational therapy. They enable occupational scientists and occupational therapists to gain warranted assertions on the relationships between occupations and their consequences (cf. Biesta & Burbules, 2003) and the "situatedness of occupation" (Madsen & Josephsson, 2017, p. 412). Occupational therapists can use the information provided by narratives to plan and enact interventions with their clients. Occupational scientists can use narrative inquiry to gain a deeper understanding of how situational elements in which people are embedded shape occupations and are in turn shaped by them. Furthermore, occupational scientists may explore how beliefs, emotions, and experiences shape the performance of occupations.

Narrative inquiry contributes to the body of knowledge of occupational science and occupational therapy through its ability to present the development of occupations over time. It has, thereby, the potential to reveal the transformative capacity of occupations, which occupations are meaningful, according to the definition of Ikiugu et al. (2015), and why "psychologically rewarding occupations" are important for people's long-term aims as they induce positive mood (Ikiugu et al., 2015, p. 47).

Summarized, narrative inquiry is a way to obtain holistic pictures of occupations and consequently underpins the meaning of occupations for people's lives. As pointed out by Bonsall (2012), narrative inquiry can thus help to increase the recognition of occupational science and occupational therapy by other disciplines.

Critiquing Narrative Studies

When critiquing a study that uses narrative inquiry as a research design, you can assess the research process for adherence to the qualitative touchstones by Clandinin and Caine (2012; Textbox 8.4). In the understanding of a Deweyan pragmatist, a research study is a Deweyan inquiry (Morgan, 2014) consisting of several actions such as designing the study,

---

Textbox 8.4   Questions to Think About Answering When Reading Narrative Studies

1 Is there *sufficient description and justification* of why narrative inquiry was used as the research design for the study?
2 Are all persons involved in the research process *named and adequately described* (e.g., academic peers)?
3 Do the researchers sufficiently *outline their own perspectives, experiences, and beliefs* in relation to the research subject?
4 Are the *ethical principles* and the *research relationship* sufficiently presented?
5 Are the *framework conditions* described with regard to the invitation to participate in the study, the way of communication and joint work between study participants and researchers?
6 Did the researchers use *different data* to collect the narratives?
7 Are the participants' narratives connected to their *situational elements*?
8 Does the publication include details of the time, place and social environment in which the experiences described took place, in order to be able to *relate the narratives to other contexts*?
9 Are the narratives in such a *quality* that they reflect the experiences of both the study participants and the researchers, and the situations and environments in which they were experienced?
10 Did the researchers focus the narratives on the *target audience*, paying attention not only to an academic audience, but also to the participants and the practical and social impacts their research can have?

---

defining the research aim(s), creating the research question(s), carrying out the interview(s) and transcription(s), writing the participants' narrative(s) and, if required, translating them. In terms of the preceding discussion, warranted assertions emerge from a research process at the point when meaning is assigned to the outcome of the process and the associated actions which had been carried out therein. It is important to bear in mind that assertions gained "are always only warranted in relation to concrete inquiries" (Biesta & Burbules, 2003, p. 67). Consequently, a detailed description of the research process is essential in order to be able to understand the findings and thus essential for the quality of a study.

Jens' Personal Journey

When Jens first started thinking about his PhD project, it was to follow on from his master's thesis, in which he had used narrative inquiry to explore the experiences of young transgender adults (Schneider et al., 2019). He had obtained informative narratives of his participants about their occupational transitions. Drawing on this experience, he also considered narrative inquiry to be an appropriate research design for his doctoral thesis. The use of narrative inquiry in his doctoral study required a much more intensive engagement with this research design than was possible for the master's study.

Jens became increasingly aware of the diversity and complexity of various narrative inquiry approaches in the field. This process of engaging with narrative inquiry was both a fascinating and an educational experience. A major question during that time was which philosophical worldview should become the theoretical foundation of his narrative inquiry. After some detours, he came across publications by Clandinin and colleagues and he saw how they grounded narrative inquiry in Dewey's understanding of experience. Jens had already read about Deweyan pragmatism in connection with transactional perspectives on occupation (Cutchin & Dickie, 2013b) and had become increasingly curious about the connection between narrative inquiry, Deweyan pragmatism, and occupation. He was fascinated by how Dewey's concept of inquiry can be used to understand the acquisition of warranted assertions in daily life and research as well as the central role that actions and occupations serve in the acquisition of these warranted assertions. In addition, Dewey's theory of inquiry and the transactional understanding of the world allowed him and the co-authors of the current chapter to explore how the performance of occupations is transacted with the environment and vice versa.

Preparation for the interviews and undertaking them did not present any challenges. The interviews were unstructured, and the participants talked freely about the occupations and experiences that were meaningful to them during their gender transition process. They did this in a surprisingly structured and detailed way, so that Jens rarely had to ask questions. One reason why the participants told their narratives in this way might be that transgender people in Germany have to undergo assessments before the start of gender-affirming measures and are, therefore, often used to telling their life stories. Furthermore, observations by researchers revealed that transgender people start to inform others about their issues at a later stage of their gender transition process with the aim to improve the situation for transgender people on a social, political, and health and social care level (Beagan et al., 2012; Budge et al., 2017; Daley & Hynes, 2020; Schneider, 2022). These transgender people are thus familiar to talk about their lives. The information content of the stories surprised Jens because many sensitive and intimate experiences were shared. He was, therefore, able to learn about study participants' situational elements and how they cope with them via occupations. Jens found it very gratifying that the participants were willing to share their experiences with him in such depth. During the two and a half years when Jens was transcribing the interviews, preparing the next interview rounds, creating intermediate texts, and writing the final narratives, he found it challenging to keep the individual stories short due to the rich details and interesting aspects that he would have liked to include. As the stories revealed rich and nuanced information, narrative inquiry acted as an appropriate design to address the research question and aims. Stories were created in an accessible way while conveying rich information that was achieved by reading the stories again and again, and by removing information less relevant to the question and aims.

Summary

Narrative inquiry is a research design that is used by occupational scientists, occupational therapists, and occupational therapy researchers to explore how people experience meaningful occupations. It enables understanding of the "transformative capacity" and "the situatedness of occupation" (Madsen & Josephsson, 2017, p. 412) as well as the 'situational elements' that frame the performance of occupations and how the performance and meaning of occupations change over the course of time. Although, or even because, there are no general rules for conducting narrative inquiries, the research methods can largely be selected and adapted to meet the research aim(s). The 'qualitative touchstones for narrative inquiry' by Clandinin and Caine (2012) assist in ensuring the quality of a narrative inquiry. Narrative inquiry can be theoretically grounded in Deweyan pragmatism which acts as a key philosophical frame to understand experience, knowledge acquisition, and the role of actions and occupations in the research process, as well as in participants' and researchers' lives. Narrative inquiry is, therefore, a particularly suitable research design for both occupational science and occupational therapy research.

References

Adams, N., Pearce, R., Veale, J., Radix, A., Castro, D., Sarkar, A., & Thom, K. C. (2017). Guidance and ethical considerations for undertaking transgender health research and institutional review boards adjudicating this research. *Transgender Health, 2*(1), 165–175. https://doi.org/10.1089/trgh.2017.0012

Alsaker, S., Josephsson, S., & Dickie, V. A. (2013). Exploring the transactional quality of everyday occupations through narrative-in-action: Meaning-making among women living with chronic conditions. In M. P. Cutchin & V. A. Dickie (Eds.), *Transactional perspectives on occupation* (pp. 65–78). Springer. https://doi.org/10.1007/978-94-007-4429-5

Asaba, E., Laliberte Rudman, D., Mondaca, M., & Park, M. (2015). Visual methodologies: Photovoice in focus. In S. Nayar & M. Stanley (Eds.), *Qualitative research methodologies for occupational science and therapy* (pp. 155–173). Routledge.

Baum, C. M., & Edwards, D. (2008). *Activity card sort (ACS)* (2nd ed.). American Occupational Therapy Association.

Beagan, B. L., De Souza, L., Godbout, C., Hamilton, L., MacLeod, J., Paynter, E., & Tobin, A. (2012). "This is the biggest thing you'll ever do in your life": Exploring the occupations of transgendered people. *Journal of Occupational Science, 19*(3), 226–240. https://doi.org/10.1080/14427591.2012.659169

Biesta, G. J. J., & Burbules, N. C. (2003). *Pragmatism and educational research*. Rowman & Littlefield.

Birch, L. J. (2011). *Telling stories: A thematic narrative analysis of eight women's PhD experiences* [Doctoral dissertation, Victoria University]. VU Research Repository. https://vuir.vu.edu.au/19398/1/Lesley_Birch.pdf

Bonsall, A. (2012). An examination of the pairing between narrative and occupational science. *Scandinavian Journal of Occupational Therapy, 19*(1), 92–103. https://doi.org/10.3109/11038128.2011.552119

Brinkmann, S., & Kvale, S. (2015). *Interviews: Learning the craft of qualitative research interviewing* (3rd ed.). SAGE.

Budge, S. L., Chin, M. Y., & Minero, L. P. (2017). Trans individuals' facilitative coping: An analysis of internal and external processes. *Journal of Counseling Psychology, 64*(1), 12–25. https://doi.org/10.1037/cou0000178

Caine, V., Estefan, A., & Clandinin, D. J. (2013). A return to methodological commitment: Reflections on narrative inquiry. *Scandinavian Journal of Educational Research, 57*(6), 574–586. https://doi.org/10.1080/00313831.2013.798833

Clandinin, D. J., & Caine, V. (2012). Narrative inquiry. In A. A. Trainor & E. Graue (Eds.), *Reviewing qualitative research in the social sciences: A guide for researchers and reviewers* (1st ed., pp. 166–179). Routledge. https://doi.org/10.4324/9780203813324

Clandinin, D. J., & Connelly, F. M. (2000). *Narrative inquiry: Experience and story in qualitative research*. Jossey-Bass.

Clandinin, D. J., & Rosiek, J. (2007). Mapping a landscape of narrative inquiry. In D. J. Clandinin (Ed.), *Handbook of narrative inquiry: Mapping a methodology* (pp. 35–75). SAGE.

Clark-Ibáñez, M. (2007). Inner-city children in sharper focus: Sociology of childhood and photo-elicitation interviews. In G. C. Stanczak (Ed.), *Visual research methods: Image, society, and representation* (pp. 167–196). SAGE.

Cutchin, M. P., & Dickie, V. A. (2013a). *Transactional perspectives on occupation*. Springer.

Cutchin, M. P., & Dickie, V. A. (2013b). Transactional perspectives on occupation: An introduction and rationale. In M. P. Cutchin, & V. A. Dickie (Eds.), *Transactional perspectives on occupation* (pp. 1–10). Springer.

Daley, V., & Hynes, S. H. (2020). A phenomenological study of occupational participation for people who identify as transgender. *Annals of International Occupational Therapy*, *3*(3), 127–135. https://doi.org/10.3928/24761222-20200309-04

De Jong, D. C., Pike, G., West, S., Valerius, H., Kay, A., & Ellis, S. (2021). Shared music, shared occupation: Embedding music as a socio-altruistic collective- and co-occupation in occupational therapy education. *Journal of Occupational Science*, *28*(3), 374–378. https://doi.org/10.1080/14427591.2020.1793808

Dewey, J. (1929). *Experience and nature*. George Allen & Unwin. (Original work published 1925)

Dewey, J. (1938). *Logic: The theory of inquiry*. Henry Holt and Company.

Dewey, J. (1941). Propositions, warranted assertibility, and truth. *The Journal of Philosophy*, *38*(7), 169–186. https://doi.org/10.2307/2017978

Dewey, J. (1997). *Logic: Experience and education*. Touchstone (Original work published 1938)

Dewey, J., & Bentley, A. (1949). *Knowing and the known*. Beacon Press.

Dwyer, R., Davis, I., & Emerald, E. (2017). *Narrative research in practice: Stories from the field*. Springer.

Dwyer, R., & Emerald, E. (2017). Narrative research in practice: Navigating the terrain. In R. Dwyer, I. Davis, & E. Emerald (Eds.), *Narrative research in practice: Stories from the field* (pp. 1–25). Springer.

Fisher, A. G., & Marterella, A. (2019). *Powerful practice: A model for authentic occupational therapy*. Center for Innovative OT Solutions.

Harper, D. (2002). Talking about pictures: A case for photo elicitation. *Visual Studies*, *17*(1), 13–26. https://doi.org/10.1080/14725860220137345

Hartman, L. R., Mandich, A., Magalhães, L., & Orchard, T. (2011). How do we 'see' occupations? An examination of visual research methodologies in the study of human occupation. *Journal of Occupational Science*, *18*(4), 292–305. https://doi.org/10.1080/14427591.2011.610776

Hemmingsson, H., Forsyth, K., Haglund, L., Keponen, R., Ekbladh, E., & Kielhofner, G. (2017). Talking with clients: Assessments that collect information through interviews. In R. R. Tayler (Ed.), *Kielhofner's model of human occupation: Theory and application* (5th ed., pp. 275–290). Wolters Kluwer.

Ikiugu, M. N., Hoyme, A. K., Mueller, B. A., & Reinke, R. R. (2015). Meaningful occupation clarified: Thoughts about the relationship between meaningful and psychologically rewarding occupations. *South African Journal of Occupational Therapy*, *45*(1), 47–50. https://dx.doi.org/10.17159/2310-3833/2015/v45no1a8

Jackendoff, R. (2009). *Language, consciousness, culture: Essays on mental structure*. MIT Press.

Josephsson, S., & Alsaker, S. (2015). Narrative methodology: A tool to access unfolding and situated meaning in occupation. In S. Nayar, & M. Stanley (Eds.), *Qualitative research methodologies for occupational science and therapy* (pp. 70–83). Routledge.

Josephsson, S., Asaba, E., Jonsson, H., & Alsaker, S. (2006). Creativity and order in communication: Implications from philosophy to narrative research concerning human occupation. *Scandinavian Journal of Occupational Therapy*, *13*(2), 86–93. https://doi.org/10.1080/11038120600691116

Labov, W., & Waletzky, J. (1967). Narrative analysis: Oral versions of personal experiences. In J. Helm (Ed.), *Essays on the verbal and visual arts* (pp. 12–44). University of Washington Press.

Lisahunter. (2017). If you see what I mean? Visual narratives – Stories told through, with and by visual images. In R. Dwyer, I. Davis, & E. Emerald (Eds.), *Narrative research in practice: Stories from the field* (pp. 89–116). Springer.

Madsen, J., & Josephsson, S. (2017). Engagement in occupation as an inquiring process: Exploring the situatedness of occupation. *Journal of Occupational Science*, *24*(4), 412–424. https://doi.org/10.1080/14427591.2017.1308266

Miettinen, R. (2000). The concept of experiential learning and John Dewey's theory of reflective thought and action. *International Journal of Lifelong Education*, *19*(1), 54–72. https://doi.org/10.1080/026013700293458

Morgan, D. L. (2014). Pragmatism as a paradigm for social research. *Qualitative Inquiry*, *20*(8), 1045–1053. https://doi.org/10.1177/1077800413513733

O'Bryan, J. (2017). Where words fail: Storying audio-visual data. In R. Dwyer, I. Davis, & E. Emerald (Eds.), *Narrative research in practice: Stories from the field* (pp. 117–130). Springer.

Patterson, W. (2013). Narratives of events: Labovian narrative analysis and its limitations. In M. Andrews, C. Squire, & M. Tamboukou (Eds.), *Doing narrative research* (2nd ed., pp. 27–46). SAGE.

Patton, M. Q. (2015). *Qualitative research & evaluation methods integrating theory and practice* (4th ed.). SAGE.

Polkinghorne, D. E. (1995). Narrative configuration in qualitative analysis. *International Journal of Qualitative Studies in Education*, *8*(1), 5–23. https://doi.org/10.1080/0951839950080103

Polkinghorne, D. E. (2005). Language and meaning: Data collection in qualitative research. *Journal of Counseling Psychology*, *52*(2), 137–145. https://doi.org/10.1037/0022-0167.52.2.137

Riessman, C. K. (2008). *Narrative methods for the human sciences*. SAGE.

Riessman, C. K. (2013). Concluding comments. In M. Andrews, C. Squire, & M. Tamboukou (Eds.), *Doing narrative research* (2nd ed., pp. 255–260). SAGE.

Schneider, J. (2022). *Narratives on meaningful occupations of transmen during their gender transition process* [Doctoral dissertation, University of Brighton]. The University of Brighton research portal (accessible to the public from January 2024). https://research.brighton.ac.uk/en/studentTheses/narratives-on-meaningful-occupations-of-transmen-during-their-gen

Schneider, J., Page, J., & van Nes, F. (2019). "Now I feel much better than in my previous life": Narratives of occupational transitions in young transgender adults. *Journal of Occupational Science*, *26*(2), 219–232. https://doi.org/10.1080/14427591.2018.1550726

Seal, K. (2014). *Living the struggle against obesity: Common threads in the life-narratives of women who have regained weight* [Doctoral dissertation, University of Brighton]. The University of Brighton research portal. https://research.brighton.ac.uk/files/4754728/Living%20the%20Struggle%20Against%20Obesity%20-%20Common%20Threads%20in%20the%20Life-Narratives%20of%20Women%20Who%20Have%20Regained%20Weight%20(Klara%20Sea~1.pdf

Squire, C. (2013). From experience-centred to socioculturally-orientated approaches to narrative. In M. Andrews, C. Squire, & M. Tamboukou (Eds.), *Doing narrative research* (2nd ed., pp. 47–71). SAGE.

Squire, C., Andrews, M., & Tamboukou, M. (2013). Introduction: What is narrative research? In M. Andrews, C. Squire, & M. Tamboukou (Eds.), *Doing narrative research* (2nd ed., pp. 1–23). SAGE.

Squires, A. (2009). Methodological challenges in cross-cultural qualitative research: A research review. *International Journal of Nursing Studies*, *46*, 277–287.

Taylor, J. A. (2008). *The construction of identities through narratives of occupations* [Doctoral dissertation, University of Salford]. https://usir.salford.ac.uk/id/eprint/1946/1/Whole_thesis_Final_version.pdf

Taylor, J., & Kay, S. (2015). The construction of identities in narratives about serious leisure occupations. *Journal of Occupational Science*, *22*(3), 260–276. https://doi.org/10.1080/14427591.2013.803298

Van Nes, F., Abma, T., Jonsson, H., & Deeg, D. (2010). Language differences in qualitative research: Is meaning lost in translation? *European Journal of Ageing*, *7*(4), 313–316. https://doi.org/10.1007/s10433-010-0168-y

Vincent, B. W. (2018). Studying trans: Recommendations for ethical recruitment and collaboration with transgender participants in academic research. *Psychology and Sexuality*, *9*(2), 102–116. https://doi.org/10.1080/19419899.2018.1434558

Williams, G. (1984). The genesis of chronic illness: Narrative re-construction. *Sociology of Health & Illness*, *6*(2), 175–200. https://doi.org/10.1111/1467-9566.ep10778250

Additional Resources

Burwash, S. C. (2013). Doing occupation: *A narrative inquiry into occupational therapists' stories of occupation-based practice* [Doctoral dissertation, University of Alberta]. ERA: Education and research archive. https://era.library.ualberta.ca/items/4544bca2-2de9-41f4-a92f-721c25e1051c

Clandinin, D. J. (2022). *Engaging in narrative inquiry* (2nd ed.). Routledge. https://doi.org/10.4324/9781003240143

9 Ethnography

Suzanne Huot and Anne-Cécile Delaisse

Ethnography is one of the oldest qualitative methodologies, with roots dating back to the late 1800s and early 1900s. It is essentially the study of a group or culture. Here, culture should be interpreted broadly as the "acquired knowledge that people use to interpret their world and generate social behavior" (Spradley & McCurdy, 1984, p. 2). Cultures do not only exist at national or regional scales or in relation to ethno-racial groups; a classroom, a group of professionals, or a neighborhood, for instance, can be also considered as having their own cultures. In this chapter, we explain ethnographic methodology and its fit for the study of human occupation. In doing so, we draw upon examples from two critical ethnographies exploring the experiences of French-speaking immigrants living in a Canadian metropolitan area.

Drawing on the work of others, Bryman (2001) has provided a comprehensive definition of ethnography that highlighted five central features of the approach. First, researchers must immerse themselves in the society or group they are interested in studying. Second, by engaging in fieldwork, researchers collect descriptive data. Third, the data collected must reflect the culture of those being studied. Fourth, the perspective of the research participants and the meanings they attach to their social worlds must be at the center. Finally, findings must be made relevant for target audiences.

There is a diverse range of approaches to ethnography, including critical ethnography (Jamal, 2005; Madison, 2012), feminist ethnography (Huisman, 2008; Manning, 2018), focused ethnography (Knoblauch, 2005; Stahlke Wall, 2014), institutional ethnography (Kearney et al., 2019; Prodinger et al., 2015), and autoethnography (Gouzouasis & Yanko, 2018; Holman Jones et al., 2016), among others. Within this ethnographic school of inquiry, particular methodological styles may be adopted depending on the purpose of specific research studies. This chapter will address ethnographic research as a broad school of inquiry characterized by particular features that distinguish it from other methodologies.

A range of ethnographic studies examining diverse topics are available within the occupation-focused literature (e.g., Delaisse et al., 2021; Lavalley et al., 2022; Prodinger et al., 2015; Simaan, 2017). For example, Aldrich et al.'s (2020) collaborative ethnography of people's experiences of long-term unemployment in the United States (St. Louis, Missouri) and Canada (London, Ontario) drew on a range of methods to examine how participants' engagement in daily occupations were shaped by social policies and dominant discourses. Ethnography is particularly well suited to studying occupation by focusing on everyday lived experiences and the contexts within which these are embedded.

DOI: 10.4324/9781003456216-9

Background

Modern ethnography is typically traced back to traditions within social and cultural anthropology and sociology. It is important to note that ethnography was initially used by researchers during the colonial era to study 'non-Western' populations (Bejarano et al., 2019). Researchers currently using this methodology should be aware of this history and reject extractive approaches and misrepresentations of (formerly) colonized populations that can characterize some ethnographic studies (Bejarano et al., 2019; Simaan, 2017). In this chapter, we discuss ways scholars have suggested mitigating colonial power dynamics in ethnographic research.

Ethnography provides a close study of a culture shared and performed by a group, through occupations, within a specific spatial and temporal context (Hammersley & Atkinson, 2007; Van Maanen, 2004). This methodology provides the opportunity to study participants' historically and socially situated experiences (Lecompte, 2002). As cultures are internally diverse, communities studied in ethnographic research are viewed as a collection of individuals rather than monoliths whose "often contentious interactions constitute the fabric of a culture full of hitherto unnoticed diversity" (Lecompte, 2002, p. 292). Therefore, this methodology is particularly useful for examining people's engagement in daily occupations and considering how their 'doing, being, and becoming' (Rebeiro, 2001; Wilcock, 1999, 2006) are shaped by and serve to reproduce culture (Bailliard et al., 2013).

Hallmarks of ethnographic research include prolonged engagement and participant observation, whereby researchers immerse themselves in fieldwork by entering naturalistic settings where the group of interest is located. The field of ethnographic research is co-constructed by the researcher with the study partners and participants (cf. Huot, 2018); meaning that it is not always a pre-existing, discretely bounded space that is accessed by the researcher. Instead, it involves a process of determining which spaces are relevant to include in the study and in what ways.

Epistemology, Ontology, Axiology

Early ethnographies were situated within a positivist paradigm, but contemporary ethnographic studies have been expanded through the adoption of constructivist, interpretivist, and critical theory paradigm positions. This chapter focuses primarily on research located within these latter paradigms that are ontologically relativist and acknowledge the existence of multiple realities experienced by diverse populations (Guba & Lincoln, 2004). The researcher is thereby involved in co-creating the data with participants and, as a result, should reflect on the ways their own axiology (e.g., values and ethics) shape the design and conduct of the study. In particular, it is important for researchers to consider how their values inform what they are aiming to achieve through their work (Bressers et al., 2020). In migration research for example, this may include a commitment to open borders with the aim for research to support occupational justice for immigrant populations. Understanding of research participants' experiences and occupations are developed in relation to their contexts through fieldwork and additional forms of data collection. Findings generated are located within the relevant current and historical social contexts and analyzed in relation to these.

Epistemologically, data are transactional, intersubjective, and value-mediated. Knowledge is understood as co-constructed through interactions between researcher and participants (Guba & Lincoln, 2004). Viewing knowledge in this way leads to the adoption of diverse methods (e.g., observational, participatory, visual, dialogical) to overcome misapprehensions and to promote more informed understandings between the parties involved.

Further, addressing the role of the researcher through ongoing reflexivity is vital, as "what can be known is inextricably intertwined with the interaction between a *particular* investigator and a *particular* object or group" (Guba & Lincoln, 2004, p. 26). Our positionality as researchers shaped the studies discussed in this chapter. Suzanne is a Canadian-born Francophone of European settler ancestry. She has never lived abroad and has no personal experience of international migration. Her interest in this topic stems from having lived in Francophone minority communities (FMCs) all her life and being motivated to make these communities more receptive to immigration. Anne-Cécile is an international student from France. In this study, she was both an insider as a French-speaking foreigner and an outsider as a researcher. Given the diversity of the participants in this research, her positionality as a white woman implied that some participants' experiences resonated more closely with her than others.

Topic and Questions Best Suited for Ethnographic Studies

Ethnographic research is well suited to studies of cultures as performed through occupations or occupations of a group, that can be considered a cultural 'unit' based on shared identity markers in a specific context. Examples within occupational science include Simaan's (2017) decolonial ethnography exploring how olive growers' occupations are shaped by land colonization in Palestine; Lavalley et al.'s (2022) ethnography exploring the changing nature of a senior center as it shifted toward inclusion of increasing numbers of Spanish-speaking members; and Aldrich et al.'s (2020) collaborative ethnography that studied the ways discourses and policies influenced the daily occupations of people experiencing long-term unemployment.

Our research centers on the FMC in Metro Vancouver, British Columbia. Canada has two official languages, but the majority of the national population is Anglophone. French speakers are mainly located within the province of Quebec, while French speakers outside of this province constitute FMCs, together with the institutions representing and serving them. Approximately 28% of French-speakers in British Columbia were born abroad and of these 50% were born in Europe, 22% in Asia, 18% in Africa, and 10% in the Americas (Office of the Commissioner of Official Languages, 2020). Immigration generates demographic, social, and cultural change within communities. Given the changes occurring within the region's FMC, the two ethnographic studies we draw on in this chapter addressed the integration experiences of French-speaking immigrants, with a specific focus on their social participation and engagement in occupations with others outside their homes.

The first study examined the role of Francophone community spaces within the FMC (Delaisse et al., 2021). The three main objectives were to critically examine:

1 Why and how French-speaking immigrants participate in different Francophone community spaces, and the factors that shape their involvement;
2 French-speaking immigrants' motivations and expectations for participating in community spaces, and the role of their participation in activities within these spaces for their long-term integration and social inclusion (taking into account the intersecting markers of language, race, ethnicity, gender, and immigration category among others); and
3 The role of the structural context in shaping French-speaking immigrants' participation in daily activities, including Metro Vancouver's geographic and socio-historic context, and the institutional context of three selected community sites (e.g., discourses, programs, practices).

The second study explored the concept of community cohesion in relation to growing diversity within the FMC as a result of immigration (Huot et al., 2020b). The three main objectives critically addressed:

1 How community cohesion has been conceptualized and addressed in national stake-holders' documents attending to FMCs, particularly with respect to immigration;
2 Understandings of the ways community members (i.e., those born in Canada and abroad) perceive community cohesion and experience everyday life in FMCs; and
3 Stakeholder awareness of the implications of growing diversity stemming from immi-gration upon community cohesion through a focus on specific spaces (e.g., workplaces, schools), occupations (e.g., employment, parenting), and issues (e.g., racism, precarity).

The research objectives of these studies were worded to reflect the critical positioning of the ethnographies and are phrased in ways that support the use of diverse methods to explore the interrelationships of relevant issues (e.g., structural, personal) in different ways (e.g., discourse analysis, participant observations, go-along interviews) and at different scales (e.g., neighborhood, municipal, provincial, national).

As ethnographies focus on the culture a group of people share, they address the con-texts within which groups of individuals are embedded. Research questions, problems, and objectives are framed to address what is happening within the research field of interest (e.g., Francophone institutions, associations, religious spaces) and why it is happening. This approach enables emphasis to be placed on contextual images and patterns (e.g., values, symbols, norms, beliefs) within the field or site. Research questions from the two example studies outlined in this chapter, as well as other ethnographies, are included in Textbox 9.1

Textbox 9.1   Examples of Ethnographic Research Questions

1 How do local policies and practices influence the social production and meaning of occupations in people's everyday lives?
2 What are the characteristics of current discursive and demographic Francophone minority community contexts?
3 How do community members perceive and experience community cohesion, social inclusion, and social participation?
4 How was the community, as a whole, responding to new community members from a population that had been historically marginalized? (Lavalley et al., 2022, p. 3)
5 How do settler-colonialism and the military occupation influence the daily occu-pations of olive growing communities in the oPt [occupied Palestinian territory], such as travelling to and from grove and press, accessing land, harvesting, planting and maintaining groves? (Simaan, 2017, p. 511)
6 What means do communities adopt to enable their usual occupations to continue, given that humans are occupational beings who adapt what they do and their environment in response to changes in circumstances? (Simaan, 2017, p. 511)

A key consideration when designing an ethnographic study is how the research field will be defined. As noted above, the research field is not simply an objective pre-existing space entered from the outside by researchers; it is, instead, defined by researchers in relation to their objectives (Nast, 1994). This relates, in part, to how the cultural group being studied is defined. Contemporary understandings of culture recognize that it is dynamic and interwoven rather than static, unchanging, bounded, and monolithic. As processes of globalization have accelerated, the blending and hybridity of cultures have become increasingly visible making it progressively difficult to study cultural groups as 'isolated' within or outside one's own society. It is essential for ethnographers to acknowledge that particular cultures are socially constructed and are constantly evolving in relation to the social context. Ethnography is useful for examining how culture is lived, produced, and reproduced; and, from an occupational perspective, for exploring how the process of cultural change influences, and is influenced by, occupation.

Recruitment and Sampling

A key feature of ethnography is the immersive fieldwork undertaken that typically includes participant observation. Researchers must, therefore, co-construct the 'field' by determining, often in collaboration with research partners and/or participants, where fieldwork will occur (i.e., what spaces are relevant for the community/cultural group being studied) and with whom (Huot, 2018). We chose to study the experiences of Francophone immigrants. 'Francophone' was defined as people whose mother tongue or first official language is French. However, we found that some people did not self-identify as Francophone and we later adopted the term 'French-speaking' to be more inclusive. 'Immigrants' was used broadly to include all classes and categories of people who migrated to Canada (e.g., international students, refugees, asylum seekers, temporary foreign workers). We chose to focus on Vancouver because it has one of the most immigrant-rich FMCs in the country and is one of the main immigrant-receiving metropolitan centers in Canada. However, British Columbia has been understudied given its official language population accounts for only 1.3% of the total population (Statistics Canada, 2017). Once the group and field of interest are defined, partnerships are developed, and institutional ethics approval is obtained, participants can be recruited.

We included two different participant groups for these studies: French-speaking immigrants residing in Metro Vancouver and key informants from the area's FMC. The first group constituted the main population of interest and included French-speaking adults who emigrated from a range of countries. To obtain a diversity of perspectives, we included participants who had resided in Canada for varying lengths of time and who had different immigration statuses. This helped to provide insight into the dimensions of integration that occur over time. As we aimed to explore the interrelationships between immigrants and the broader social locale within which they were embedded, we also recruited key informants who could provide details regarding the socio-historical context. This second group of participants included employees, members of the board or directors, or representatives of governmental and nonprofit organizations geared toward serving the FMC including, but not restricted to, those providing immigrant settlement and integration services. We prioritized purposeful sampling for both participant groups.

Successful recruitment is dependent on access to the cultural group and entry into the field. This can be achieved using different techniques. For instance, a gatekeeper can be approached to assist with recruitment. Standard techniques for recruitment such as the

---

Textbox 9.2   Entering the Field: Potential Strategies

1 Use the Internet to explore what organizations, services, and programs are available within the community and to identify potential partners
2 Arrange meetings with contacts from community organizations to discuss research and obtain their insights and feedback on the study
3 Regularly attend community events, festivals, meetings, and forums to meet community members
4 Volunteer for community organizations and programs to meet community members and reciprocally contribute to the community
5 Get involved with community initiatives to build trust and rapport

---

dissemination of study information can also be used, but may not generate the most purposeful group of participants. In our studies, word-of-mouth was the most successful strategy for recruitment. Community members appreciated hearing about the study directly and being able to begin developing a rapport with the researchers prior to volunteering to participate. Within our research we adopted a range of strategies to gain entry into the field. Potential strategies are summarized in Textbox 9.2.

Participants in both groups (i.e., immigrants and key informants) were recruited through a variety of means. We conducted meetings with gatekeepers within the community before beginning formal data collection. In the first study, we formally partnered with three community sites: a church, a community organization, and a provincial association. In the second study, we formed a research advisory committee that met twice a year. Community partners assisted with recruitment by emailing the study recruitment flyer to their clients and members. Recruitment was facilitated primarily through direct contact with potential participants. The researchers (Anne-Cécile in particular) spent time in community spaces, participating in community activities and events in order to meet community members and inform them of the study. As observations continued within the community sites (further described below), initial participants were recruited. Reflecting the iterative nature of ethnography, additional recruitment was withheld to allow for preliminary data generation and analysis so that further recruitment could be purposefully informed by the preliminary analysis. We then sought to recruit additional participants. Recruitment took a more targeted approach using word-of-mouth to locate people who could provide further insight. For instance, we aimed to ensure women and men were included from each of the partnering sites (Study 1). Recruitment of community members in the second study adopted similar methods. Key informant participants were recruited mainly through personal communication. Having been immersed in the field though ongoing data collection, recruitment was facilitated by the familiarity of the researchers.

There is no standard for the number of participants that should be included in an ethnographic study. The decision to stop recruiting is informed by a number of considerations, including the approaches to data collection selected (e.g., the range of methods used, the number of sessions conducted), practical constraints (e.g., time and resources), and success in identifying information rich participants, among others. In Study 1, we recruited 26 participants (20 immigrants, 6 key informants), and engaged in 39 individual data collection sessions. This resulted in a large volume of rich textual, observational, and visual data. The second study sought to include 11 key informants and 24 community members in Metro Vancouver (with similar numbers being recruited in three additional cities from different provinces to inform a comparative analysis).

Data Collection

Within ethnographic research, a variety of methods may be utilized. We used a critical ethnographic approach, adapted from Carspecken (1996), to design both studies and select the data collection methods. An ethnographic approach is intended to study action occurring within social sites and to understand that action by exploring the locales and social systems within which those sites are embedded. The social system is not understood as existing separately from human activity; rather, it is comprised by patterned human activity, meaning that its existence depends on its continual reproduction. Moreover, our critical ethnographies applied a critical theory lens aimed at uncovering how spaces and the study participants' experiences were shaped by social power relations (Carspecken, 1996; Jamal, 2005).

We used a range of methods engaged in over a course of stages to complete these studies. In the first study, we began at the micro scale with observations and then completed interviews with participants to understand their experiences in relation to what we had observed. We then conducted the key informant interviews to better understand the macro context. In the second study, we reversed the order, beginning with an exploration of the broader context through critical discourse analysis of documents produced by national stakeholders and then narrowing to the community level with key informant interviews, before conducting interviews with community members about their personal experiences. A summary of these methods is included in Table 9.1.

Critical Discourse Analysis

In the second study, we wanted to begin by identifying the dominant discourse(s) related to notions of community cohesion and diversity related to policy priorities for Francophone immigration to Canada. Following consultation with the advisory committee, we prioritized the analysis of documents from five key national stakeholders with influence on FMCs throughout the country. These included the Ministry of Immigration, Refugees and Citizenship Canada, the Ministry of Canadian Heritage, the Office of the Commissioner for Official Languages of the Canadian government, the *Fédération des communautés francophones et acadienne*, and the *Société Nationale de l'Acadie*. We included 86 documents published between 2010 and 2021. We used an approach to critical discourse analysis informed by Bacchi's (2009) 'What's the problem represented to be' approach to interrogate the texts and respond to the following questions in our analysis guide:

Table 9.1 Data collection methods across the two critical ethnographies

1	Critical discourse analysis (document and text analysis)
2	Observations (participant observation)
3	Interviewing methods (in-depth, key informant)
4	Participatory methods (occupational mapping and go-alongs)

Author created

1 What is/are the problem(s) or challenge(s) represented to be in the document?
2 What presuppositions or assumptions underlie this representation of the 'problem'?
3 How has this representation of the 'problem' come about?
4 What is left unproblematic in this problem representation?
5 How/where has this representation of the 'problem' been produced, disseminated, and defended?
6 What is/are offered up as the solution(s)?
7 What effects are produced by this representation of the 'problem'?

Each of these sections also included related sub-questions to support a critical analysis of the texts. Examples and quotations drawn from the documents were included in the guides as support for our analysis and interpretation of the dominant discourses identified.

Observations

In the first study, we began with observations, conducting at least six formal observations within each of the three partnering community sites over a period of approximately 11 months. The decision was informed mainly by the frequency of events occurring within the partnering community spaces and through consultation with community partners. We wanted to ensure a minimum number of observations over the course of the ethnographic fieldwork to include key community events (e.g., Black History month and National Francophone Immigration Week programming), but additional observations were possible in some spaces when the frequency of events was more consistent (e.g., weekly church service). For this method, we developed an observation guide where information could be recorded, including: date, time, location, organizer, location description, map or sketch of location, type of activity, target audience, participants, general atmosphere, social and physical interactions and dynamics, verbal and social interactions and dynamics, languages spoken, themes, subjects, issues and questions raised, additional observations, and research reflections. As the second study builds on the first, we did not conduct additional formal observations within the community. Instead, we adopted a participatory approach to data collection through the use of occupational mapping (further described below) to inform our understanding of the field; that is, how participants represent the FMC and other spaces they frequent within the community, as well as the types of occupations they engage in within those spaces.

Interviewing Methods

In both studies, we used interviewing methods to generate data with the two groups of participants. In-depth interviews were conducted with the primary participants (Francophone immigrants) in each of the studies. In the first study, interviews addressed French-speaking immigrants' participation in the community sites. In the second study, we interviewed community members of the FMC about their perceptions of their communities' openness to diversity, their interactions with community members, and their lived experiences related to their intersectional identities within the FMC.

Interviews are an ideal method for gaining an in-depth understanding of everyday experiences from individuals' perspectives, while also getting insight into the role of broader structures in shaping these experiences (Longhurst, 2010). The interviews helped us understand Francophone immigrants' experiences of participation in FMCs, as well as the opportunities and/or limitations that various physical and virtual spaces provide to facilitate their participation in occupations—and thus their integration and social inclusion—in the community. Specifically, interview data were useful for understanding participants' agency in these processes in relation to broader social structures such as the community institutions and power dynamics in FMCs and Canadian society.

Key informant interviews were conducted with representatives from the community. In the first study, key informant interviews were conducted after the interviews with immigrant participants and included representatives of various community spaces (e.g., executive director, front-line staff) in order to examine the relationship between the social sites of interest and other related sites. We interviewed representatives from the three participating community spaces, as well as three additional stakeholders from organizations that were emphasized in the interviews with immigrant participants. These interviews served to help contextualize the experiences of the Francophone immigrants in relation to the broader social structures within which they were embedded.

In the second study, key informant interviews were conducted following the completion of the critical discourse analysis, but before in-depth interviews with immigrant participants. Questions focused on key informants' perspectives (e.g., how they understood their roles; how they defined community cohesion; and what they saw as challenges to, enablers of, and promising practices for enhancing social inclusion, participation, and community cohesion within the FMCs). One aim of these interviews was to understand whether and how these organizations adopt and/or resist the dominant discourses identified through our critical discourse analysis.

Participatory Approaches

In both studies, we also used different participatory approaches to complement the interviews and provide the primary participants with additional ways to express themselves and share their experiences and perspectives. These methods provided different ways for the researchers to immerse themselves in the field.

In the first study, we conducted follow-ups to the in-depth interviews using a 'go-along' approach (Gardner, 2011). In this style of participatory interview, the researcher accompanies participants "on their natural outings while actively exploring their physical and social practices by asking questions, listening, and observing" (Gardner, 2011, p. 1249). Data generated through this approach complement the in-depth interview data by enabling further ethnographic observation, as well as opening possibilities to capture participation in additional community spaces and occupations. The go-along approach also enables a less formal conversation in a naturalistic setting.

In the second study we used occupational mapping (Huot & Laliberte Rudman, 2015) to identify where respondents engaged socially, shedding light on the formal and informal spaces characterizing the local Francophonie. The occupational maps outlining daily routines generated spatial information to complement the interviews. This elicitation method asks participants to draw a map in response to a prompt (e.g., create a map indicating where you go during a typical week and describe what you do in those places and whom you interact with there). In addition to the visual map, the process is recorded to generate a transcript of the session.

Data Analysis

Approaches to analysis must be selected for every method used and the types of data collected. The methods described above generated forms of textual, observational, and visual data. The approach we developed for analyzing each of these is outlined below, reflecting Creswell's (2013) assertion that:

> Data analysis is not off-the-shelf; rather, it is custom-built, revised, and "choreographed" (Huberman & Miles, 1994). The processes of data collection, data analysis, and report writing are not distinct steps in the process—they are interrelated and often go on simultaneously in a research project. Qualitative researchers often "learn by doing" (Dey, 1993, p. 6) data analysis.
>
> (p. 182)

The process outlined contributed to our immersion in the data and served to deepen our understanding of the participants' experiences and how these were situated within and shaped by the broader context. However, beyond the analysis of individual types of data stemming from different methods, it is important to recognize that findings are generated from an integration of these forms of analysis. For instance, in Study 1, the analysis of observations informed the types of questions asked during interviews with immigrant participants, and the analysis of those interviews informed the questions that were asked of key informants. Similarly, in the second study, findings from the critical discourse analysis were taken up in key informant interviews, and analysis of those interviews shaped the guide for interviews with immigrant participants. Likewise, the go-alongs and occupational maps were not analyzed in isolation from the broader data set as the analysis of these data-sets informed the analysis and interpretation of the interviews by providing additional insight and context into participants' lives.

The different forms of data collected must all be managed throughout the study. Each session was digitally recorded and transcribed verbatim. Each transcript was entered into analysis software (NVivo), which was used for the open and theoretical coding stages described below. Maps were photographed and saved electronically as PDF documents. They were then narratively described, and sample maps inspired by the originals were included in dissemination to protect participant anonymity. Interrogation guides for the critical discourse analysis and observation tables were completed electronically and saved in a folder where they could be reviewed as needed to inform ongoing analyses. Development of the interrogation guide was informed by the analysis sheets described by Laliberte Rudman and Dennhardt (2014) and Bacchi's (2009) approach to critical discourse analysis of policy (Textbox 9.3). The observation table (Table 9.2) contains several columns and rows that can be expanded as needed to include relevant details. Field notes maintained throughout both studies were reviewed in their entirety to inform the ongoing progress of the study.

Textual Data

Documents from national stakeholders included in the critical discourse analysis were one form of textual data. Digital recordings of dialogic data generation sessions (e.g., interviews) held with immigrant participants and key informants were transcribed verbatim providing another form of textual data.

Textbox 9.3   Document Interrogation Guide

1 How is the 'problem' of community cohesion represented within the documents?
2 What assumptions are made about 'diversity,' 'immigration,' and 'community cohesion'?
3 What has shaped this particular representation of the problem? (e.g., prevailing political context, etc.)
4 What 'silences' remain within the documents?
5 In what ways has this representation of the 'problem' been promulgated?
6 What are the proposed 'solutions' to the 'problem'?
7 What are the potential impacts and consequences of this 'problem' framing?

Table 9.2 Observation table

Type of information	Context and description (descriptive data about context – 'context notes,' and comments – 'thick description'	Field notes (taken from memory after observation)
Date		
Location		
Time/observation schedule		
Organization(s) involved and their role(s)		
Location description		
Simple map or sketch of location		
Type of activity		
Target audience/to whom is activity geared		
Participants		
General atmosphere		
Social and physical interactions and dynamics		
Verbal social interactions and dynamics		
Languages spoken or used		
Themes, subjects, issues, questions asked during the activity		
Other observations		

Author created

Following the completion of the interrogation guide for each of the documents included in the critical discourse analysis of Study 2, analysis of the full data set began. Particular attention was paid to how community cohesion was described and envisioned within the documents. Following stakeholder-specific analysis (i.e., documents from each of the included Ministries, etc.), discursive emphases and trends were compared across the stakeholders in order to understand points of convergence and divergence in the shaping of community cohesion within FMCs. For instance, we noted whether government and non-governmental stakeholders adopted similar discourses and emphasized similar issues, or not.

To analyze transcripts in both studies, we began by reading each individually to engage in a process of 'whole-text analysis' (Sandelowski, 1995) in order to familiarize ourselves with the data. We developed a sense of each individual transcript before beginning any coding or comparison across transcripts.

All transcripts were entered into NVivo. Using a low-level coding approach (Carspecken, 1996), the initial stage of open coding entailed a line-by-line approach that remains close to the transcript and is not highly abstracted. These initial 'raw' codes (e.g., child care, transportation) were used to include the participants' opinions as they were voiced. Each transcript was coded in its entirety. The process remained iterative and inductive. As analysis was conducted concurrently with ongoing data generation, insights developed over the course of the study served to inform further data generation and analysis.

Following open coding, the transcripts were again analyzed in full using high-level, theoretical codes that required more abstraction and interpretation. In this stage, the code was based on more than the transcript alone (Carspecken, 1996), and we applied concepts from the theoretical framework guiding the studies (e.g., production of space, third space, intersectionality) (e.g., Delaisse et al., 2020, Delaisse et al., 2021). Given that we conducted *critical* ethnographies, findings stemmed from the data themselves (i.e., 'pure' induction) and from the critically informed analysis and interpretation processes. Once the coding of transcripts was complete, the individual codes were reorganized into categories. Each category was then explored by examining its component codes, and findings were further elaborated following this analysis process.

Observational Data

Participant observation occurred in multiple sites during the first study as part of the observation sessions and go-alongs (e.g., skateboard park, supermarket, clothing store). The observation tables for each formal observation were completed, which also included a section for a reflexive memo. These observation tables were reviewed to inform the interview guides and were incorporated into the broader study analysis by providing specific examples from the field. For instance, while participants discussed their personal experiences during the interviews, it was challenging to gauge particular community dynamics from these interviews alone. During the observations we noted racialized socio-spatial separations within the community (i.e., some events were attended primarily by immigrants from Europe, while others were attended mainly by African immigrants) and were able to ask key informants about how they sought to ensure diversity among their members and client-base. Thus, the analysis of completed observation tables served to highlight themes, issues, and areas of inquiry that were addressed in subsequent interviews and, ultimately, emphasized in analyses of the textual data.

Visual Data

Analysis of the occupational maps from Study 2 were analyzed similar to those generated in other studies (Aldrich et al., 2020; Huot & Laliberte Rudman, 2015; Huot et al., 2020a). The occupational maps were first analyzed on their own. Their contents were identified and described (e.g., types of places, presence of roads). In addition to exploring what was included on the maps and how things were presented, we also considered what was absent (e.g., presence of large blank spaces on the map in general or absence of specific places such as grocery stores). Key places and occupations included were itemized.

Additionally, we asked participants to include virtual spaces and these were often added to the map of physical spaces through an itemized list specifying their purpose (e.g., using particular apps to connect with family members, using Zoom to participate in virtual workshops, etc.). We then compared and contrasted the maps. The maps were not considered in isolation from other forms of data. The insights drawn from the analysis of textual and observational data informed our understanding of the maps. Likewise, our analysis of the maps contributed to our interpretation of the textual and observational data. This was possible because the different types of data collected enabled us to incorporate a range of perspectives into the analysis and the participants to address their experiences in a variety of ways.

Findings

Ethnographic findings should address details regarding the researchers' prolonged engagement in the field, how they accessed the population and entered the sites of interest, their exit from the field, and how the voices of participants and researcher are represented within the text (Bryman, 2001). The researchers' ongoing engagement in reflexivity should also be documented including a discussion of researchers' positionality with respect to the study. For instance, in what ways are the researchers 'insiders' and/or 'outsiders' to the cultural group being studied? 'Insider' and 'outsider' categories are dynamic throughout the research process and researchers should detail who they are and how this shaped the conduct of the study (Manning, 2018; Rose, 2020). These issues reflect important considerations characteristic of the alternative paradigms that aim to understand the multiple realities experienced by research participants, as well as the role of the researcher in co-constructing interpretations of these experiences with them. The presentation of findings should ultimately reflect the ontological and epistemological positioning of the study.

These two critical ethnographies addressed individual experiences of social participation and community cohesion embedded within the particular socio-historic context of Metro Vancouver. Individual experiences were emphasized throughout the in-depth interviews, go-alongs, and occupational mapping. The ways that participation and cohesion within FMCs are framed by, and are embedded within, the social structure has material implications for the daily lives of immigrants who are affected by the government policies, strategies, and action plans developed to address these issues. The broader context within which immigrants' experiences were embedded was, therefore, highlighted through the critical discourse analysis, observations, and key informant interviews. Findings that stemmed from the various forms of data collected were integrated to present a comprehensive discussion in response to the research objectives. Illustrative examples from the data were included to support our interpretations, such as direct quotations from transcripts and stakeholder documents, sample maps, and descriptions taken from the observation tables.

Rigor and Ethics

The rigor of a study is dependent on the type of ethnography being conducted as well as its guiding philosophical principles. As we conducted critical ethnographies, we were guided by Jamal's (2005) argument that a critical ethnography must satisfy three conditions. First, it must be organized in a way that ensures approaches to data collection and analysis are consistent with the study aims. This ensures a coherent approach with a clear connection established between the ontological and epistemological positions guiding the work, and the methodology and methods used to carry out the study. For instance, the methods of data generation, analysis, and interpretation we selected were inductive, theoretically informed, and dialogical to reflect our emphasis on the co-construction of knowledge.

Second, the work must be conceived as a starting point for changing the conditions of oppressive and unfair regulations. While critical ontology strives to improve the lives of those within vulnerable positions in society, this is done by recognizing that vulnerability is not an individual problem. Instead, people are impacted by dominant social forces. Our studies did not seek to 'fix' the participants to make them more amenable to existing Canadian society; rather, we learned from their experiences to better understand the challenges and barriers they faced and to convey that understanding to a wider audience, including policy-makers and community leaders.

Third, the work must acknowledge and discuss the limits of its own claims. While the intent of our research is not to produce generalizable findings, insights drawn from the study may be transferable to other FMCs because they highlight the challenges and opportunities faced by a particular group of people. Indeed, this is why the second study compared the context of Metro Vancouver with those in three other FMCs in different Canadian provinces. Nonetheless, the dialogical nature of the data generation procedures should be emphasized throughout so that people can locate the research within the particular context in which it was conducted.

Best Practice

Ethnography has been criticized for perpetuating post-colonial dynamics of knowledge extraction from oppressed people for the benefit of privileged (often 'Western') researchers (Bejarano et al., 2019). In order for research to truly challenge colonialism, scholars have suggested 'decoloniality' (Ramugondo, 2018) to work "toward a vision of human life that is not dependent upon or structured by the forced imposition of one ideal of society over those that differ" (Mignolo, 2007, p. 459). Good intentions, awareness, or even critical approaches to post-colonial dynamics do not prevent researchers from reproducing them through their own work, especially as they operate in institutions that are rooted in coloniality (Manning, 2018). There is a need to move beyond the critique of colonialism commonly found in academia and to turn the critique to ourselves as researchers and implement real changes in our work; given that decolonization cannot happen from research conducted in a colonial way (Bejarano et al., 2019; Huff et al., 2022; Manning, 2018; Simaan, 2017).

Authors discuss different ethical considerations when conducting research in a post-colonial context. On the one hand, most authors emphasize the importance of reflexivity (i.e., critical reflection and transparency about one's positionality and its impact on the research process and products) as well as reciprocity through service to the community to balance the benefits of the research, rather than simply 'extracting' knowledge (Huisman, 2008; Manning, 2018). On the other hand, 'decolonial' scholars suggest that research must also be as collaborative as possible and include the community from the initiation and planning of the research to its conduct and publication (Bejarano et al., 2019; Huisman, 2008). They also invite researchers to aim at concrete and direct benefits for the community under study; for example, through activism (Bejarano et al., 2019; Huisman, 2008).

Application to Occupational Science

Ethnography is well suited for research focusing on occupations as this methodology examines the performance of culture; that is, what people do and what shapes their 'doing' within a specific context (Tedlock, 2000). Moreover, the emphasis on contextualizing people's experiences and the possibility to observe and participate in people's occupations are in line with the transactional approach introduced in occupational science. The ethnographic process is in itself transactional as researchers enter and acknowledge their co-construction of the field (Bailliard et al., 2013; Huot, 2018).

Furthermore, occupational scientists have increasingly called for studies that attend to how occupations are dialectically related to the context within which they are socially situated. Research integrating social theory into studies of occupation have also critiqued the emphasis on individualism within the discipline and have called for research to consider the socially transformative potential of occupation (Laliberte Rudman, 2021; Schiller et al., 2022). An ethnographic approach allows researchers to attend to the situated nature of occupation by considering how individuals' motivations and opportunities for, and experiences of, occupation are mediated by their intersecting identities within and across different places and social positions. For example, our ethnographic studies allowed us to situate French-speaking immigrants' experiences and their occupational possibilities (Laliberte Rudman, 2010) in their broader social context. Our deep immersion in the field and the variety of methods we used were key to examining the structural barriers and enablers (e.g., access to services, language barriers, resources of Francophone community sites, etc.) to immigrants' occupational engagement; rather than considering integration as an individual problem to be resolved. The rich data collected allowed us to identify how power dynamics embedded in society (e.g., Anglo-dominance, racism etc.) operate in immigrants' daily occupations. Our ethnographies contribute to the growing number of migration studies within occupational science that make the implied role of occupation within discussions of immigrant integration more explicit (e.g., Trimboli et al., 2019; Rivas-Quarneti et al., 2018).

Application to Occupational Therapy

Some ethnographies may have more direct applications to therapeutic practice than others depending on their focus. Ethnographies examining diverse issues are presented within a range of occupational therapy journals. For example, Lavalley (2022) conducted a six-month ethnography examining occupation at a community level. He used "interviews, observations, document review, group mapping activities and collaborative analysis to explore occupations of a senior center as the community and staff welcomed older adult Spanish speakers" (Lavalley, 2022, p. 1). One aim of this work was to inform potential roles that occupational therapists could fulfil within this space. Another example includes a nine-month ethnography of a collaboration adopting a community-based participatory research approach conducted by Magasi et al. (2021). Their objective was "to understand the group dynamics and relational processes of a CBPR [community-based participatory research] team in the context of an intervention development study focused on health management for people with disabilities (PWD)" (Magasi et al., 2021, p. 1). They used interviews and participant observation to conduct the study with nine participants who were part of the collaborative team. In a third example, Huff et al. (2022) called for the necessity of adopting methodologies that decolonize occupation-based research. They shared ethnographic research conducted in Tanzania in partnership with a local non-governmental organization to examine "gendered occupations and women's experiences of gender inequities" (Huff et al., 2022, p. 115). These examples highlight various ways that ethnographic research can inform occupational therapy practice in different locations around the world.

The global acceleration of international migration has led to increasingly diverse societies. Occupational therapists often have to work with clients whose worldviews, beliefs, values, and norms may differ from their own. To provide holistic, client-centered, and culturally safe care, therapists must recognize that culture is context dependent and shaped by dominant discourses and social power relations. Ethnographic research is well suited to studies of culture that can provide a broader context for better understanding individual experiences and occupations.

Critiquing Ethnographic Studies

All studies generate only partial knowledge and should be critically appraised when considering how findings may inform research, education, or clinical practice. The questions featured in Textbox 9.4 reflect strategies recommended by Carspecken (1996) for ensuring methodological quality in ethnography. The application of common techniques to ensure rigor (e.g., member checking) will vary based on the ontological and epistemological positioning of a study; however, similar techniques are often used.

Textbox 9.4   Critiquing Ethnographic Studies – Questions to Ask

1 Did the research use a *flexible observation schedule*?
2 Was *prolonged engagement* practiced with the participants?
3 Were the same participants *interviewed repeatedly*?
4 Were participants encouraged to *use and explain the terms* they use in naturalistic contexts?
5 Did the researcher use a *low-inference vocabulary* and add interpretations later?
6 Were *consistency checks* conducted between observed activity and what was said in interviews?

Author Reflections

Having moved to Vancouver only a year before undertaking the first ethnographic study described above, Suzanne was initially uncertain whether she could develop sufficient community support for the research. However, she used the foundation developed through her doctoral study (Huot, 2014) to inform the process to building collaborative relationships with community members. She became involved with the provincial Francophone migration network and had informal, individual meetings with community stakeholders. Given the paucity of research conducted with the local FMC due to structural factors such as the lack of a French-language university in the province, community organizations were eager to partner and support the study. Anne-Cécile was recruited to coordinate these ethnographies and led the majority of the data collection and analysis with mentorship from Suzanne and additional research team members. Their commitment to the quality of this study led to the development of strong rapport and trust with community members.

This contributed to the first ethnography, and was instrumental to the second ethnography because we had become familiar to key community stakeholders.

This school of inquiry encouraged us to use multiple data collection strategies and to spend an extended period of time with the participants, which promoted a depth of understanding that may not otherwise have been possible. The focus in ethnography on the relationship between individuals and the larger contexts that shape and are reproduced by daily practices was particularly useful for our theoretical interests in understanding the spatiality of occupation in relation to international migration (Delaisse et al., 2020). This approach enabled us to examine the experiences of individual immigrants and to explore how these experiences were related to broader contextual factors including governmental immigration policies, eligibility for government-funded services provided by community organizations, and systems of oppression such as racism and sexism, among others. Critically exploring the FMC context informed our increasing awareness of the structural barriers hindering the expression of identities and engagement in occupations for members of minority communities. As noted in the occupation-based literature, identity is not solely something that we are; it is also something that we *do* (Laliberte Rudman, 2002). Indeed, completing this research was a consciousness raising experience that enabled us to identify and begin working to address challenges Francophone immigrants and the FMC were experiencing within a broader Anglo-dominant context. This outcome reflects the aims of critical ethnography to increase awareness of social systems and structures among those involved.

Summary

While maintaining the key characteristics of participant observation, fieldwork, and prolonged engagement, ethnography has greatly evolved from its early beginnings. This has presented new and interesting research opportunities to study a range of groups and cultures (e.g., the culture of virtual communities). The range of methods utilized enable research participants to both 'show and tell' occupation. For occupational scientists and occupational therapists, this school of inquiry and its methodologies support approaches to study how occupations are culturally situated and how they are shaped by the broader social context within which engagement takes place.

References

Aldrich, R. M., Laliberte Rudman, D., Park, N. E., & Huot, S. (2020). Centering the complexity of long-term unemployment: Lessons learned from a critical occupational science inquiry. *Societies*, *10*(3), 65. https://doi.org/10.3390/soc10030065

Bacchi, C. (2009). *Analysing policy: What's the problem represented to be?* Pearson.

Bailliard, A. L., Aldrich, R. M., & Dickie, V. A. (2013). Ethnography and the transactional study of occupation. In M. P. Cutchin & V. A. Dickie (Eds.), *Transactional perspectives on occupation* (pp. 157–168). Springer Netherlands. https://doi.org/10.1007/978-94-007-4429-5_13

Bejarano, C. A., Juárez, L. L., García, M. A. M., & Goldstein, D. M. (2019). *Decolonizing ethnography: Undocumented immigrants and new directions in social science.* Duke University Press.

Bressers, G., Brydges, M., & Paradis, E. (2020). Ethnography in health professions education: Slowing down and thinking deeply. *Medical Education*, *54*(3), 225–233. https://doi.org/10.1111/medu.14033

Bryman, A. (2001). Introduction: A review of ethnography. In A. Bryman (Ed.), *Ethnography* (Vol. 1, pp. ix–xxxix). SAGE.

Carspecken, P. F. (1996). *Critical ethnography in educational research: A theoretical and practical guide*. Routledge.

Creswell, J. W. (2013). *Qualitative inquiry and research design*. SAGE.

Delaisse, A.-C., Huot, S., & Veronis, L. (2020). Conceptualizing the role of occupation in the production of space. *Journal of Occupational Science, 28*(4), 550–560. https://doi.org/10.1080/14427591.2020.1802326

Delaisse, A.-C., Huot, S., Veronis, L., & Mortenson, B. (2021). Occupation's role in producing inclusive spaces: Immigrants' experiences in linguistic minority communities. *OTJR: Occupation, Participation and Health, 41*(2), 124–131. https://doi.org/10.1177/1539449220981952

Dey, I. (1993). *Qualitative data analysis: A user-friendly guide for social scientists*. Routledge.

Gardner, P. J. (2011). Natural neighborhood networks – Important social networks in the lives of older adults aging in place. *Journal of Aging Studies, 25*(3), 263–271. https://doi.org/10.1016/j.jaging.2011.03.007

Gouzouasis, P., & Yanko, M. (2018). Reggio's arpeggio: Becoming pedagogical through autoethnography. In W. Parnell & J. M. Iorio (Eds.), *Meaning making in early childhood research: Pedagogies and the personal* (pp. 56–70). Routledge.

Guba, E. G., & Lincoln, Y. S. (2004). Competing paradigms in qualitative research: Theories and issues. In S. Nagy Hesse-Biber & P. Leavy (Eds.), *Approaches to qualitative research: A reader on theory and practice* (pp. 17–38). Oxford University Press.

Hammersley, M., & Atkinson, P. (2007). *Ethnography: Principles in practice* (3rd ed). Routledge.

Holman Jones, S., Adams, T. E., & Ellis, C. (2016). *Handbook of autoethnography*. Routledge.

Huberman, A. M., & Miles, M. B. (1994). Data management and analysis methods. In N. K. Denzin & Y. S. Lincoln (Eds.), *Handbook of qualitative research* (pp. 428–444). SAGE.

Huff, S., Laliberte Rudman, D., Magalhães, L., Lawson, E., & Kanyamala, M. (2022). Enacting a critical decolonizing ethnographic approach in occupation-based research. *Journal of Occupational Science, 29*(2), 115–129. https://doi.org/10.1080/14427591.2020.1824803

Huisman, K. (2008). "Does this mean you're not going to come visit me anymore?": An inquiry into an ethics of reciprocity and positionality in feminist ethnographic research. *Sociological Inquiry, 78*(3), 372–396. https://doi.org/10.1111/j.1475-682X.2008.00244.x

Huot, S. (2014). Ethnography: Understanding occupation through an examination of culture. In S. Nayar & M. Stanley (Eds.) *Qualitative research methodologies for occupational science and therapy* (pp. 84–100). Routledge.

Huot, S. (2018). Co-constructing the field for a critical ethnography of immigrants' experiences in a Canadian Francophone minority community. *Qualitative Research*, 146879411876978. https://doi.org/10.1177/1468794118769785

Huot, S., Aldrich, R., Laliberte Rudman, D., & Stone, M. (2020a). Picturing precarity through occupational mapping: Making the (im)mobilities of long-term unemployment visible. *Journal of Occupational Science, 29*(4), 529–544. https://doi.org/10.1080/14427591.2020.1821244

Huot, S., & Laliberte Rudman, D. (2015). Extending beyond qualitative interviewing to illuminate the tacit nature of everyday occupation: Occupational mapping and participatory occupation methods. *OTJR: Occupation, Participation & Health, 35*(3), 142–150. https://doi.org/10.1177/1539449215576488

Huot, S., Veronis, L., Sall, L., Piquemal, N., & Zellama, F. (2020b). *Favoriser la cohesion communautaire dans un contexte de diversité* [Facilitating community cohesion in a context of diversity]. Fédération des communautés francophones et acadiennes du Canada [Federation of Canadian Francophone and Acadian communities]. https://immigrationfrancophone.ca/images/documents/Bibliotheque/Favoriser-cohesion-identitaire.pdf

Jamal, S. (2005). Critical ethnography: An effective way to conduct anti-racism research. In G. J. S. Dei & J. Singh (Eds.), *Critical issues in anti-racist research methodologies* (pp. 225–240). Peter Lang.

Kearney, G. P., Corman, M. K., Hart, N. D., Johnston, J. L., & Gormley, G. J. (2019). Why institutional ethnography? Why now? Institutional ethnography in health professions education. *Perspectives on Medical Education, 8*(1), 17–24. https://doi.org/10.1007/s40037-019-0499

Knoblauch, H. (2005). Focused ethnography. *Forum: Qualitative Social Research*, 6(3). https://doi.org/10.17169/fqs-6.3.20

Laliberte Rudman, D. (2002). Linking occupation and identity: Lessons learned through qualitative exploration. *Journal of Occupational Science*, 9(1), 12–19. https://doi.org/10.1080/14427591.2002.9686489

Laliberte Rudman, D. (2010). Occupational terminology: Occupational possibilities. *Journal of Occupational Science*, 17(1), 55–59. https://doi.org/10.1080/14427591.2010.9686673

Laliberte Rudman, D. (2021). Mobilizing occupation for social transformation: Radical resistance, disruption, and re-configuration. *Canadian Journal of Occupational Therapy*, 88(2), 96–107. https://doi.org/10.1177/00084174211020836

Laliberte Rudman, D., & Dennhardt, S. (2014). Critical discourse analysis: Opening possibilities through deconstruction. In S. Nayar & M. Stanley (Eds.) *Qualitative research methodologies for occupational science and therapy* (pp. 137–154). Routledge.

Lavalley, R. (2022). Occupation's role in inclusion of Spanish-speaking older adults in a senior center. *OTJR: Occupation, Participation and Health*, 43(1), 74–80. https://doi.org/10.1177/15394492221093311

Lavalley, R., Womack, J. L., & Bailliard, A. (2022). A live community growing together: Communal occupation of a senior centre welcoming Spanish-speaking elders. *Journal of Occupational Science*. https://doi.org/10.1080/14427591.2020.1816209

Lecompte, M. (2002). The transformation of ethnographic practice: Past and current challenges. *Qualitative Research*, 2(3), 283–299. https://doi.org/10.1177/146879410200200301

Longhurst, R. (2010). Semi-structured interviews and focus groups. In N. Clifford, S. French & G. Valentine (Eds.), *Key methods in geography* (pp. 103–115). SAGE.

Madison, D. (2012). Introduction to critical ethnography: Theory and method. In *Critical ethnography: Method, ethics, and performance* (pp. 1–16). SAGE. https://doi.org/10.4135/9781452233826

Magasi, S., Angell, A. M., Papadimitriou, C., Ramirez, R. D., Ferlin, A., Reis, J. P., & Wilson, T. (2021). Inside an occupational therapy–disability community partnership to promote mental health management: Ethnography of a research collaboration. *American Journal of Occupational Therapy*, 75(4), 7504180050. https://doi.org/10.5014/ajot.2021.045468

Manning, J. (2018). Becoming a decolonial feminist ethnographer: Addressing the complexities of positionality and representation. *Management Learning*, 49(3), 311–326. https://doi.org/10.1177/1350507617745275

Mignolo, W. D. (2007). Delinking. *Cultural Studies*, 21(2–3), 449–514. https://doi.org/10.1080/09502380601162647

Nast, H. J. (1994). Women in the field: Critical feminist methodologies and theoretical perspectives. *Professional Geographer*, 46(1), 54–66. https://doi.org/10.1111/j.0033-0124.1994.00054.x

Office of the Commissioner of Official Languages. (2020). *Infographic: The French presence in British Columbia*. www.clo-ocol.gc.ca/en/statistics/infographics/french-presence-british-columbia

Prodinger, B., Laliberte Rudman, D., & Shaw, L. (2015). Institutional ethnography: Studying the situated nature of human occupation. *Journal of Occupational Science*, 22(1), 71–81. https://doi.org/10.1080/14427591.2013.813429

Ramugondo, E. (2018). Healing work: Intersections of decoloniality. *World Federation of Occupational Therapists Bulletin*, 74(2), 83–91.

Rebeiro, K. L. (2001). Enabling occupation: The importance of an affirming environment. *Canadian Journal of Occupational Therapy*, 68(2), 80–89. https://doi.org/10.1177/000841740106800204

Rivas-Quarneti, N., Movilla-Fernández, M.-J., & Magalhães, L. (2018). Immigrant women's occupational struggles during the socioeconomic crisis in Spain: Broadening occupational justice conceptualizations. *Journal of Occupational Science*, 25(1), 6–18. https://doi.org/10.1080/14427591.2017.1366355

Rose, J. (2020). Dynamic embodied positionalities: The politics of class and nature through a critical ethnography of homelessness. *Ethnography*, 23(4), 451–472. https://doi.org/10.1177/1466138120913061

Sandelowski, M. (1995). Qualitative analysis: What is it and how to begin. *Research in Nursing and Health, 18*(4), 371–375. https://doi.org/10.1002/nur.4770180411

Schiller, S., van Bruggen, H., Kantartzis, S., Laliberte Rudman, D., Lavalley, R., & Pollard, N. (2022). "Making change by shared doing": An examination of occupation in processes of social transformation in five case studies. *Scandinavian Journal of Occupational Therapy.* https://doi.org/10.1080/11038128.2022.2046153

Simaan, J. (2017). Olive growing in Palestine: A decolonial ethnographic study of collective daily-forms-of-resistance. *Journal of Occupational Science, 27*(1), 510–523. https://doi.org/10.1080/14427591.2017.1378119

Spradley, J. P., & McCurdy, D. W. (1984). *Conformity and conflict: Readings in cultural anthropology.* Little, Brown and Company.

Stahlke Wall, S. (2014). Focused ethnography: A methodological adaptation for social research in emerging contexts. *Forum: Qualitative Social Research, 16*(1). https://doi.org/10.17169/fqs-16.1.2182

Statistics Canada. (2017). *British Columbia [Province] and Canada [Country]* (table). *Census Profile.* 2016 Census. Statistics Canada Catalogue no. 98-316-X2016001. Ottawa. www12.statcan.gc.ca/census-recensement/2016/dp-pd/prof/index.cfm?Lang=E (accessed June 7, 2022).

Tedlock, B. (2000). Ethnography and ethnographic representation. In N. Denzin & Y. Lincoln (Eds.), *Handbook of qualitative research* (pp. 455–473). SAGE.

Trimboli, C., Rivas-Quarneti, N., Blankvoort, N., Roosen, I., Simó Algado, S., & Whiteford, G. (2019). The current and future contribution of occupational therapy and occupational science to transforming the situation of forced migrants: Critical perspectives from a think tank. *Journal of Occupational Science, 26*(2), 323–328. https://doi.org/10.1080/14427591.2019.1604408

Van Maanen, J. (2004). An end to innocence: The ethnography of ethnography. In S. Nagy Hesse-Biber & P. Leavy (Eds.), *Approaches to qualitative research: A reader on theory and practice* (pp. 427–446). Oxford University Press.

Wilcock, A. A. (1999). Reflections on doing, becoming and becoming. *Australian Occupational Therapy Journal, 46*(1), 1–11. https://doi.org/10.1046/j.1440-1630.1999.00174.x

Wilcock, A. A. (2006). *An occupational perspective of health* (2nd ed.). SLACK.

Additional Resources

Aldrich, R. M., & Callanan, Y. (2011). Insights about research discouraged workers. *Journal of Occupational Science, 18*(2), 153–166. https://doi.org/10.1080/14427591.2011.575756

Cook, K. E. (2005). Using critical ethnography to explore issues in health promotion. *Qualitative Health Research, 15*(1), 129–138. https://doi.org/10.1177/1049732304267751

Lavalley, R., & Bailliard, A. (2021). A communal perspective of occupation: Community change in a senior center welcoming Spanish-speaking immigrants. *Journal of Occupational Science, 28*(1), 29–41. https://doi.org/10.1080/14427591.2020.1775111

10 Critical Discourse Analysis

Debbie Laliberte Rudman and Silke Dennhardt

Variants of discourse analysis, alone or in combination with other methodologies, have increasingly been employed in occupation-focused research over the past few decades. Although examples of studies cover a range of substantive areas and research purposes, the focus on how discourses—that is, ways of writing and talking about a phenomenon—shape possibilities for how groups of people can and do act in their everyday life, hold them together as studies employing discourse analysis. For example, Ballinger and Payne (2000b, 2002) combined critical discourse analysis and ethnography to interrogate how risk was understood and enacted in a community day hospital, pointing to how a dominant bio-medical discourse on risk minimizes agency for older clients and positions health care professionals as experts. Silcock et al. (2014), informed by Foucauldian concepts, conducted a critical discourse analysis of children's descriptions and demonstrations of technology use as a means to deepen understanding of how their occupational possibilities were shaped through discourses addressing play and technology. Informed by post-colonial theories, Blankvoort et al. (2021) conducted a critical discourse analysis of texts used in Dutch civic integration programs, highlighting how such texts integrated discourses of Othering based in colonial logics and promoted particular ways of being and doing as means through which migrant 'others' could be transformed into 'modern,' neoliberal citizens.

Within this chapter, we draw upon our experiences of using a particular approach to discourse analysis, specifically, critical discourse analysis. We emphasize the existence of a multiplicity of approaches to critical discourse analysis and attempt to highlight elements that constitute 'best practices' or essential elements across several variants. Throughout this chapter, we use the term 'best practice' with caution given its foundation in the 'evidence-based practice' movement, a powerful discourse within the health professions that has been critiqued for reinforcing the assumption that positivist knowledge and research is inherently 'best' (Holmes et al., 2006).

Our shared research interest lies in enhancing understanding of how occupational possibilities become shaped within specific socio-political contexts; that is, how discourses contribute to "what people take for granted as what they can and should do, and the occupations that are supported and promoted by various aspects of the broader systems and structures in which their lives are lived" (Laliberte Rudman, 2010, p. 55). Both studies used as examples in this chapter employed critical discourse analysis informed by a governmentality theoretical perspective. The first study, referred to as the 'retirement study,' examined the discursive construction of aging and retirement in media documents (Laliberte Rudman, 2005, 2006; Laliberte Rudman et al., 2009; Laliberte Rudman & Molke, 2009) to address how discourses, and the identity and occupational possibilities

DOI: 10.4324/9781003456216-10

they promote, are taken up, resisted, and negotiated by aging individuals (Laliberte Rudman, 2013, 2014, 2015a, 2015b). The second study, referred to as the 'risky driver study,' examined how risk is taken up to govern everyday occupation in information brochures for aging drivers. The study showed how risk was deployed to individualize responsibility for occupation and obscure its social and political shaping by constituting an ideal occupational subjectivity for aging drivers and outlining practices for aging individuals to responsibly govern their driving (Dennhardt, 2013; Dennhardt & Laliberte Rudman, 2012).

Background: Discourse Analysis and Critical Discourse Analysis

Discourse analysis is a broad methodological space, and debate exists regarding its defining features and what counts as a discourse analysis (Ballinger & Cheek, 2006; Hafner, 2017). The diversity of approaches labeled discourse analysis stems from interdisciplinary origins, and a multiplicity of theoretical and philosophical underpinnings. For example, definitions of discourse may refer to any instance of communication; language used in a particular field of practice; instances of talk or text that contain particular properties; or knowledge practices that produce particular problematizations, objects, and subjects (Bacchi, 2009a; Cheek, 2004; Fairclough, 2009). As for examples of diversity in research approaches, discourse analysis, as enacted in ethnomethodological research, is focused on how language is interactively used to organize social action within local contexts; for example, how communicative processes structure work within an occupational therapy clinic. Approaches located within discursive constructionism focus on how discourses are employed in interactions in ways that construct everyday reality (Holstein & Gubrium, 2011). Approaches informed by post-structural perspectives, often labeled critical discourse analysis, are concerned with how discourses enact power through shaping particular problematics and carving out possibilities for being and acting, as well as how the self and everyday life are negotiated in relation to discourses (Ainsworth & Hardy, 2004a, 2004b; Bacchi, 2016a).

Given that discourse analysis is not a unified approach, we do not provide a singular definition nor attempt to address all of its diverse approaches. Rather, in this chapter, we focus on a particular variant, specifically, critical discourse analysis, and address its potential contributions to the study of occupation and occupational therapy. We have chosen this focus because we see it as a valuable research methodology for advancing understanding of occupation as contextually situated and inherently political, as well as for enhancing the social relevance and transformative potential of occupational science and occupational therapy (Schiller et al., 2022). It is important to clarify that although critical discourse analysis always needs to be framed by a theoretical framework (Wodak & Meyer, 2016a), it is neither a fixed method nor a singular methodology but an approach to conceptualize and study discourse as a social practice. We strongly agree with Cheek (2004) that there cannot be a set of rules for critical discourse analysis and that it is important to work against framing discourse analysis as "a value free technology – a theory free method and tool to do research" (p. 1148).

Epistemological Assumptions and Methodological Implications

The addition of the word 'critical' to 'discourse analysis' signals the centrality of paradigmatic positioning to ensure methodological coherence (Wodak & Meyer, 2016a). The use of the word critical refers to inter-linked ontological and epistemological assumptions

(Farias et al., 2016; Kincheloe et al., 2018). Ontologically, critical discourse analysis studies are characterized by a position of tentative realism, in which social reality is viewed as 'reified' over time, through interactions of social, political, economic, cultural, gender, and other factors, in ways that particular structures and systems become taken as if they were real rather than socially constructed. Epistemologically, critically informed qualitative researchers assume that language is key in the shaping of social life and in the enactment of power (Kincheloe et al., 2018). Thus, how an object, such as mental health, or a social collective, such as Indigenous youth, are discursively constructed shapes the ways systems, structures, processes, and practices are constructed and enacted in relation to that phenomenon (Mumby, 2004). The primacy placed on language leads to a focus on the form, content, and structure of discourse, as well as an overarching aim to deconstruct the ways language is used to mobilize particular forms of knowledge and construct 'realities' about particular phenomenon and particular types of people (Fadyl et al., 2012). The underlying assumption, related to an axiological commitment to re-dress inequities and promote more just situations, is that deconstruction clears a space for thinking and acting otherwise in relation to a group or phenomena (Fadyl et al., 2012; Farias et al., 2016).

Critical discourse analysis, as taken up in health sciences, has been greatly influenced by the theoretical work of Foucault, in addition to other post-structural perspectives (Cheek, 2004; Hardin, 2003). As such, definitions of discourse used within critical discourse analysis draw on a post-structural view of language as a social practice, emphasizing the productive, constitutive, and value-laden nature of language (Allen & Hardin, 2001; Ballinger & Cheek, 2006). As can be seen in Textbox 10.1, such definitions focus on discourses as systems of meaning or knowledges, conveyed through talk and text, which produce particular versions of concepts, problems, objects, and subject positions (Bacchi, 2009a; Hardy & Phillips, 2004).

Overall, definitions of discourse commensurate with critical discourse analysis refer to discourse as a productive social practice, intimately tied to power, that constructs what comes to be taken-for-granted as 'real' or 'truth' in a particular socio-historical context (Hafner, 2017; Mumby, 2004). Rather than viewing language as making visible an extra-linguistic reality (e.g., the meaning associated with an occupation), there is a focus on how meaning (e.g., what is 'risky'), subjectivities (e.g., 'the unemployed'), and objects (e.g., 'a problem') are created in and through language (Ainsworth & Hardy, 2004a). This shifts the focus of analysis away from the individual and the meaning they assign to an

---

Textbox 10.1   Understanding Discourse in Critical Discourse Analysis: Example Definitions of Discourse

"practices that systematically form the objects [and subjects] of which they speak." (Foucault, 1972, p. 49)

"broad social, cultural, and historical systems of meanings, creating both the notion of the 'self' and how the 'self' constructs its world." (Hardin, 2001, p. 14)

"scaffolds of discursive frameworks, which order reality in a certain way. They both enable and constrain the production of knowledge, in that they allow for certain ways of thinking about reality while excluding others." (Cheek, 2004, p. 1142)

"socially produced forms of knowledge that constitute 'the real.'" (Bacchi, 2016a, p. 8)

occupation, towards situating individual accounts and occupations within broader discourses (Hardin, 2003). For example, Laliberte Rudman and Aldrich (2017) analyzed narrative data generated with persons experiencing long-term unemployment in ways that situated their everyday occupations and the meaning they attributed to these within neoliberal discourse emphasizing the centrality of self-reliance, being productive, and individual responsibility.

In line with their critical position, various approaches to critical discourse analysis are concerned with the power effects of discourse; that is, the ways in which power is enacted and reproduced by a range of social authorities and agencies through the discursive production of 'normalizing truths' (Allen & Hardin, 2001; Fadyl et al., 2012). Attending to such power effects, Hardy and Phillips (2004) explained that discourse both "'rules in' certain ways of talking about a topic" and "'rules out, limits and restricts other ways of talking, of conducting ourselves in relation to the topic or constructing knowledge about it" (p. 300). While realizing that there may be a number of discourses pertaining to any particular subject or object, there is a focus on the marginalizing and exclusionary effects of dominant discourses. For example, in the 'retirement study,' we examined how the dominant discourse on ideal housing for retirement living excluded aging individuals with significant physical or cognitive disabilities and those with limited financial resources (Laliberte Rudman et al., 2009).

Given that multiple, often competing, discourses exist, analysis can also attend to how people negotiate their possibilities for being and doing within the discourses accessible within their specific socio-historical conditions (Hardin, 2003; Laliberte Rudman & Aldrich, 2017). For example, in the 'retirement study,' the ways that individuals conveyed their stories of retirement were not taken as reflections of un-mediated inner feelings or a core self. Rather, the form and content of the narratives were examined in relation to how individuals actively drew upon and negotiated broader discourses of aging to shape themselves as subjects and make sense of their occupations (Laliberte Rudman, 2013, 2014, 2015a, 2015b).

Another key assumption is that discourses are themselves situated within relations of power, often serving to reproduce particular rationalities that hold dominant forms of power in place (Wodak & Meyer, 2016a). In turn, it is essential that critical discourse analysis studies situate discourses within socio-political, economic, cultural, and other contextual forces (Fadyl et al., 2012; Holstein & Gubrium, 2011). For example, in both the retirement and risky driver studies, we found that dominant discourses emphasized individual responsibility through outlining what individuals should do in order to ensure health, autonomy, and other idealized outcomes. Situating this individualizing of responsibility within the contemporary socio-political context, we have pointed to ways that dominant discourses on aging well and driving well align with the values and aims of neoliberalism, thereby reinforcing this political rationality and obscuring socio-politically produced inequities in resources and conditions required to take up such responsibilities (Dennhardt, 2013; Laliberte Rudman, 2006, 2013, 2015a).

A further essential feature of critical discourse analysis is a commitment to a critical intent. Such an intent aims to address situations of injustice through challenging dominant rationalities and ideologies, questioning the taken-for-granted ways society has come to be structured, creating space for resistance and change, and raising awareness of how discourses shape disparities (Bacchi, 2016a; Ballinger & Payne, 2000a). For example, in the retirement study, Debbie questioned the taken-for-granted 'positivity' of dominant discourses of 'positive' aging, by examining how positive aging discourses have been taken up in ways that align with broader governmental aims to retreat from programs and services for aging citizens and limit spaces for occupation for certain types of aging subjects (Laliberte Rudman, 2006, 2010). Moreover, this work has pointed to contradictions produced in the lives of retirees who attempt to enact the 'duty to age well' constructed through positive aging discourses (Laliberte Rudman, 2015a, 2015b).

Research Purposes and Critical Discourse Analysis

Critical discourse analysis studies aim to raise awareness of how discourses shape possibilities for how people understand their worlds and themselves, as well as what they view as possible and ideal ways to be and do in everyday life. This methodological approach is an appropriate choice within research studies that aim to situate individual accounts of experiences, including occupations, within broader social, political, economic, racial, and gendered contexts (Holstein & Gubrium, 2011). As articulated by Hardin (2003), critical discourse analysis enables a researcher to "move data beyond the level of the individual and into historical, social and cultural realms" (p. 544).

Research purposes that fit with critical discourse analysis encompass questioning the ways dominant discourses shape and reproduce injustices and inequities (Ainsworth & Hardy, 2004b), including injustices and inequities related to occupation. For example, in the retirement study, one research purpose was to raise awareness of the ways in which assumptions about who older workers are and what types of work they should engage in, constructed via dominant discourses of 'productive' aging, may set up inequities between older and younger workers and amongst older workers (Laliberte Rudman, 2015b). This translated in the retirement study into research questions such as: "What types of subjectivities are presented within a contemporary Canadian media source as ideal and non-ideal for aging and older workers? What practices of the self are presented as ways to work towards achieving ideal subjectivities? What forms and types of work are presented as ideal and non-ideal for aging and older workers?" In the risky driver study, research questions also addressed subject positions constructed through discourses; for example, "How is risk taken up and referred to within brochures addressing aging individuals as drivers and their families? How is the subjectivity of the 'aging driver' constituted within brochures that address the occupation of driving in later life?"

Constructing the Research Field

Since discourses are realized within and through texts (Fairclough, 1995), critical discourse analysis studies use texts as data. Texts are "any kind of symbolic expression requiring a physical medium and permitting of permanent storage" (Hardy & Phillips, 2004, p. 300). Texts can include printed materials that 'pre-exist' (e.g., newspaper articles, governmental policies, occupational therapy documentation, historical documents) or are produced in the research process (e.g., interview transcripts, photo diaries). Depending on the research questions, various types of texts are thinkable as data, such as toys (van Leeuwen, 2008), cartoons (Hardy & Phillips, 1999), games (Millington, 2011), diagnostic manuals (DSM-IV) (Crowe, 2001), promotional videos (Harris et al., 2015), service and program guidelines (Blankvoort et al., 2021), and social media (Del Casino & Brooks, 2015).

As in all qualitative research, the research field in critical discourse analysis "is not out there waiting to be described by researchers" (Cheek, 2000, p. 126) and does not exist independently from the researcher and the questions posed. A primary goal of data collection is to generate a data-rich body of texts that can be expected to offer new insights into how the social phenomenon under investigation is constituted (Phillips & Hardy, 2002). For instance, one rationale for choosing information brochures for aging drivers in the 'risky driver study' was that these texts are explicitly produced to advise aging drivers on what they, and others, should and should not do. As well, brochures were expected to contain rich data on how the occupational subjectivity of the aging driver is discursively constructed, given that texts which target a particular group of subjects need to discursively establish these subjects as somehow 'different' from the implicit main group (Castel, 1991).

Selecting and analyzing relevant texts are interwoven tasks that inform and build on each other. While gathering and selecting texts needs to be provisional and emergent in accordance with analysis, best practice involves a systematic scholarly process, grounded in a study's research questions, theoretical framework, and methodology (Fadyl et al., 2012; Phillips & Hardy, 2002). Since discourses are not a pre-existing object that can be 'revealed' by investigating a particular number of texts, there is an awareness that researchers "can only trace clues to them regardless of how much data they collect" (Phillips & Hardy, 2002, p. 74). Therefore, the challenge of data collection is not to find 'all' possible texts 'out there'; rather, to decide which texts to choose in order to best trace discourses of interest (Fadyl et al., 2012; Jäger & Maier, 2009). Such sampling choices, which require continuous documentation, should be guided by consideration of the study's research questions; for example, how do the central aims of a text align with the research questions, how much of the content of the text is relevant to the research questions, and how does the format of the text contribute to its potential relevance to the research questions. Examples of other parameters that could influence choices, depending on the research questions, could relate to when a text was produced, who the intended audience is for a text, who produced a text, and where a text was produced.

Data Analysis

As in many forms of critical qualitative inquiry, approaches to data analysis embrace a broad variety of analytic methods, with the process best described as an individualist approach that is creatively customized for each study in order to translate its theoretical underpinnings into productive analysis methods (Jørgensen & Phillips, 2002; Wodak & Meyer, 2016a). In this section, we draw primarily on the risky driver study to illustrate the analysis process constructed and enacted.

Key Features of Analysis in Critical Discourse Analysis

Integrating theory in critical discourse analysis is essential in ensuring interpretations go beyond surface meanings (Fadyl et al., 2012; Phillips & Hardy, 2002; Wodak & Meyer, 2016a). A strategy we used in both studies to facilitate theory-informed data analysis is the development of an analysis sheet (Jäger & Maier, 2009; Richardson, 2007) (see Textbox 10.2 for an example). Besides the value in facilitating theory-informed analysis, we found that analysis sheets helped to ensure transparency of the analysis process, comprehensive reading, and cross-text analysis.

Textbox 10.2   Examples of Questions Included in an Analysis Sheet

Analysis sheets guide a theory-informed reading that pushes beyond a text's superficial content, and facilitates attending to its form and function in producing content, social meaning, and power relations (Fairclough, 1995). Such sheets contain guiding questions informed by (a) framing theory, (b) research questions, and (c) tools for deconstructing texts.

Examples of questions from the 'risky driver' study:

a) informed by theory (here: governmentality):

- Problematization: What is being problematized? Where is the problem located? What social problems are to be alleviated/what social goals are to be achieved? Power relations: Who is defining the problems? Who is proposing the solutions? Who is likely to benefit from the discourse?

b) informed by research questions (here: related to the occupation 'later life driving'):

- Occupation: How is the occupation conceptualized in the text (e.g., as an individual or social occupation? as a 'right or privilege'? as a leisure activity?) Who engages in it and who does or should not? What is absent with regard to the way the occupation is constructed? What kind of relationship are subjects called to take towards their occupation?

c) informed by tools for deconstruction (here: critical linguistics; Richardson, 2007)

- Naming and reference: How are subjects within the texts named and referred to? Which adjectives and pronouns (e.g., 'us' and 'they') are used? Which qualities, attributes, and characteristics (positive/negative?) are linguistically assigned? What subject positions, social relations, and social values do the employed referential strategies construct?

Data analysis is an emergent process that should be constantly refined in response to the overall research process and understandings of the analyzed data (Hardy & Phillips, 1999; Jørgensen & Phillips, 2002). For example, initially the analysis sheet in the risky driver study did not contain questions related to the aging body. When it was found that the body was repeatedly mentioned across texts and constructed in relation to driving, a new set of questions was added to guide attention to the constructed relationship between driving and the body, self-body relationships, and the body as an object of governing (e.g., How is the body related to driving?, What kind of relationship are subjects called to take towards their bodies?).

Analysis is multilayered, employing and combining multiple level and foci of analysis (Fairclough, 1995; Jäger & Maier, 2009). Approaches to data analysis include various methods of 'deconstruction' and the use of linguistic tools (Richardson, 2007; Wodak & Meyer, 2016a). Deconstructive approaches involve a certain way of reading and investigating texts, which does not aim to find the meaning within a text nor reveal an assumed underlying 'truth.' Rather, deconstruction aims to expose and 'unsettle' implicit meanings and assumptions, including a text's taken-for-granted perspectives, categorizations, binary oppositions, its absences, and so on (Cheek, 2000). For instance, analysis investigates presuppositions that a sentence such as 'Make transportation an important consideration in choosing a retirement home' contains; such as, that aging subjects have the possibility to 'choose' a retirement home, that it is 'normal' and expected to transition to a retirement home at some future point, and that subjects can shape their future mobility positively by 'making' it a priority and preparing for it.

Given that a text's content is never independent of its form and organization, analysis also needs to attend to both what is said and the 'texture' of texts (Fairclough, 1995). Thus, the use of linguistic tools and concepts, such as syntax, mode, tense, actors, grammar, vocabulary, and so forth, is essential (Richardson, 2007). Textual analysis in the risky driver study, for example, closely attended to how subjects were linguistically categorized and separated (e.g., 'most older drivers, as a *sign of continued good judgment*,' 'other drivers *stubbornly deny*'), and how referential strategies constructed ideal and non-ideal subject positions (e.g., the subjectivity of a self-aware, responsible, 'safe' individual versus an inflexible, denying, and risky 'other').

Analysis of form and organization also attends to a text's visual elements such as layout, headings, images, symbols, and colors, considering inter-relationships between visual and other textual material. For example, in the risky driver study, accompanying images, which encompassed photos, cartoon-like, and sketchy drawings, shared many similarities (see Textbox 10.3). These recurring images were interpreted as functioning together with printed text; they employed similar discursive strategies, such as the use of biomedical expertise to shape aging bodies as inherently risky, the emphasis on personal responsibility for oneself and others, and the promotion of healthy aging as a means to continue safe driving.

Textbox 10.3   Example of Attending to Visual Images

Through systematically noting features of images included in information brochures for aging drivers, repetitive features were identified. These included:

- *an image of a medical scene*, object or symbol, such as pill containers, a stethoscope, or a woman getting an eye exam, positioning the declining aging body as inherently at risk, governed by medicine
- *an image of a driving scene, often a potentially dangerous one*, such as a cluttered traffic scene, a busy intersection, or a night scene, positioning the occupation of driving as risky and in need of specific skills
- *an image of individuals positioned close to each other*, implying a caring and loving relationship, such as images of couples and families, standing close to each other, resting the arm on another individual's shoulder, or one individual looking at another
- *an image showing or signifying an active and healthy lifestyle*, such as an aging individual riding a bike or holding an apple
- *an image showing or signifying transportation other than driving*, such as a shuttle-bus or a bus pass, implying choice
- *an educational or symbolic image*, such as a vehicle with suggested safety features, or a green and red traffic light next to a text, pointing to a 'good' practice to take up or a 'bad' one to avoid

Critical discourse analysis also involves attending to absences (Bacchi, 2016a; Wood & Kroger, 2000); that is, examining the text in terms of "what is present and what *could* have been but is *not* present" (Richardson, 2007, p. 38, emphasis in original). By drawing out what is recurrently absent when texts frame or construct a particular social issue or type of subject, analysis can address how dominant problem frames exclude alternative ways of thinking about and approaching an issue. For example, in the risky driver study, attending to absences enabled identification of the relative neglect of solutions to the 'aging driver problem' that focused on societal actions, such as altering driving environments, as opposed to individual actions.

As analysis proceeds, different levels and foci of analysis should be analytically related to each other through various forms of writing as well as through dialogue (Fairclough, 1995; Jørgensen & Phillips, 2002). In the risky driver study, continually writing analytical notes ensured that connections were made between different levels and foci. In addition to recording impressions, insights, or data-rich quotations on analysis sheets, analytical and reflexive notes were written. These notes took different forms, such as free writing, summarizing first insights across texts, or drawing visual understandings of relationships between constructs. Form and foci of notes altered as analysis moved from early to later cycles. For instance, earlier cycles of analysis involved more free and open notes about emerging ideas, while later notes focused on systematically putting things together and linking different foci of analysis. Dialogue within the research team was on-going providing a means to both articulate emerging analytical insights and consider inter-connections with broader contextual forces.

The Process of Analysis

Best practice in critical discourse analysis—as in all qualitative research—incorporates an analytic process that is iterative, interwoven, and non-linear (Jäger & Maier, 2009). Thus, while described separately, the main cycles of analysis in the risky driver study were repeated several times, sometimes separate from each other and sometimes in parallel; ultimately overlapping and feeding into each other in many ways. Main cycles of analysis included open reading, theory-informed reading, and textual analysis with specific tools within single texts, as well as across-text analysis and contextualizing findings.

Within-text analysis began with an open reading of a text, accompanied by free note writing. Early notes were broad and contained various initial impressions, and reactions, referring to various textual levels (i.e., form, function, content). To not constrain potential interpretation early in the analytical process, these initial notes attended more to "the possibility that something interesting was going on, rather than [to] an indication of what it might be" (Wood & Kroger, 2000, p. 92). Open reading also included a careful 'reading' and marking of semiotic elements included in the text, such as photographs, checkmarks, or self-tests. For instance, in 'reading' a photograph for the first time in the risky driver study, any detail of the picture was described (e.g. 'good teeth,' 'white hair,' 'woman looking up'). Though at times tedious, this strategy of detailed description facilitated stepping outside taken for granted 'ways of seeing' (Rose, 2007), drawing attention to what had come to be invisible and profoundly enhancing analysis.

Next, the text was read again, using a theory-informed lens. Focused reading, informed by governmentality, was guided by questions on the analysis sheet, such as "Who is defining the problem and who is addressed as having power to 'fix' it?" and "What practices of the self are the targeted audience called upon to participate in?" Such theory-informed analysis enabled another level of critical reading, one that also considered broader contextual conditions.

Each text was also read 'linguistically,' focusing on how particular meanings were created by form and function features. For instance, particular types of verb choices consistently repeated within and across texts were marked. Texts repeatedly called upon aging subjects to 'remain,' 'stay,' and 'continue' to be safe drivers; as well as to 'maintain,' 'preserve,' and 'keep' their body's driving fitness. Applying linguistic tools, these verbs were investigated with regard to what presuppositions and meanings these particular verb choices shared (i.e., these verbs imply that something involuntarily worsens or is lost in the absence of action to maintain it), where in a text specific verb choices were primarily used (i.e., these verbs are dominantly used when safety or the aging body is brought up); and how actors and objects were linguistically related (i.e., drivers having to watch 'their' bodies like objects). The findings of this cycle of analysis were then combined with previous and later findings of other cycles and foci of analysis, such as when analysis demonstrated how driving and the aging body become constructed as risk objects in need for self-governing.

The next main cycle of analysis contained cross-text analysis in which texts were repeatedly read 'against' each other. Analysis in this cycle focused on similarities, variations, contrasts, repetitions, connections, contradictions, and absences in content, form, and function across texts. For instance, early on in the process it was noticed that almost all texts in the risky driver study contained numerical representations, such as measures of declining body function or accident statistics. Systematically investigating this observation showed that quantification techniques served similar functions across texts; for example, establishing age-related changes in body function and driving ability as objective, calculable, and predictable 'facts' which are measurable and thus 'real.' Moreover, quantification techniques, by mainly drawing upon biomedical knowledges, also constructed driving as an individual occupation and located the problems associated with the occupation solely in aging bodies and irresponsible body 'owners' – and not, for example, in an auto-centered organization of space, time, and social relations.

Rigor

Given the diversity of theoretical underpinnings, there is no one set of quality criteria established for critical discourse analysis (Wodak & Meyer, 2016a). However, being based in critical epistemological assumptions, critical discourse analysis does not aim to produce the most 'accurate' reading, leading to a resistance to using criteria such as external validity that are grounded in an assumption of a static, objective external reality. Rather, the key aim is to produce a theoretically-informed reading that questions taken-for-granted assumptions and related practices, and situates texts within broader contextual conditions and power relations (Bacchi, 2016a; Cheek, 2004).

In our work, we have found the four considerations outlined by Ballinger (2006) to be helpful in addressing best practice in critical discourse analysis. These considerations include: coherence, systematic and careful research conduct, convincing and relevant interpretation, and accounting for the role of researchers. *Coherence*, referring to the overall fit between the elements of a study, such as its theoretical frame, research objectives and analytical foci, is particularly crucial given that critical discourse analysis is always theoretically framed. For this to be appraised, it is essential that the theoretical grounding is made explicit from the beginning of a study, and the ways in which it is drawn upon to frame the study articulated (Wodak & Meyer, 2016a).

Systematic and careful research conduct attends to recording and reporting the research process. This process should be demonstrated through careful documentation, such as a decision trail, that supports the plausibility and persuasiveness of the interpretative analysis (Ballinger, 2006; Cheek, 2004). The ultimate evaluation of the extent to which a study is *convincing and relevant*, Ballinger's third quality consideration, resides in the reader. A relevant critical discourse analysis should offer a new reading of texts through drawing on theoretical perspectives, and address the structures, strategies, and situatedness of discourses. In addition, it should present the reader with adequate textual examples to ascertain the plausibility of the theoretical interpretation. As articulated by van Dijk (1997): "Indeed, the whole point should be to provide insights into structures, strategies or other properties of discourse that could not readily be given by naïve recipients" (p. 5).

The fourth consideration in enacting best practice is the need to *account for the role of the researcher*, noting that this is often done through reflexivity (Ballinger, 2006). Reflexive researchers provide their audience with information about themselves and their perspectives, and engage in practices to reflect on their own subjectivities and their discursive positioning. As such, researchers need to be aware that their own work is shaped within a specific socio-political context, and thus must be explicit regarding the values that inform what they define as situations of injustice and inequity (Bacchi, 2016a).

To conclude this section, we provide a set of critical questions in Textbox 10.4 that we have found helpful to guide appraisal of the quality of a critical discourse analysis, and for informing 'best practice' in its conduct

---

Textbox 10.4   Reviewing and Enacting Critical Discourse Analysis Studies – Questions to Ask

1 Do the researchers locate the study epistemologically and provide information about a *theoretical framework* that informs their critical discourse analysis?
2 Do the researchers provide a *definition of discourse* and is their definition congruent with the study's theoretical framework?
3 Are *language choices* within the article in line with the underlying theory?
4 Do the authors provide a rationale for how the *body of texts was constructed*? Does their choice of texts enable them to address the study's research question?
5 Do the authors *systematically outline the strategies* used to search for and/or produce texts, as well as the criteria used to include and exclude texts?
6 Does the analysis pay attention to both *what is said* (content) and *how it is said*? Commensurate with the theoretical framework employed, does the analysis attend to the *potential effects* of particular discourses (e.g., identity possibilities, occupational possibilities)?
7 Are the findings of the critical discourse analysis *situated within aspects of the broader context* in which the discourses are produced, circulated, and negotiated? Do the findings attend to power relations and implications of these?
8 Have the researchers engaged in *reflexivity*?
9 Do the *results go beyond mere 'commenting'* on texts? Is the critical intent of the study articulated?

Ethics

As previously addressed, critical discourse analysis embodies an axiological commitment to creating more just situations (Fadyl et al., 2012). As such, critical discourse analysis itself is an ethical project given that it is an "unavoidably moralistic pursuit with explicit aims of beneficially transforming social and political systems to make them more equal and democratic" (Graham, 2018, p. 186). Enacting an ethical approach requires on-going transparency and critical reflexivity regarding the values and commitments informing the work, with such reflexivity informing decisions throughout the entire research process from selecting texts to representing findings and interpretations.

As noted, a wide range of types of texts can be included in a critical discourse analysis study. Whether or not a particular study is required to undergo an institutional ethical review process is primarily dependent on the nature of the texts included. An over-arching consideration is that review by an ethics board is not required if the texts used are public and pre-existing data; for example, both the retirement study and the risky driver study used publicly available and accessible texts that were created for public consumption and existed prior to the initiation of the research. However, the delineation of whether texts are public or not can be fuzzy and contested. For example, there is on-going debate regarding whether various types of social media texts, for example, Facebook pages, Twitter posts, or blogs, are public and open for research use or are private and require informed consent for research use (Mayr & Weller, 2016). As guidelines for the use of social media continue to evolve, knowing the current guidelines and challenges within a particular researchers' context is important to guide decision-making regarding submission for ethical review and protocol development (Mayr & Weller, 2016). In an instance where a researcher wants to use pre-existing texts that are sensitive or protected via legislation and institutional procedures, such as health care practitioner records or client medical records, institutional ethical approval is essential. In other cases, a researcher may want to conduct a critical discourse analysis of texts that are generated through a research study; in this situation, ethics approval through an institutional review board would be required in the same way it would be for any qualitative study that involves generating data with participants.

Application to Occupational Science

There have been significant calls to incorporate methodologies into occupational science that enable researchers to enhance understanding of 'occupation as situated'—that is, as shaped within and shaping economic, political cultural, gendered, and other types of social conditions; and 'occupation as political'—that is, as implicated within the enactment of social power relations (Laliberte Rudman et al., 2022). We have found that critical discourse analysis provides a methodology that enables us to enhance understanding of how injustices and inequities with regard to occupation and possibilities to engage in occupation are discursively shaped and perpetuated. Using critical discourse analysis to deconstruct taken-for-granted ideas and knowledge regarding occupation provides a means to enhance awareness of the social relations of power that shape occupational possibilities in ways that privilege some groups while simultaneously disadvantaging others (Laliberte Rudman, 2010). Such work can advance understanding of how occupation is governed, negotiated, and enacted at societal, collective, and individual levels, and inform actions aimed at supporting occupational rights.

Critical discourse analysis also provides a means to build upon the large body of qualitative research that has focused on understanding the meaning of occupation in the lives of individuals. Rather than locating meaning purely within individuals, critical discourse analysis provides a means to attend to questions "concerning the broad cultural and the institutional contexts of meaning making and social order" (Holstein & Gubrium, 2011, p. 342). By situating the meaning given to occupation by individuals within the contexts in which they live, scholars can advance understanding of how contextual features are embedded within how people view, and actively negotiate, themselves and their occupations. For example, Laliberte Rudman and Aldrich (2017) examined how the occupational possibilities of persons experiencing long-term employment were negotiated in relation to broader discourses permeating policies and employment support services, pointing to how these discourses created contractions and tensions that resulted in being 'stuck' in moving forward in various occupations tied to relationships, work, family, schooling, and leisure.

Application to Occupational Therapy

Critical discourse analysis offers a promising methodology to understand how occupational therapy practice and professional knowledge is shaped within broader socio-political and institutional frames. Such research is important as occupational therapy practice is not only shaped by broader discourses, but actively and constantly shapes itself and its assumptions, relations, and contexts through the discourses it produces and enacts. As one example, Njelesani et al. (2015) critically problematized how assumptions regarding 'normal' occupations and occupational possibilities serve to diminish client-centered practice approaches. Ballinger and Payne's (2000a) critical discourse analysis of health care practices addressing falling in later life raised critical questions related to how the predominant use of biomedical discourses of health and illness and "a focus on falling may be at odds with the profession's self-proclaimed 'holistic' practices as occupational therapists" (p. 568). Understanding how specific discourses shape professional practice, in turn, can create possibilities for alternative viewpoints, other practices, and resistance of dominant discourses constraining occupational therapy and other forms of health care practice (Ceci & Purkis, 2009; Njelesani et al., 2015).

Authors' Reflections

Our introductions to critical discourse analysis occurred within our doctoral dissertations. Finding that our view on the topics we were interested in—'positive' aging and risk—were commensurate with a critical paradigm, critical discourse analysis, informed by a governmentality frame, enabled us to address questions regarding the socio-political shaping of occupational possibilities in relation to these topics. It is clear to us that critical discourse analysis would not fit well for researchers who are looking for a research approach that meticulously outlines what should be done and how it should be done, as critical discourse analysis demands engaging in a systematic, on-going process of ensuring a congruence between paradigm, theory, methodology, and methods. For Debbie, this methodology was particularly attractive as it provided a means for her to 'dig under' the assumptions that she had begun to question within her daily life, and in her work as an occupational therapist, regarding what it means to age 'successfully' and what occupations are appropriate, and inappropriate, for people as they age. This methodology has continued to offer a way within her program of research to unpack what is taken-for-granted regarding the occupations that particular groups facing inequities, such as the long-term unemployed and migrants, should and should not do.

For Silke, it was her interest in risk, its connection to power, and how risk discourses shape possibilities to engage in occupation, that led her to critical discourse analysis. Working as an occupational therapist she encountered how concerns about 'safety' were able to justify or deny almost any change in work practice. She observed how institutional fears of accountability seemed to increasingly shift the focus from needs- to risk-assessments, overruling individual needs and wishes, such as living independently, and without questioning such new practices by professionals. This methodology has continued to offer her a way within occupational therapy education to use research to engage students in critical thinking about taken-for granted truths within the profession and for re-thinking practices.

Within this reflection section, we highlight two additional challenges: (a) the 'unsettling' effect of questioning dominant ways of understanding a phenomenon, and (b) the difficulty of stepping outside of and/or resisting being drawn into the discourses one is attempting to de-construct.

In questioning particular discourses, one begins to see that one's work is also a discursive production. Various types of knowledge one takes for granted and acts upon, in unnoticed ways, are also discursively produced. This might not only unsettle one's certainty in the knowledge one has long drawn upon in one's professional, and perhaps personal life, but can also have a paralyzing effect in that one might fear to construct anything—given that any text produced itself is a discourse. For example, in de-constructing discourses of 'positive' aging that increasingly inform health care practices, Debbie struggled with deconstructing aspects of such discourses that align with the value she, and occupational therapy, places on active engagement in occupations as a means to health. Debbie was also concerned that any alternative ways of writing and thinking about aging she produced within her own texts might inadvertently perpetuate aspects of positive aging discourses she had critiqued as marginalizing and exclusionary. It is our stance that in doing critical discourse analysis one needs to come to terms with operating within an ontological position in which that which is taken as 'real' (including the knowledge created through one's analysis) is viewed as constructed and 'tentative' (Ainsworth & Hardy, 2004a). While this does not enable claims of 'scientific' certainty, it creates a sense of freedom as what is taken-for-granted is seen as always changeable. It also means that best practice encompasses on-going critical reflexivity regarding the power relations implicated within the texts one produces. As stated by Bacchi (2016a):

> Such a practice reflects recognition that each of us is immersed in the governing knowledges, in the 'unexamined ways of thinking' of our age and that those among us trained as 'experts' or professionals have a responsibility to reflect on the political implications of the knowledges we employ.

(p. 10)

Further, critical discourse analysis is not about proving a discourse 'wrong,' 'right,' or replacing it with a 'better' one, as all discourses are constructions tied to particular viewpoints, values, and aims. We have both found it challenging, at times, to avoid being drawn into the discourses we are analyzing. For instance, Silke, at the very beginning of the analysis noticed inconsistencies within what was presented as objective, scientifically derived 'facts' regarding aging drivers. She felt compelled to carve out the inconsistencies and faults of logic within them. By feeling the need to 'prove them wrong,' Silke had been drawn into the powerful logic of the texts, endeavoring to replace one 'truth' with another 'truth,' struck by the authoritative ways texts provided information. Engaging in reflexivity, taking a step back and referring to her theoretical framework, allowed her to shift analysis back to the see *effects* of these constructed 'truths'; that is, to focus on *how* particular facts about driving in later life become constructed as a given 'truth' and what power effects and constraints on occupational possibilities these constructions have.

Stepping outside the logic of discourses which are part of the taken-for-granted reality in which our lives are lived is a related challenge. For example, it is difficult to question a construction of aging drivers as inherently increasingly risky in their driving or to question the promotion of continued engagement in volunteer work as a means to age well because being safe and having something meaningful to do are values we share too. This is why we both realize the importance of employing a theoretical framework in our work to guide all aspects of critical discourse analysis. Using a governmentality framework provided us with a means to question such constructions, push beyond their apparent truthfulness, and focus on their power effects. Such constructions are powerful because they are unquestioned, even by those who do not benefit from them. By opening up the possibility of alternative viewpoints, discourse analysis offers us "possibilities for critical resistance, challenge and change" (Fook, 2002, p. 89).

Summary

Critical discourse analysis demands that researchers take a stance and articulate the values and ideas that guide their analysis. Given the long-standing predominance of objectivist or positivist models of science within and outside of the occupation-based literature, choosing to do critical discourse analysis can be challenging. Despite this challenge, it is imperative that researchers who take up this methodology ensure that their theoretical underpinnings are commensurate with a critical paradigmatic understanding of discourse as a social practice and that their research purposes encompass a critical intent. Indeed, Cheek (2004) has argued that critical discourse analysis exists at the margins of qualitative research, contending that this marginal position fruitfully allows critical discourse analysis to be used to transform understandings and question health care practices. As illustrated through the increasing number of critical discourse analysis studies addressing occupation, we contend that critical discourse analysis studies have and can continue to make vital contributions to advancing understandings of occupation. Moreover, critical discourse analysis can be employed to question and extend practices of both occupational scientists and occupational therapists through opening up new spaces for thinking and doing differently.

References

Ainsworth, S., & Hardy, C. (2004a). Critical discourse analysis and identity: Why bother? *Critical Discourse Studies*, 1(2), 225–259. https://doi.org/10.1080/1740590042000302085
Ainsworth, S., & Hardy, C. (2004b). Discourse and identities. In D. Grant, H. C. Oswick, & L. Putnam (Eds.), *The Sage handbook of organizational discourse analysis* (pp. 153–174). SAGE.
Allen, D., & Hardin, P. K. (2001). Discourse analysis and the epidemiology of meaning. *Nursing Philosophy*, 2(2), 163–176. https://doi.org/10.1046/j.1466-769X.2001.00049.x
Bacchi, C. (2009a). *Analysing policy: What's the problem represented to be?* Pearson.
Bacchi, C. (2016a). Problematization in health policy: Questioning how 'problems' are constituted in policies. *SAGE Open, April–June*, 1–16. https://doi.org/10.1177/2158244016653986

Ballinger, C. (2006). Demonstrating rigour and quality? In L. Finlay & C. Ballinger (Eds.), *Qualitative research for allied health professionals: Challenging choices* (pp. 235–246). John Wiley & Sons.

Ballinger, C., & Cheek, J. (2006). Discourse analysis in action: The construction of risk in a community day hospital. In L. Finlay & C. Ballinger (Eds.), *Qualitative research for allied health professionals: Challenging choices* (pp. 200–217). John Wiley & Sons.

Ballinger, C., & Payne, S. (2000a). Discourse analysis: Principles, applications and critique. *British Journal of Occupational Therapy*, *63*(12), 566–572. https://doi.org/10.1177/030802260006301202

Ballinger, C., & Payne, S. (2000b). Falling from grace or into expert hands? Alternative accounts about falling in older people. *British Journal of Occupational Therapy*, *63*(12), 573–579. https://doi.org/10.1177/030802260006301203

Ballinger, C., & Payne, S. (2002). The construction of risk of falling among and by older people. *Ageing and Society*, *22*(2), 305–324. https://doi.org/10.1017/S0144686X02008620

Blankvoort, N., van Hartingsveldt, M., Laliberte Rudman, D., & Krumeich, A. (2021). Decolonising civic integration: A critical analysis of texts used in Dutch civic integration programmes. *Journal of Ethnic and Migration Studies*, *47*(15), 3511–3530. https://doi.org/10.1080/1369183X.2021.1893668

Castel, R. (1991). From dangerousness to risk. In G. Burchell, C. Gordon, & P. Miller (Eds.), *The Foucault effect: Studies in governmentality* (pp. 281–298). University of Chicago Press.

Ceci, C., & Purkis, M. (2009). Bridging gaps in risk discourse: Home care case management and client choices. *Sociology of Health and Illness*, *31*(2), 201–214. https://doi.org/10.1111/j.1467-9566.2008.01127.x

Cheek, J. (2000). *Postmodern and poststructural approaches to nursing research*. SAGE.

Cheek, J. (2004). At the margins? Discourse analysis and qualitative research. *Qualitative Health Research*, *14*(8), 1140–1150. https://doi.org/10.1177/1049732304266820

Crowe, M. (2001). Constructing normality: A discourse analysis of the DSM-IV. *Journal of Psychiatric and Mental Health Nursing*, *7*(1), 69–77. https://doi.org/10.1046/j.1365-2850.2000.00261.x

Del Casino, V. J., & Brooks, C. F. (2015). Talking about bodies online: Viagra, You Tube, and the politics of public(ized) sexualities. *Gender, Place & Culture*, *22*(4), 474–493. https://doi.org/10.1080/0966369X.2013.879106

Dennhardt, S. (2013). *Governing occupation through constructions of risk: The case of the aging driver* [Unpublished doctoral thesis. The University of Western Ontario]. London, Ontario, Canada.

Dennhardt, S., & Laliberte Rudman, D. (2012). When occupation goes 'wrong': A critical reflection on risk discourses and their relevance in shaping occupation. In G. E. Whiteford & C. Hocking (Eds.), *Occupational science: Society, inclusion and participation* (pp. 117–136). Wiley-Blackwell.

Fadyl, J. K., Nicholls, D. A., & McPherson, K. M. (2012). Interrogating discourse: The application of Foucault's methodological discussion to specific inquiry. *Health*, *17*(5), 478–494. https://doi.org/10.1177/1363459312464073

Fairclough, N. (1995). *Critical discourse analysis: The critical study of language*. Longman.

Fairclough, N. (2009). A dialectical-relational approach to critical discourse analysis in social research. In R. Wodak & M. Meyer (Eds.), *Methods of critical discourse analysis* (2nd ed., pp.162–186). SAGE.

Farias, L., Laliberte Rudman, D., & Magalhaes, L. (2016). Illustrating the importance of critical epistemology to realize the promise of occupational justice. *OTJR: Occupation, Participation and Health*, *36*(4), 234–243. https://doi.org/10.1177/1539449216665561

Fook, J. (2002). *Social work: Critical theory and practice*. SAGE.

Foucault, M. (1972). *The archaeology of knowledge*. Pantheon.

Graham, P. (2018). Ethics in critical discourse analysis. *Critical Discourse Studies*, *15*(2), 186–203. https://doi.org/10.1080/17405904.2017.1421243

Hafner, C. A. (2017). Discourse analysis/critical discourse analysis. In D. Wyse, N. Selywn, E. Smith, & L. E. Suter (Eds.), *The BERA/SAGE handbook of educational research* (pp. 812–829). SAGE.

Hardin, P. K. (2001). Theory and language: Locating agency between free will and discursive marionettes. *Nursing Inquiry, 8*(1), 11–18. https://doi.org/10.1046/j.1440-1800.2001.00084.x

Hardin, P. K. (2003). Constructing experience in individual interviews, autobiographies and on-line accounts: A poststructuralist approach. *Journal of Advancing Nursing, 41*(6), 536–544. https://doi.org/10.1046/j.1365-2648.2003.02565.x

Hardy, C., & Phillips, N. (1999). No joking matter: Discursive struggle in the Canadian refugee system. *Organization Studies, 20*(1), 1–24. https://doi.org/10.1177/0170840699201001

Hardy, C., & Phillips, N. (2004). Discourse and power. In D. Grant, C. Hardy, C. Oswick & L. Putnam (Eds.), *The Sage handbook of organizational discourse* (pp. 299–316). SAGE.

Harris, R., Wathen, C. N., MacGregor, J. C. D., Dennhardt, S., Naimi, A., & Ellise, K. S. (2015). 'Blaming the flowers for wilting': Idealized aging in a health charity video. *Qualitative Health Research, 26*(3), 377–386. https://doi.org/10.1177/1049732315570121

Holmes, D., Perron, A., & O'Byrne, P. (2006). Evidence, virulence, and the disappearance of nursing knowledge: A critique of evidence-based dogma. *Worldviews on Evidence-Based Nursing, 3*(3), 95–102. https://doi.org/10.1111/j.1741-6787.2006.00058.x

Holstein, J. A., & Gubrium, J. F. (2011). The constructionist analytics of interpretive practice. In N. K. Denzin & Y. S. Lincoln (Eds.), *The SAGE handbook of qualitative research* (pp. 341–357). SAGE.

Jäger, S., & Maier, F. (2009). Theoretical and methodological aspects of Foucauldian critical discourse analysis and dispositive analysis. In R. Wodak & M. Meyer (Eds.), *Methods of critical discourse analysis* (2nd ed., pp. 34–61). SAGE.

Jørgensen, M., & Phillips, L. J. (2002). *Discourse analysis as theory and method.* SAGE.

Kincheloe, J. L., McLaren, P., Steinberg, S. R., & Monzo, L. D. (2018). Critical pedagogy and qualitative research: Advancing the bricolage. In N. Crossley (Ed.), *Key concepts in critical social theory* (pp. 235–259). SAGE.

Laliberte Rudman, D. (2005). Understanding political influences on occupational possibilities: An analysis of newspaper constructions of retirees. *Journal of Occupational Science, 12*(3), 149–160. https://doi.org/10.1080/14427591.2005.9686558

Laliberte Rudman, D. (2006). Shaping the active, autonomous and responsible modern retiree: An analysis of discursive technologies and their connections with neoliberal political rationality. *Ageing and Society, 26,* 181–201. https://doi.org/10.1017/S0144686X05004253

Laliberte Rudman, D. (2010). Occupational possibilities. *Journal of Occupational Science, 17*(1), 55–59. https://doi.org/10.1080/14427591.2010.9686673

Laliberte Rudman, D. (2013). Enacting the critical potential of occupational science: Problematizing the 'individualizing of occupation'. *Journal of Occupational Science, 20*(4), 298–313. https://doi.org/10.1080/14427591.2013.803434

Laliberte Rudman, D. (2014). Reflecting on the socially situated and constructed nature of occupation: A research program addressing the contemporary restructuring of retirement. In D. Pierce (Ed.), *Occupational science for occupational therapy* (pp. 143–156). Slack.

Laliberte Rudman, D. (2015a). Embodying positive aging and neoliberal rationality: Talking about the aging body within narratives of retirement. *Journal of Aging Studies, 34*(1), 10–20). https://doi.org/10.1016/j.jaging.2015.03.005

Laliberte Rudman, D. (2015b). Situating occupation in social relations of power: Occupational possibilities, ageism and the retirement choice. *South African Journal of Occupational Therapy, 45*(1), 27–33. http://dx.doi.org/10.17159/2310-3833/2015/v45no1a5

Laliberte Rudman, D., & Aldrich, A. (2017). Discerning the social in individual stories of occupation through critical narrative inquiry. *Journal of Occupational Science, 24*(4), 470–481. https://doi.org/10.1080/14427591.2017.1369144

Laliberte Rudman, D., Aldrich, R. M., & Kiepek, N. (2022). Evolving understandings of occupation. In M. Egan & G. Restall (Eds.), *Promoting occupation participation: Collaborative relationship-focused occupational therapy* (pp. 12–30). Canadian Association of Occupational Therapists.

Laliberte Rudman, D., Huot, S., & Dennhardt, S. (2009). Shaping ideal places for retirement: Occupational possibilities within contemporary media. *Journal of Occupational Science, 16*(1), 18–24. https://doi.org/10.1080/14427591.2009.9686637

Laliberte Rudman, D., & Molke, D. (2009). Forever productive: The discursive shaping of later life workers in contemporary Canadian newspapers. *WORK: A Journal of Prevention, Assessment & Rehabilitation, 32*(4), 377–390. https://doi.org/10.3233/WOR-2009-0850

Millington, B. (2011). Use it or lose it: Ageing and the politics of brain training. *Leisure Studies, 31*(4), 429–446. https://doi.org/10.1080/02614367.2011.589865

Mumby, D. K. (2004). Discourse, power and ideology: Unpacking the critical approach. In D. Grant, H. C. Oswick & L. Putnam (Eds.), *The SAGE handbook of organizational discourse analysis* (pp. 217–259). SAGE.

Mayr, P., & Weller, K. (2016). Think before you collect: Setting up a data collection approach for social media studies. In L. Sloan & A. Quan-Haase (Eds.). *The SAGE handbook of social media research methods* (pp. 108–124). SAGE.

Njelesani, J., Teachman, G., Durocher, E., Hamdani, Y., & Phelan, S. K. (2015). Thinking critically about client-centred practice and occupational possibilities across the life span. *Scandinavian Journal of Occupational Therapy, 22*(4), 252–259. https://doi.org/10.3109/11038128.2015.1049550

Phillips, N., & Hardy, C. (2002). *Discourse analysis: Investigating processes of social construction.* SAGE.

Richardson, J. E. (2007). *Analysing newspapers: An approach from critical discourse analysis.* Palgrave Macmillan.

Rose, G. (2007). *Visual methodologies: An introduction to the interpretation of visual materials* (2nd ed.). SAGE.

Schiller, S., van Bruggen, H., Kantartzis, S., Laliberte Rudman, D., Lavalley, R., & Pollard, N. (2022). 'Making change by shared doing': An examination of occupational possibilities in social transformation in five case studies. *Scandinavian Journal of Occupational Therapy*, 1–14. https://doi.org/10.1080/11038128.2022.2046153

Silcock, M., Hocking, C., & Payne, D. (2014). Childhood constructions of contemporary technology: Using discourse analysis to understand the creation of occupational possibilities. *Journal of Occupational Science, 21*(3), 357–370. https://doi.org/10.1080/14427591.2013.832647

van Dijk, T. A. (1997). Editorial: Analysing discourse analysis. *Discourse & Society, 8*(1), 5–6. https://doi.org/10.1177/0957926597008001001

van Leeuwen, T. (2008). Representing social actors with toys. In T. van Leeuwen (Ed.), *Discourse and practice: New tools for critical discourse analysis* (pp. 149–162). Oxford University Press.

Wodak, R., & Meyer, M. (2016a). Critical discourse analysis: History, agenda, theory and methodology. In R. Wodak & M. Meyer (Eds.), *Methods of critical discourse analysis* (3nd ed., pp. 1–22). SAGE.

Wood, L. A., & Kroger, R. O. (2000). *Doing discourse analysis: Methods for studying action in talk and text.* SAGE.

Additional Resources

Bacchi, C. (2009b). *Analysing policy: What's the problem represented to be?* Pearson.

Bacchi, C. (2016b). *Poststructural policy analysis, a guide to practice.* Springer.

Grant, D., Hardy, C., Oswick, C., & Putnam, L. (Eds.). (2004). *The SAGE handbook of organizational discourse.* SAGE.

Kendall, G., & Wickham, G. (1999). *Using Foucault's methods.* SAGE.

Parker, I., & Bolton Discourse Network. (1999). *Critical textwork: An introduction to varieties of discourse and analysis.* Open University Press.

Wodak, R., & Meyer, M. (2016b). *Methods of critical discourse analysis* (3rd ed.). SAGE.

11 Participatory Action Research

Tanya Elizabeth Benjamin-Thomas and
Debbie Laliberte Rudman

Participatory action research is a research approach or methodological umbrella that embodies central tenets of equitable participation and social transformation (Benjamin-Thomas et al., 2018). More specifically, equitable participation within participatory action research seeks to involve community members as co-researchers within the research process, in both decision-making processes and the conduct of research and action; for example, identifying and exploring issues that they deem as relevant and needing to be changed, as well as informing decisions regarding methodologies, methods, and ways forward for mobilizing social transformation. Co-researchers are supported in contributing to various activities (e.g., data collection, data analysis, knowledge mobilization and action), while acknowledging that equitable contributions require openness to on-going negotiation given potential constraints on participation in the context of other life demands (Kemmis et al., 2014). Social transformation within participatory action research goes beyond the identification of issues and seeks to mobilize action steps aimed at changing contextual conditions identified as problematic. Through working towards social transformation, there is also an ongoing process of personal transformation of knowledge and skills of research team and extended community members (Benjamin-Thomas et al., 2018).

The origins of participatory action research include Northern and Southern traditions. Within the Global North, Kurt Lewin, in the late 1930s and 1940s, developed action research, which sought to address issues of discrimination and social equity through democratic participation of those experiencing marginalization within research and action (Glassman & Erdem, 2014). Within the Global South, Paulo Freire (1993) and Fals Borda (2006) worked to address the emancipation of the oppressed through shared dialogue and the raising of critical consciousness as the means for sociopolitical transformation (Fine & Barreras, 2001; Glassman & Erdem, 2014; Kemmis et al., 2014). These diverse approaches share a commitment to shift away from relations with participants as research subjects to be *researched on* towards relations as collaborators and co-researchers to *research with* (Heron & Reason, 1997). In addition, these foundational approaches created spaces for shared dialogue and critical reflexivity among people experiencing oppression and marginalization as a means to inform and enact social change.

Within occupation-based scholarship, starting in the late 1990s, there have been ongoing dialogues highlighting the potential of participatory action research in addressing community development and sustainable community change (Law 1997; Suarez-Balcazar et al., 2005; Taylor et al., 2004; Townsend et al., 2000). For example, Law (1997) discussed how participatory action research, at the time, was situated as an alternate methodology within the field of health sciences that was dominated by quantitative, experimental

DOI: 10.4324/9781003456216-11

research. Within Law's early example of participatory action research, parents of children with disabilities explored and addressed barriers to participation experienced by children with disabilities, recommended policy changes, and worked towards facilitating change within their own communities. Taylor et al. (2004) also argued for greater incorporation of participatory action research pointing to its potential to guide creation of innovative, sustainable models of occupational therapy service delivery and contribute evidence on program-related outcomes. These authors presented two case exemplars of how participatory action research was used to work alongside people with chronic health conditions to build and evaluate relevant occupational therapy programs.

Participatory action research has also been put forward as an appropriate methodology for occupation-based scholarship given that its underlying values parallel those of client-centered occupational therapy, which prioritizes collaborative relationships with clients through the sharing and negotiation of power as the means to explore first-hand experiences to address occupation-based issues (Cockburn & Trentham, 2002; Letts, 2003; Townsend et al., 2000) and changes in occupation-based service delivery (Turcotte et al., 2019). It has also been linked to health promotion goals, where clients are positioned as active participants in managing their own health through capacity building (Albuquerque & Farias, 2022; Cockburn & Trentham, 2002). Further, such scholarship has positioned participatory action research as consistent with the core values of occupational therapy that focus on meaningful engagement in tasks and activities within the research process (Cockburn & Trentham, 2002; Letts, 2003; Townsend et al., 2000).

More recently, participatory action research has been increasingly positioned as a vehicle for mobilizing occupation-based social transformation (Benjamin-Thomas et al., 2021; Farias et al., 2017) through creating spaces for understanding occupation as situated and addressing situations of occupational injustices (Benjamin-Thomas & Laliberte Rudman, 2018). For example, Kramer-Roy's (2011) work utilized participatory action research to engage Pakistani families of children with disabilities to identify and address support needs from an occupational justice perspective, specifically exploring how cultural and familial expectations impacted occupational balance of family members. Similarly, Blakeney and Marshall (2009) used participatory action research to explore and address how water quality impacts occupational participation within a specific community.

The promise of participatory action research can be further mobilized through positioning participatory action research as an *occupational process* through embodying a variety of occupations within the research process, as well as an *occupation-based process* where research is informed by an occupational lens (Benjamin-Thomas et al., 2021). As such, occupation-centered participatory action research can provide a space for collective generation of contextually relevant knowledge through occupational participation as a means to deepen understanding of the socio-political production of occupational injustices and mobilize praxis. For example, Crabtree et al. (2016a, 2016b), utilized a participatory action research approach to explore issues of occupational justice experienced among prison inmates, positioning interviews with inmates as a means to engage in co-occupation addressing experiences of occupational deprivation. This participatory action research created a space to explore strengths, weaknesses, and elements valued by prison inmates participating within an occupational therapy informal education program as a means to mobilize change.

In the participatory filmmaking project, Tanya strove to design and enact an occupation-centered participatory action research (Benjamin-Thomas et al., 2021). As one example, she integrated culturally relevant visual illustrations of various occupations to support child co-researchers in understanding the construct of 'occupation' which lacked literal translation in the local language. Additionally, child co-researchers engaged in various occupations within the participatory action research process such as guided walks in the community, shared dialogues, creating and editing their participatory film, and playing local games. Centering occupation within the participatory action research process facilitated the building of relationships among the group as well as participatory explication and action addressing situations of occupational injustices experienced by children with disabilities within their community.

Epistemology, Ontology, Axiology

Participatory action research has been inextricably linked to values centralized within critical, transformative, and/or participatory paradigms (Kemmis et al., 2014). These paradigmatic underpinnings challenge traditional boundaries that separate the researcher from the researched thereby supporting the essential positioning of community members as co-researchers. In addition, these paradigmatic underpinnings acknowledge researcher and co-researcher values as central in informing the research process, and inform framing injustices as contextually shaped and constructed that, in turn, promote generation of actions that address larger contextual forces. More specifically, shared ontological, epistemological, and axiological assumptions of critical, transformative, and participatory paradigms central to participatory action research are that new knowledge is generated through shared dialogue among collectives experiencing marginalization and that injustices must be acknowledged, situated, and prioritized to inform social change.

However, as participatory action research has become widely implemented, critiques have been raised regarding tendencies in the health, educational, and social sciences to treat participatory action research as a set of methods divorced from critical, transformative, or participatory paradigmatic underpinnings (Brydon-Miller, 2008; Kemmis, 2006; Sandwick et al., 2018). Such research often fails to enact equitable participation or commit to social transformation, and may inadvertently reproduce oppressive power relations (Laliberte Rudman, 2019). For example, community members may not be embraced as co-researchers; rather, positioned as objects of data collection (Corrado et al., 2020; Laliberte Rudman, 2019). As well, such studies may de-politicize and individualize inequities and thereby fail to enhance understandings that can inform actions aimed at social transformation (Hickey & Mohan, 2005; Laliberte Rudman, 2019). As noted by Kemmis (2006), the risk is that participatory research that fails to address the sociopolitical production of inequities is "more likely to reproduce rather than transform irrational, unjust and alienating consequences" (p. 46). Indeed, best practice in participatory action research, as in all qualitative research, requires coherence amongst philosophical underpinnings, methodology, methods, research aims, and outcomes. Within the context of participatory action research, moving forward with its participatory and transformative intent requires coherence with critical, transformative, and/or participatory paradigmatic underpinnings (Farias et al., 2017; Kemmis, 2006; Sandwick et al., 2018).

The participatory filmmaking project was informed by critical paradigmatic values (Crotty 1998; Ponterotto, 2005), which situated the occupational injustices experienced by children with disabilities and their communities as shaped by contextual forces. It challenged the dichotomy between knowledge generation and action by situating them within the same continuum; and acknowledged the relationship between the researcher and participants through positioning children with disabilities as co-researchers and created a space for shared critical reflexivity. Freire's (1993) work on critical pedagogy was a theoretical perspective that underpinned this work, which emphasized the need for critical dialogue and shared reflections among co-researchers to facilitate the raising of critical consciousness among co-researchers and extended community members and address social transformation. Other theoretical underpinnings within this participatory action research were critical disability perspectives (Devlin & Pothier, 2006; Meekosha & Shuttleworth, 2009) that seek to rethink disability related assumptions and challenge deficit-focused discourses; and the critical occupational science perspective (Laliberte Rudman, 2018; Njelesani et al., 2013) that highlights the situated and political nature of occupation. Overall, critical paradigmatic values informed the uptake of these specific theoretical perspectives that aligned with the paradigm and the intent to work towards social transformation which, in turn, informed the uptake of specific research methods and methodologies (e.g., participatory filmmaking, group discussions) that embodied values of equitable collaboration.

Research Purpose, Topics, or Problems Best Suited for Participatory Action Research Studies

The research purpose within a participatory action research needs to reflect tenets of equitable participation and social transformation. Further, it is important to have space for co-researchers to shape the research focus depending on what they deem as important and relevant to be explored and addressed, given the underlying assumption that they are the experts regarding their lives and contexts. In turn, research questions or research purposes within participatory action research need to be broad and open ended so community co-researchers can take the lead in narrowing the foci of interest to explore and address. As Glassman and Erdem (2014) pointed out, "The goal of research is not hypothesis testing with objective measures but to participate in the realities and experiences of the community and collaborate, learn, and move toward social change in order to improve the human condition" (p. 214).

The purpose of the participatory filmmaking project was to work with children with disabilities as co-researchers in exploring their first-hand experiences about their lives pertaining to occupation, explicating the situated nature of their everyday experiences related to occupation and occupational injustices, and working alongside them and community stakeholders in mobilizing change to address situations of occupational injustices. Through the process of working alongside child co-researchers, they identified, discussed, and explicated situations of occupational injustices at individual and community levels. More specifically, they focused on issues of marginalization with school, home, and community settings, and issues of teasing and bullying. They also discussed larger community problematics such as issues of occupational degradation, community violence, and substance abuse (Benjamin-Thomas et al., 2021; Benjamin-Thomas et al., 2022).

The purposes that can be addressed using participatory action research in occupational science and occupational therapy are diverse as illustrated with a few examples in Table 11.1.

Recruitment and Sampling

The process of participatory action research is an on-going cycle of knowledge generation, reflection, and action (Kemmis et al., 2014). This means that recruitment, data collection, and devising actions or implementing actions often occur more than once. The cyclical

Table 11.1 Research purposes identified within exemplar occupation-based participatory action research projects

Authors	National location of research	Focus
Bennet et al. (2016)	Australia	Engaging occupational therapists as co-researchers in a cyclical participatory action research process, this study sought to identify barriers and enablers to knowledge translation and implement action strategies to build capacity among occupational therapy clinicians for knowledge translation.
Gonçalves & Malfitano (2020)	Brazil	This study used participatory workshops to explore the representations that young dwellers of a Brazilian favela in Rio de Janeiro have about that place; exploring how these representations impact their urban mobility and possibilities for social participation.
Pettican et al. (2022)	England	Using the World Café method, the aim of this first phase of a participatory action research was to explore the nature and value of participation in a community-based football league for people with experience of mental distress, generating knowledge to inform accessible sport development.
Suarez-Balcazar et al. (2005)	United States of America	With active involvement of community residents, a needs assessment process was implemented in this participatory action research study to identify the service needs of an underserved Hispanic population as well as set action agendas to meet their needs.

Author created

process enables on-going co-learning of co-researchers through a process of 'looking, thinking, and acting' (Koch et al., 2005), engaging in on-going critical reflexivity to deepen understanding, analyze situations, and generate and enact informed actions towards social change. In the following sections, we primarily address the initial cycle of a participatory action research project; for example, focusing on recruiting co-researchers for the participatory action research team, while also pointing to the need for on-going attention to such activities through each participatory action research cycle.

Participatory action research challenges traditional research boundaries by positioning community members as knowledge producers and change agents, as well as challenging taken for granted assumptions regarding who can participate as co-researchers (Glassman & Erdem, 2014). For example, participatory action research projects in occupational science and occupational therapy have involved co-researchers who are older adults (Trentham & Neysmith, 2018; Turcotte et al., 2019), people, including children, with disabilities (Benjamin-Thomas et al., 2021; Van Niekerk et al., 2006), prison inmates (Crabtree et al., 2016a), young people experiencing poverty (Gonçalves & Malfitano, 2020), caregivers of people with disabilities and chronic conditions (Taylor et al., 2004), and occupational therapy clinicians (Bennett et al., 2016; Wilding & Whiteford, 2008).

In instances where a participatory action research project is initiated by community members, recruitment activities may involve these community members reaching out for involvement from researchers. Most often, however, given the nature of funding mechanisms, many researchers may be involved in recruiting co-researchers from a community. It is imperative for recruitment of co-researchers within participatory action research to be grounded in reciprocity (Maiter et al., 2008), where relationships are central to establishing trust and collaborations, as well as for mobilizing sustainable forms of transformation. More specifically, recruitment processes within participatory action research are ideally carried out through local organizations, institutions, groups, or committees run by or serving the community of interest in a study and should mobilize community members in identifying processes and sites for recruitment.

Whether community or researcher initiated, it is important to consider that participatory action research might be carried out by researchers or academics who are outsiders to the community of focus. This kind of work can be positioned as cross-cultural research which mandates the importance of embracing cultural humility (Tervalon & Murray-Garcia, 1998) even before the initiation of the project. Cultural humility involves openness to interacting with individuals or collectives from diverse cultures; self-awareness of one's own strengths, values, beliefs, behaviors, and appearance to others; having a humble attitude; having supportive interactions; and engaging in reflexivity of one's thoughts, feelings, and actions (Foronda et al., 2016).

More specifically, within the recruitment phase, it is important to utilize culturally and linguistically relevant recruitment materials and events so community members have the opportunity to make informed decisions about their involvement within the process. It is also important to recruit co-researchers embodying shared experiences in relation to the broad focus of research so that shared dialogue and reflexivity can mobilize critical consciousness and transformation (Kemmis et al., 2014).

The participatory filmmaking project used a multi-step recruitment process to identify a community in which there was a group of children who could work together in the project. This started based on Tanya's previous connection with a community health department of a local medical college and hospital that served approximately 82 rural communities in the south of India. Following ethical approval, Tanya visited four villages with an occupational therapist from this local institution who had identified potential villages based on village demographics, and a community that could host the project was identified.

Recruitment efforts were carried out using culturally and linguistically relevant posters with the help of a community health aide, who was a member of the village and worked for the local collaborating institution. The community health aide visited the houses of children with disabilities who fit the inclusion criteria and handed out recruitment posters along with the letter of information in the local language, and the parents and children were invited to a recruitment meeting. The recruitment meeting was conducted within the village and attended by parent(s) of eight children with six children present. During this meeting, Tanya presented the details of the project, went through the letter of information, and addressed attendees' questions. Parents of six children were interested and provided written consent for their child's involvement. The parents of some children expressed needing additional time and were asked to contact the local health aide if they were interested at a later point. This meeting was followed up with a subsequent session with just the children to share information about the research and to obtain their consent for involvement. Tanya had completed her undergraduate education within this institution, thus had an established relationship, was familiar with the villages it serves, and was fluent in speaking the local language, all of which played a central role in building relationships and collaboration.

Crabtree et al. (2016b) enacted a more cyclical approach to recruitment in their project conducted in a prison setting. First, they recruited three co-researchers, who were former participants of an informal education program within a prison setting. In turn, the co-researchers were involved in recruiting 27 prison residents who completed an informal educational program within the prison setting who they then engaged in interviews for data generation.

Data Collection Methods and Methodologies

Participatory action research is situated as a research approach or methodological umbrella that embodies a variety of methods and methodologies. Broadly, methods, such as interviews, refer to procedures used to generate information; while methodologies, such as participatory filmmaking, encompass theoretical and paradigmatic underpinnings that guide how specific methods are to be used (Schwandt, 2001). Given the philosophical underpinnings of participatory action research which point to prioritizing the need for shared dialogue and critical reflexivity, participatory action research has been closely linked to qualitative methods and methodologies (Kidd & Kral, 2005). However, participatory action research can involve a variety of qualitative and quantitative methods and methodologies, such as interviews (Suarez-Balcazar et al., 2005; Taylor et al., 2004), go along interviews with opportunities for show and tell (Pettican et al., 2022), focus groups or group meetings (Suarez-Balcazar et al., 2005; Benjamin-Thomas et al., 2019b), photo elicitation or photovoice (St. John et al., 2018), participatory filmmaking (Benjamin-Thomas et al., 2019b), or surveys (Suarez-Balcazar et al., 2005). Flexibility in methodologies and methods is required in order to enable on-going design of projects based on co-researcher dialogue and decision-making.

Increasingly, mixed-methods research involving quantitative and qualitative methods and methodologies are also being utilized within participatory action research (Akwataghibe et al., 2021; Fine et al., 2003; Shearn et al., 2022; Suarez-Balcazar et al., 2005). For example, Shearn et al. (2022) carried out a mixed-methods participatory action research with 47 young people and other community collaborators, to contribute to the design of services for young people to develop capabilities and avenues to live the life they value. This participatory action research included three stages. Stage one incorporated exploratory qualitative workshops with young people that focused on identifying capabilities that young people in the town valued. Workshops included a variety of creative activities and discussions, such as creating avatars, critiquing newspaper headlines, creating illustrations, completing worksheets, modeling with building blocks and paper, and going on story walks. In stage two, data collection methods switched to quantitative surveys. The youth participants were trained in creating surveys and research ethics with support from adult facilitators, and then gathered data through the survey developed. Once data were collected, adult facilitators and young people worked to understand their data and make relevant suggestions. In stage three, the focus was to co-design services for young people through a single five-hour workshop, which included discussions as well as the use of materials for developing, prototyping, and communicating ideas generated.

Overall, participatory action research often utilizes a variety of methods and methodologies to support knowledge generation and action. Irrespective of whether the methods and methodologies utilized are explicitly labeled as 'participatory,' researchers need to continually work towards addressing the sharing and negotiation of power to facilitate equitable engagement of community members as co-researchers in choosing, designing, and carrying out methodologies and methods incorporated into the participatory action research cycles. As such, there is a need to identify and address barriers for participation, such as hierarchical power differentials, as well as pragmatic challenges such as restricted time and resources. Moreover, to involve community members as co-researchers and equitable partners in the research process, training on research-related skills as part of a commitment to capacity building is essential (Koch et al., 2005). Additionally, all members of the research team need to be oriented to the central tenets of participatory action research so that these are utilized throughout the research process.

Within the participatory filmmaking project (Benjamin-Thomas et al., 2019b), child co-researchers were provided two methodological options—digital storytelling or participatory filmmaking. We differentiated these methodologies based on whether child co-researchers wanted to work on creating individual video narratives (i.e., digital storytelling) or a group video (participatory filmmaking). Child co-researchers decided to utilize participatory filmmaking as a research methodology as they preferred to work on a group project. They were then provided training on camera use (e.g., how to hold a camera, turning it on and off, focusing an image, rule of thirds, recording video clips, panning videos, the importance of lighting). Child co-researchers also engaged in discussions on visual research ethics that encompassed the importance of consent, confidentiality, and issues of identity. All research personnel, including the photographer and local occupational therapist, engaged in discussions to better understand and apply the central tenets of equitable collaboration and social transformation within participatory action research.

Data generation within participatory action research goes beyond knowledge generation regarding issues of concern to encompass information addressing the research process. To guide ethical research practices, all members within a participatory action research project are called to engage in critical reflexivity, defined as a "continuous process of critical scrutiny and interpretation, not just in relation to the research methods and the data but also to the researcher, participants, and the research context" (Guillemin & Gillam, 2004, p. 275). These reflexive processes, and resulting notes, can encompass attention to the tensions, challenges, and solutions experienced and enacted through the research process, which can also be considered as data used to guide ethical ways of doing participatory action research. As such, engaging in shared reflexivity is a form of research, where the research process, and researchers' and co-researchers' experiences are considered new knowledge (Enosh & Ben-Ari, 2016).

Within the participatory filmmaking project, Tanya engaged in reflexivity through maintaining a journal to think about and address ongoing tensions within the research process in relation to ethical issues and pragmatics, as well as consider how her positionality, experiences, and assumptions influenced key decisions made and outcomes within the research. She also engaged in shared dialogic reflexivity with the co-facilitator who was the volunteer photographer to identify tensions and barriers in relation to fully enacting tenets of equitable collaboration and transformation. Finally, all child co-researchers engaged in dialogic shared reflexivity to identify challenges in relation to participation and on-going tensions and issues in relation to confidentiality and harm.

Data Analysis

Within participatory action research, data analysis is ideally a collaborative process completed amongst co-researchers in a participatory fashion (Corrado et al., 2020); thus, data analysis needs to be adapted to meet needs, resources, and skills of co-researchers. Within any form of research, data analysis is informed by specific theoretical underpinnings, and all co-researchers need to gain familiarity with the theoretical underpinnings of the specific participatory action research in which they are involved. This familiarity can be informed through ongoing dialogues with co-researchers where types of questions forwarded for discussions are informed by specific theoretical underpinnings. Moreover, approaches to data analysis should align with the various forms of data; for example, textual, verbal, artistic representations, body maps, and other forms that may be generated through a participatory action research project given the diversity of methods that may be integrated. At the same time, all approaches to data analysis should be enacted in ways that enable co-researcher input and participation.

Data analysis is not necessarily separate from the data generation phase, especially within qualitative participatory action research projects. Data analysis starts during the process of data generation, where co-researchers are engaged in collective dialogue on shared experiences surrounding issues they want to address, which may or may not be supported through additional activities such as photography, drawings, or guided walks. Co-researchers both identify issues and need to consider how such issues are contextually shaped and informed, as means to identify and mobilize actions. Data analysis within participatory action research may occur in stages with varying levels of co-researcher involvement depending on co-researcher interests and resources (e.g., time). It is an ongoing process that includes engaging in dialogue with co-researchers and revisiting topics identified for further discussion and explication throughout the research process. For example, when engaging in thematic analysis of textual data, not all co-researchers will necessarily be involved in in-depth line by line coding of all data generated; therefore, it is important to bring these ideas and codes back to all co-researchers for further dialogic analysis. Additionally, the process of transcribing and translating discussions, and writing up of information, also inform ideas for analytical considerations (Saldaña, 2016). If co-researchers need specific skill sets in relation to data analysis, training needs to be incorporated within the participatory action research process.

Within the participatory filmmaking project, data analysis encompassed a participatory thematic analysis carried out in collaboration with child co-researchers and an additional layer of theoretical analysis carried out by Tanya. These are labelled as layers, rather than stages or phases, as each layer of analysis was interwoven with the other. Participatory thematic analysis encompassed the process of creating the participatory film. Specifically, child co-researchers identified issues they wanted addressed. They then engaged in shared dialogue using their captured videos to explicate the causes and consequences of issues, and potential solutions addressing these issues. This dialogic process, stirred through questions posed by Tanya, was informed by the theoretical underpinnings of this work, thus interweaving with theoretical analysis. This participatory analysis informed the key content and messages highlighted within a short film created by child co-researchers which can be accessed on YouTube (https://youtu.be/sPyiQCj82Qs).

Another layer of theoretical analysis was carried out to further explicate issues discussed by child co-researchers, such as this theoretical analysis was intricately informed by the participatory analysis. The theoretical analysis, led by Tanya and involving on-going reflexive dialogue with Debbie, involved multiple, iterative, whole-text readings of all transcripts and reflexive notes along with a simultaneous coding process where smaller codable moments were identified (Saldaña, 2016). An analysis guide with questions informed by the theoretical underpinnings, specifically critical disability and critical occupational science perspectives, supported this coding process (see Textbox 11.1 for selected examples of questions included in this guide). All codes were re-arranged, grouped, and presented as themes (Charmaz, 2006; Miles et al., 2014); and were further refined during the process of writing and dialogue.

Textbox 11.1   Example Guiding Questions for Supporting Theoretical Analysis

Questions Informed by a Critical Occupational Science Perspective

What are some themes relevant to the occupational justice framework highlighted within this transcript? (e.g., When and how are reduced opportunities for children with disabilities to participate in meaningful occupations addressed? Are issues related to restricted or absent occupational participation of children with disabilities seen as an injustice? And how?)

What are some themes related to the situated nature of occupation and/or occupational justice? (e.g., What are some cultural, economic and socio-political factors shaping occupational injustices experienced by children with disabilities?)

Questions Informed by Critical Disability Perspectives

How is impairment and disability conceptualized? (e.g., How are impairments and disabilities talked about within transcripts? Where is disability located, in individual, in context, in both?)

How are children with disabilities positioned within this context? (e.g., What are some disability related experiences as well as expected outcomes in relation to children with disabilities within that context? Do children with disabilities have a voice within their community?)

Rigor and Ethics

Ethically, it is important to consider that participatory action research, although holding great promises for addressing injustices and mobilizing social transformation, can also perpetuate harm if it is not carried out in ways that acknowledge its central tenets and principles (Brydon-Miller, 2008; Sandwick et al., 2018). A good quality participatory action research needs to embody practices that work towards the goals of equitable research collaboration and social transformation (Benjamin-Thomas et al., 2018). Also, good quality participatory action research demonstrates coherence between paradigmatic values, theoretical underpinnings, methods and methodologies used, and outcomes addressed (Ravenek & Laliberte Rudman, 2013). Addressing equitable participation within participatory action research is both an ethical commitment and a marker of rigor, as the research process is as important as the research outcome (Cargo & Mercer, 2008; Gubrium et al., 2015).

Research practices need to embody flexibility so community members are provided with a space to participate as much as they would like within the different phases of the research and action processes. Research practices should be enacted in ways that share and negotiate power and build capacity among all members of the research team through challenging existing hierarchies and ensuring access to required resources. It is important to think through and consider early on in the project what collaboration looks like and the roles each member is comfortable and interested in taking on, and to constantly re-visit this with co-researchers throughout the participatory action research process (Kemmis et al., 2014). At times, as further addressed in the personal reflection section of this chapter, remaining aligned with participatory action research tenets and doing research in flexible, collaborative ways may be challenging given particular institutional rules and expectations, including those of research ethics review boards (Elwood, 2007). As one example, requirements for informed signed consent from 'participants' are misaligned with positioning community members as co-researchers and working in an on-going process of designing and enacting participatory action research.

Significant harm can result through participatory action research processes that stop at generating knowledge and awareness of inequities and their socio-political production, failing to work with co-researchers and communities to generate ways forward in addressing such inequities (Brydon-Miller, 2008; Sandwick et al., 2018). As such, participatory action research needs to be located within a knowledge to action continuum that moves research into "an ongoing community-building enterprise" (Potts & Brown, 2015, p. 37) that seeks to mobilize sustainable forms of social change and transformation. In working towards goals of social transformation, personal transformation of all members of the team will also be ideally reflected through acquired skills and expanded knowledge as well a changed awareness of issues explicated within the participatory action research (Benjamin-Thomas et al., 2018).

Additionally, sincerity within the research process is central for a rigorous participatory action research and ethical research practices. Sincerity is marked by "honesty and transparency about the researcher's biases, goals, and foibles as well as about how these played a role in the methods, joys, and mistakes of the research" (Tracy, 2010, p. 841). Sincerity can be addressed through engaging in individual and shared reflexivity about one's positionality, cultural values, assumptions, and experiences, and its influence within the research process, as well as identify ongoing tensions and challenges experienced within the research process and the forces that shape such tensions.

Application to Occupational Science

Participatory action research blurs the line between research and practice, embracing praxis in which knowledge generation, theoretical understandings, and action are positioned to be within the same continuum. Addressing knowledge generation in relation to occupation and its situated nature, utilization of participatory action research within occupational science is a response to calls for methodological expansions (Bailliard, 2015; Magalhães et al., 2019) that acknowledge different ways of knowing and creates a space for perspectives on occupation seldom heard within occupation-based scholarship, such as the studies highlighted in Table 11.1 and throughout this chapter. Participatory action research is also positioned as a vehicle for further mobilizing occupational science as a socially relevant and transformative science (Farias et al., 2019; Hocking, 2012) that encompasses commitments to addressing situations of injustices in relation to occupation (Farias et al., 2019). Due to the space for methodological innovations within participatory action research, where creative and culturally relevant methods and methodologies are often utilized, it can push for further methodological developments within occupation-based scholarship. Finally, participatory action research has been situated as an occupation-based and occupational process (Benjamin-Thomas et al., 2021) embodying a variety of occupations, which urges occupation-based scholars to take up this approach to further expand situated understandings on occupation as means to address occupational injustices.

Application to Occupational Therapy

Utilizing participatory action research within occupational therapy can expand the focus of interventions from individual to community levels (Albuquerque & Farias, 2022). More specifically, participatory action research can be mobilized within community-based occupational therapy interventions (Cockburn & Trentham, 2002; Suarez-Balcazar et al., 2005) through involving community members in prioritizing population-based interventions, goals, and evaluation strategies. Participatory action research has also been utilized to work with occupational therapy clinicians to explore and address barriers to enacting population or community-based practice commensurate with occupational therapy values and the occupational needs of communities. This research approach embodies a potential for expanding focus on emergent areas of occupational practice such as working with physically displaced communities, communities experiencing homelessness, or collectives experiencing occupational injustices due to marginalization or forced participation in occupations, through community collaboration and innovation (Fazio, 2017).

Critiquing Literature and Best Practice

Drawing from various sources, Benjamin-Thomas et al. (2018) developed a set of six participatory action research principles along with guiding questions to support critical analysis of completed participatory action research, as well as those that are ongoing or in the proposal phase. Table 11.2 offers an adapted version of these guiding principles and questions, along with best practice recommendations.

Table 11.2 Guiding questions to guide critical analysis of participatory action research and best practice recommendations

Participatory action research principle	Guiding questions	Best practice
Research problem is identified by co-researchers and situated	Do the authors frame the 'problem' in broader social, economic, or political forces? If so, how? What have the authors problematized? In what ways have they made these things problematic? Who was involved in stating and framing the research problem?	Research problem needs to be located as contextually shaped and situated. Community co-researchers need to be involved in identifying specific problems to be explored and addressed.
Key terms are clearly conceptualized and align with participatory action research's key tenets	What terminology is used to describe the nature of research? How is participatory action research described in the article? How are participation and action defined? Does the article reflect an intent for both participation and action? If so, how?	Definition of the terminology used needs to reflect commitments to equitable participation of community members and an agenda for addressing social change/transformation .

(Continued)

Table 11.2 (Continued)

Participatory action research principle	Guiding questions	Best practice
Coherence of paradigm, theories, methodologies and methods, and outcomes	Is this research situated within a specific paradigm? How do these paradigmatic values support the central tenets of participatory action research? Is this research informed by specific theoretical underpinnings and are they consistent with the goals of participatory action research? What methods and methodologies are used, and are they coherent with paradigm and theoretical underpinnings?	A good quality participatory action research is underpinned by critical, transformative, and/or participatory paradigmatic assumptions that inform the utilization of participatory methods and methodologies to support involvement of community members as co-researchers as means to work towards addressing social transformation. Research needs to demonstrate coherence between paradigmatic values, methods, and methodologies used, and outcomes addressed.
Power sharing and co-researcher involvement	Who is involved in the research team? What steps or phases of the research study are they involved in? How are the community members positioned (co-researchers, partners, informants, participants, etc.)? Was/were the community member(s) provided with choice regarding what aspects of the study they would be involved in? Are community members involved in designing the study? If so, how? Are community members involved in carrying out the study? If so, how? Are community members involved in interpreting the data? If so, how? Are community members involved in disseminating the knowledge? If so, how? Are community members involved in action steps arising through the participatory action research process? If so, how? Are researchers and community members working in a 'collaborative equitable partnership' at all stages of the research process? If so, how is this demonstrated/accomplished?	Community members need to be provided with a space to make decisions regarding their participation and involvement in various aspects of the research process depending on their interests. The participatory action research process should encompass decision-making processes that attend to sharing of power amongst all members of the research team. Resources should be provided to support equitable participation and capacity building.

(Continued)

Table 11.2 (Continued)

Participatory action research principle	Guiding questions	Best practice
Transformation addressed at personal to social levels	What action components is the study addressing? Do they address both personal and social transformation? What evidence/description is provided to demonstrate such actions and their effects?	Best practice within participatory action research will mobilize avenues for transformation which can be situated along a continuum from personal to social transformation.
Engagement in critical reflexivity	How was reflexivity described in the study? What evidence is provided to demonstrate on-going reflexivity used within the participatory action research process?	Best practice demonstrates that all members of the research team including community co-researchers engaged in critical reflexivity addressing ongoing tensions, challenges and positionality, within the research process.

Author created

Authors' Reflections

Tanya

My interests in participatory action research are rooted within my experience as an occupational therapist working among children with disabilities in rural India. I was sensitized to how children with disabilities were denied opportunities for occupational participation within home, school, and community settings, and how contextual forces such as disability-related stigma, lack of support within school systems, lack of awareness about disabilities, etc., shaped and informed such situations of exclusion. I was motivated to get further equipped in research-related skills as means to address change at the systems level. In the first year of my PhD, I started exploring research approaches that worked towards addressing injustices and mobilizing social change. I learnt about participatory action research and its commitment to inclusion, equity, and justice both within the research process and as a research outcome.

Utilizing participatory action research within a PhD dissertation came with various challenges and tensions in relation to execution of the project in ways that aligned with tenets of equitable participation of co-researchers and addressing sustainable forms of social transformation. I was made aware of the time-consuming, messy realities of carrying out participatory action research, with ongoing tensions and challenges shaped by context (Baum et al., 2006; Klocker, 2012). For instance, during the planning phase, tensions were based on expectations in academia and the misfit of some processes and expectations with participatory action research values. There were set expectations for a research protocol outlining the methodology of choice, specific research question, as well as activities planned prior to initiating the participatory action research project. Ideally, within a participatory action research project many of these details would be generated in collaboration with community co-researchers. Additionally, language used within ethics applications reflects power differentials (e.g., participants versus co-researchers), and participatory action research challenges those existing boundaries that position academics as researchers and community members as research participants. These tensions were navigated with the support of Debbie who urged me to think about alternate ways of approaching academic structures and procedures in ways that aligned with the central tenets of participatory action research but also adhered to academic expectations. For example, within my dissertation and ethics proposal I sketched out different research plans based on the various methodological options that were to be provided to co-researchers.

When executing this participatory action research, although we sought to work towards creating an equitable space for engagement of all co-researchers, who were children with disabilities, we faced further challenges. In particular, one of the child co-researchers, who was diagnosed with a speech and hearing impairment, experienced barriers to full engagement in all of the research activities as his hearing aid was not working. Written forms of communication were attempted but not successful, and sign language was not possible given lack of knowledge among facilitators as well as the child co-researcher involved. Although this child co-researcher was able to answer close-ended questions non-verbally, it was ultimately not possible to engage him in detailed discussions addressing specific topics. Additionally, there were two child co-researchers living within a residential institution for children with disabilities, and it was difficult to get them to participate alongside other co-researchers from the same village as they were not familiar with the group and felt uncomfortable. In this instance, we attempted to include these two children through creating a smaller work group, particularly as there were also time constraints as they were in the village only for a short period of time. Ultimately, we cannot claim that all of the co-researchers had equitable opportunities to participate or for their perspectives to be integrated within the participatory film created through this participatory action research.

There were also tensions with mobilizing the action phase. I was fully committed to mobilizing action through collaboration with community stakeholders serving the community; however, there were international geographical boundaries with my physical location in Canada after the research phase, and the project being in India. Further, this project was carried out as a student research project requiring independent work, in turn, creating challenges to local ownership and leadership. Barriers to local ownership during the research phase came with implications for the action phase as well. At the same time, informed by this participatory action research, various actions were mobilized in collaboration with the children, local institution, and collaborators. These actions included a public showing of the video created by the children within their community and new program developments in the village such as a tree planting program. Ongoing health education efforts carried out through the local institution were also expanded, such as incorporating content on teasing and bullying, which were identified through this participatory action research, within school health education efforts. However, there was still a personal tension when thinking about the immediate needs of child co-researchers that came to light through the course of this participatory action research, which were left unaddressed. For instance, one child co-researcher was out of school and expressed a desire to get an education, while another child co-researcher was on the verge of being dismissed from school. These were just two examples among other immediate needs discussed by child co-researchers. There was a sense of sadness knowing that their work has the potential to stir community change, but their immediate needs still remain unaddressed. I came to realize that action and transformation processes cannot be constrained with time. It needs to be acknowledged as an ongoing process with rippling effects that may or may not come to be realized. Researchers and practitioners need to hold on to the commitment for mobilizing change even when the project and/or funding for the research has come to an end.

Overall, this participatory action research was built on the principle of reciprocity, and the relationship I shared with child co-researchers is what I found most rewarding. I enjoyed working alongside and spending time with child co-researchers through participating in meaningful occupations such as playing local games, having guided walks, engaging in group discussions, and storytelling, amongst many others. As the project was coming to an end, I found it important to wrap up the project with child co-researchers, families, and extended community members, especially since I was travelling back to Canada to finish my PhD education. The dissemination process initiated the farewell process, but there were also additional sessions after dissemination where child co-researchers asked me to visit the village, play games, and spend time as a way of ending this process. These last few sessions worked as a reminder that this phase of the project was coming to an end. Additionally, specific activities were carried out to facilitate the exiting process, such as, writing notes to one another, playing games for the last time that child co-researchers enjoyed doing as a group, and spending time in locations that were special for the group within their village. These shared occupations that were embedded throughout this project are what brought a sense of community within the group.

Debbie

In my role as a PhD supervisor, I have had the opportunity to work with many developing scholars who are committed to enacting occupation-based scholarship that spans the knowledge to action continuum. The challenges of spanning this continuum within the timeline of a PhD dissertation, along with the institutional rules and procedures for completion of a doctorate, are numerous (Farias et al., 2017; Gibbon, 2002). In addition, given the time commitment required for participatory action research, the unpredictability of its process and outcomes, and the focus on social transformation, concerns have been raised regarding the risks incurred by emerging activist-scholars who are challenged to meet increasing funding, publication, and other metrics to obtain tenure and other forms of academic security within neoliberal contexts (Denzin, 2009; Richter et al., 2020). Working with Tanya, and other PhD students, had led me to focus on participatory action research as an on-going process, that can be initiated and carried out in diverse ways, responsive to both the institutional demands that doctoral students and scholars must negotiate and the contextual specificities of co-researchers and their socio-political conditions. In particular, the guiding participatory action research principles presented in this chapter (see Table 11.2), which were generated through collaboration among several doctoral students and faculty, have been particularly helpful in mentoring students in carrying out this form of research in ethical ways aligned with an on-going commitment of working towards equitable participation and social transformation.

Moving forward, using participatory action research may require doctoral students and scholars to think outside typical funding sources and typical formats for research articles considering; for example, writing papers that address critical reflexivity processes, methods for engaging community members as co-researchers, and challenges to realizing equitable participation and ways forwards in negotiating these. Moreover, as a community of scholars, given the relevance, utility, and commensurability of participatory action research with occupation-focused scholarship and social transformation, occupational scientists and occupational therapists have a role to play in transforming the institutional barriers, within and outside universities, that work against conducting participatory action research that is aligned with critical, participatory, and transformative paradigms. This can involve working with institutional ethics boards to enhance understanding of what it means to work with community members as co-researchers rather than as research subjects, and collaboratively discussing how ethics forms and procedures can be attuned to this form of research. It can also involve advocating with and for doctoral students and emerging scholars to adapt timelines and evaluation procedures to support engagement in participatory action research.

Conclusion

In this chapter we have positioned and discussed participatory action research as a research approach that embodies a variety of methods and methodologies underpinned by critical, transformative, and/or participatory paradigms. The range of methods and methodologies utilized within participatory action research need to be taken up in ways that align with tenets of equitable participation of community members as co-researchers along with a commitment to enacting sustainable social transformation through addressing contextual forces shaping situations of injustices. The uptake of participatory action research within occupational science and therapy has potential to mobilize disciplinary commitments to addressing global issues relevant to occupation and expand focus of interventions from individual to community/population levels.

References

Akwataghibe, N. N., Ogunsola, E. A., Popoola, O. A., Agbo, A. I., & Dieleman, M. A. (2021). Using participatory action research to improve immunization utilization in areas with pockets of unimmunized children in Nigeria. *Health Research Policy and Systems, 19*(2), 1–14. https://doi.org/10.1186/s12961-021-00719-9

Albuquerque, S., & Farias, L. (2022). Occupational therapists' perceptions of the need to enact health promotion in community development through occupational justice. *Cadernos Brasileiros de Terapia Ocupacional, 30*(spe), e3070. https://doi.org/10.1590/2526-8910.ctoAO23253070

Bailliard, A. L. (2015). Video methodologies in research: Unlocking the complexities of occupation. *Canadian Journal of Occupational Therapy, 82*(1), 35–43. https://doi.org/10.1177%2F0008417414556883

Baum, F., MacDougall, C., & Smith, D. (2006). Participatory action research. *Journal of Epidemiology & Community Health, 60*(10), 854–857. https://doi.org/10.1136/jech.2004.028662

Benjamin-Thomas, T. E., & Laliberte Rudman, D. (2018). A critical interpretive synthesis: Use of the occupational justice framework in research. *Australian Occupational Therapy Journal, 65*(1), 3–14. https://doi.org/10.1111/1440-1630.12428

Benjamin-Thomas, T. E., Corrado, A. M., McGrath, C., Laliberte Rudman, D., & Hand, C. (2018). Working towards the promise of participatory action research: Learning from ageing research exemplars. *International Journal of Qualitative Methods, 17*(1), 1–13. https://doi.org/10.1177%2F1609406918817953

Benjamin-Thomas, T. E., Laliberte Rudman, D., Gunaseelan, J., Abraham, V. J., Cameron, D., McGrath, C., & Vinoth Kumar, S. P. (2019b). A participatory filmmaking process with children with disabilities in rural India: Working towards inclusive research. *Methodological Innovations, 12*(3), 2059799119890795. https://doi.org/10.1177/2059799119890795

Benjamin-Thomas, T. E., Rudman, D. L., & Thomas, D. M. (2021). Enacting contextually responsive scholarship: Centring occupation in participatory action research with children in India. *South African Journal of Occupational Therapy, 51*(4), 22–31. http://dx.doi.org/10.17159/2310-3833/2021/vol51n4a4

Benjamin-Thomas, T. E., Rudman, D. L., McGrath, C., Cameron, D., Abraham, V. J., Gunaseelan, J., & Vinothkumar, S. P. (2022). Situating occupational injustices experienced by children with disabilities in rural India within sociocultural, economic, and systemic conditions. *Journal of Occupational Science, 29*(1), 97–114. https://doi.org/10.1080/14427591.2021.1899038

Bennett, S., Whitehead, M., Eames, S., Fleming, J., Low, S., & Caldwell, E. (2016). Building capacity for knowledge translation in occupational therapy: Learning through participatory action research. *BMC Medical Education, 16*(257), 1–11. https://doi.org/10.1186/s12909-016-0771-5

Blakeney, A. B., & Marshall, A. (2009). Water quality, health, and human occupations. *American Journal of Occupational Therapy, 63*(1), 46–57. https://doi.org/10.5014/ajot.63.1.46

Brydon-Miller, M. (2008). Ethics and action research: Deepening our commitment to principles of social justice and redefining systems of democratic practice. In P. Reason & H. Bradbury (Eds.), *The SAGE handbook of action research: Participative inquiry and practice* (pp. 199–2010). SAGE.

Cargo, M., & Mercer, S. L. (2008). The value and challenges of participatory research: Strengthening its practice. *Annual Review of Public Health, 29*, 325–350. https://doi.org/10.1146/annurev. publhealth.29.091307.083824

Charmaz, K. (2006). *Constructing grounded theory: A practical guide through qualitative analysis.* SAGE.

Cockburn, L., & Trentham, B. (2002). Participatory action research: Integrating community occupational therapy practice and research. *Canadian Journal of Occupational Therapy, 69*(1), 20–30. https://doi.org/10.1177/000841740206900102

Corrado, A. M., Benjamin-Thomas, T. E., McGrath, C., Hand, C., & Laliberte Rudman, D. (2020). Participatory action research with older adults: A critical interpretive synthesis. *The Gerontologist, 60*(5), e413–e427. https://doi.org/10.1093/geront/gnz080

Crabtree, J. L., Wall, J. M., & Ohm, D. (2016a). Critical reflections on participatory action research in a prison setting: Toward occupational justice. *OTJR: Occupation, Participation and Health, 36*(4), 244–252. https://doi.org/10.1177%2F1539449216669132

Crabtree, J. L., Ohm, D., Wall, J. M., & Ray, J. (2016b). Evaluation of a prison occupational therapy informal education program: A pilot study. *Occupational Therapy International, 23*(4), 401–411. https://doi.org/10.1002/oti.1442

Crotty, M. (1998). *The foundations of social research: Meaning and perspective in the research process.* SAGE.

Denzin, N. K. (2009). *Qualitative inquiry and social justice: Toward a politics of hope.* Left Coast Press.

Devlin, R., & Pothier, D. (2006). Introduction: Toward a critical theory of dis-citizenship. In. D. Pothier & R. Devlin (Eds.), *Critical disability theory: Essays in philosophy, politics, policy, and law* (pp. 1–24). UBC Press.

Elwood, S. (2007). Negotiating participatory ethics in the midst of institutional ethics. *ACME: An International Journal for Critical Geographies, 6*(3), 329–338.

Enosh, G., & Ben-Ari, A. (2016). Reflexivity: The creation of liminal spaces—Researchers, participants, and research encounters. *Qualitative Health Research, 26*(4), 578–584. https://doi.org/1 0.1177%2F1049732315587878

Fals Borda, O. (2006). Participatory (action) research in social theory: Origins and challenges. In P. Reason & H. Bradbury (Eds.), *Handbook of action research* (pp. 27–37). SAGE.

Farias, L., Laliberte Rudman, D., Magalhães, L., & Gastaldo, D. (2017). Reclaiming the potential of transformative scholarship to enable social justice. *International Journal of Qualitative Methods, 16*(1), 1–10. https://doi.org/10.1177/1609406917714161

Farias, L., Laliberte Rudman, D., Pollard, N., Schiller, S., Serrata Malfitano, A. P., Thomas, K., & van Bruggen, H. (2019). Critical dialogical approach: A methodological direction for occupation-based social transformative work. *Scandinavian Journal of Occupational Therapy, 26*(4), 235–245. https://doi.org/10.1080/11038128.2018.1469666

Fazio, L. S. (2017). *Developing occupation-centered programs with the community* (3rd ed.). SLACK.

Fine, M., & Barreras, R. (2001). To be of use. *Analysis of Social Issues and Public Policy, 1*, 175–182.

Fine, M., Torre, M. E., Boudin, K., Bowen, I., Clark, J., Hylton, D., Martinez, M., Roberts, R. A., Smart, P., & Upegui, D. (2003). Participatory action research: From within and beyond prison bars. In P. M. Camic, J. E. Rhodes, & L. Yardley (Eds.), *Qualitative research in psychology: Expanding perspectives in methodology and design* (pp. 173–198). American Psychological Association. https://doi.org/10.1037/10595-010

Foronda, C., Baptiste, D. L., Reinholdt, M. M., & Ousman, K. (2016). Cultural humility: A concept analysis. *Journal of Transcultural Nursing*, *27*(3), 210–217. https://doi.org/10.1177%2F1043659615592677

Freire, P. (1993). *Pedagogy of the oppressed*. Penguin Books.

Gibbon, M. (2002). Doing a doctorate using a participatory action research framework in the context of community health. *Qualitative Health Research*, *12*(4), 546–558. https://doi.org/10.1177%2F104973202129120061

Glassman, M., & Erdem, G. (2014). Participatory action research and its meanings: Vivencia, praxis, conscientization. *Adult Education Quarterly*, *64*(3), 206–221. https://doi.org/10.1177%2F0741713614523667

Gonçalves, M. V., & Malfitano, A. P. S. (2020). Brazilian youth experiencing poverty: Everyday life in the favela. *Journal of Occupational Science*, *27*(3), 311–326. https://doi.org/10.1080/14427591.2020.1757495

Gubrium, A., Harper, K., & Otañez, M. (Eds.). (2015). Introduction. In *Participatory visual and digital research in action* (pp. 15–37). Left Coast Press.

Guillemin, M., & Gillam, L. (2004). Ethics, reflexivity, and "ethically important moments" in research. *Qualitative Inquiry*, *10*(2), 261–280. https://doi.org/10.1177%2F1077800403262360

Heron, J., & Reason, P. (1997). A participatory inquiry paradigm. *Qualitative Inquiry*, *3*(3), 274–294. https://doi.org/10.1177%2F107780049700300302

Hickey, S., & Mohan, G. (2005). Relocating participation in a radical politics of development. *Development & Change*, *36*(2), 237–262. https://doi.org/10.1111/j.0012-155X.2005.00410.x

Hocking, C. (2012). Occupations through the looking glass: Reflecting on occupational scientists' ontological assumptions. In G. E. Whiteford & C. Hocking (Eds.), *Occupational science: Society, inclusion, participation* (pp. 54–66). Wiley-Blackwell.

Kemmis, S. (2006). Participatory action research and the public sphere. *Education Action Research*, *14*(4), 459–476. https://doi.org/10.1080/09650790600975593

Kemmis, S., McTaggart, R., & Nixon, R. (Eds.). (2014). *The action research planner: Doing critical participatory action research*. Springer.

Kidd, S. A., & Kral, M. J. (2005). Practicing participatory action research. *Journal of Counseling Psychology*, *52*(2), 187–195. https://psycnet.apa.org/doi/10.1037/0022-0167.52.2.187

Klocker, N. (2012). Doing participatory action research and doing a PhD: Words of encouragement for prospective students. *Journal of Geography in Higher Education*, *36*(1), 149–163. https://doi.org/10.1080/03098265.2011.589828

Koch, T., Mann, S., Kralik, D., & van Loon, A. M. (2005). Reflection: Look, think and act cycles in participatory action research. *Journal of Research in Nursing*, *10*(3), 261–278. https://doi.org/10.1177%2F174498710501000304

Kramer-Roy, D. (2011). Occupational injustice in Pakistani families with disabled children in the UK: A PAR study. In F. Kronenberg, N. Pollard, & D. Sakellariou (Eds.), *Occupational therapy without borders volume 2: Towards an ecology of occupation-based practices* (pp. 385–393). Elsevier Churchill Livingston.

Law, M. (1997). Changing disabling environments through participatory action research: A Canadian experience. In S. E. Smith, D. G. Willms, & N. A. Johnson (Eds.), *Nurtured by knowledge: Learning to do participatory action-research* (pp. 34–58). The Apex Press.

Laliberte Rudman, D. (2018). Occupational therapy and occupational science: Building critical and transformative alliances. *Cadernos Brasileiros de Terapia Ocupacional*, *26*(1), 241–249. https://doi.org/10.4322/2526-8910.ctoEN1246

Laliberte Rudman, D. (2019). Transformative scholarship: Possibilities and challenges for radical forms of participation. *Japanese Journal of Occupational Science, 13*, 21–31.

Letts, L. (2003). Occupational therapy and participatory research: A partnership worth pursuing. *American Journal of Occupational Therapy, 57*(1), 77–87. https://doi.org/10.5014/ajot.57.1.77

Magalhães, L., Farias, L., Rivas-Quarneti, N., Alvarez, L., & Malfitano, A. P. S. (2019). The development of occupational science outside the Anglophone sphere: Enacting global collaboration. *Journal of Occupational Science, 26*(2), 181–192. https://doi.org/10.1080/14427591.2018.15 30133

Maiter, S., Simich, L., Jacobson, N., & Wise, J. (2008). Reciprocity: An ethic for community-based participatory action research. *Action Research, 6*, 305–325. https://doi.org/10.1177 %2F1476750307083720

Miles, M. B., Huberman, A. M., & Saldaña, J. (2014). *Qualitative data analysis: A methods sourcebook*. SAGE.

Meekosha, H., & Shuttleworth, R. (2009). What's so 'critical' about critical disability studies? *Australian Journal of Human Rights, 15*(1), 47–75. https://doi.org/10.1080/13232 38X.2009.11910861

Njelesani, J., Gibson, B. E., Nixon, S., Cameron, D., & Polatajko, H. (2013). Toward a critical occupational approach to research. *International Journal of Qualitative Methods, 12*, 207–220. https://doi.org/10.1177/160940691301200109

Pettican, A., Speed, E., Bryant, W., Kilbride, C., & Beresford, P. (2022). Levelling the playing field: Exploring inequalities and exclusions with a community-based football league for people with experience of mental distress. *Australian Occupational Therapy Journal, 69*(3), 290–300. https:// doi.org/10.1111/1440-1630.12791

Ponterotto, J. (2005). Qualitative research in counseling psychology: A primer on research paradigms and philosophy of science. *Journal of Counseling Psychology, 52*(2), 126–136. https://doi. org/10.1037/0022-0167.52.2.126

Potts, K. L., & Brown, L. (2015). Becoming an anti-oppressive researcher. In S. Strega & L. Brown (Eds.), *Research as resistance: Revisiting critical, indigenous, and antioppressive approaches* (2nd ed., pp. 17–42). Canadian Scholars' Press.

Ravenek, M. J., & Laliberte Rudman, D. (2013). Bridging conceptions of quality in moments of qualitative research. *International Journal of Qualitative Methods, 12*(1), 436–456. https://doi. org/10.1177%2F160940691301200122

Richter, J., Faragó, F., Swadener, B. B., Roca-Servat, D., & Eversman, K. A. (2020). Tempered radicalism and intersectionality: Scholar-activism in the neoliberal university. *Journal of Social Issues, 76*(4), 1014–1035. https://doi.org/10.1111/josi.12401

Saldaña, J. (2016). *The coding manual for qualitative researchers*. SAGE.

Sandwick, T., Fine, M., Greene, A.C., Stoudt, B.G., Torre, M.E., & Patel, L. (2018). Promise and provocation: Humble reflections on critical participatory action research for social policy. *Urban Education, 52*(4), 472–502. https://doi.org/10.1177%2F0042085918763513

Schwandt, T. A. (2001). *Dictionary of qualitative inquiry*. SAGE.

Shearn, K., Brook, A., Humphreys, H., & Wardle, C. (2022). Mixed methods participatory action research to inform service design based on the Capabilities Approach, in the North of England. *Children & Society, 36*(4), 450–471. https://doi.org/10.1111/chso.12496

St John, B. M., Hladik, E., Romaniak, H. C., & Ausderau, K. K. (2018). Understanding health disparities for individuals with intellectual disability using photovoice. *Scandinavian Journal of Occupational Therapy, 25*(5), 371–381. https://doi.org/10.1080/11038128.2018.1502349

Suarez-Balcazar, Y., Martinez, L. I., & Casas-Byots, C. (2005). A participatory action research approach for identifying health service needs of Hispanic immigrants: Implications for occupational therapy. *Occupational Therapy in Health Care, 19*(1–2), 145–163. https://doi.org/10.1080/ J003v19n01_11

Taylor, R. R., Braveman, B., & Hammel, J. (2004). Developing and evaluating community-based services through participatory action research: Two case examples. *American Journal of Occupational Therapy, 58*(1), 73–82. https://doi.org/10.5014/ajot.58.1.73

Tervalon, M., & Murray-Garcia, J. (1998). Cultural humility versus cultural competence: A critical distinction in defining physician training outcomes in multicultural education. *Journal of Health Care for the Poor and Underserved, 9*(2), 117–125. https://doi.org/10.1353/hpu.2010.0233

Townsend, E., Birch, D. E., Langley, J., & Langille, L. (2000). Participatory research in a mental health clubhouse. *The Occupational Therapy Journal of Research, 20*(1), 18–44. https://doi.org/10.1177%2F153944920002000102

Tracy, S. J. (2010). Qualitative quality: Eight "big-tent" criteria for excellent qualitative research. *Qualitative Inquiry, 16*, 837–851. https://doi.org/10.1177%2F1077800410383121

Trentham, B. L., & Neysmith, S. M. (2018). Exercising senior citizenship in an ageist society through participatory action research: A critical occupational perspective. *Journal of Occupational Science, 25*(2), 174–190. https://doi.org/10.1080/14427591.2017.1402809

Turcotte, P. L., Carrier, A., & Levasseur, M. (2019). Community-based participatory research remodelling occupational therapy to foster older adults' social participation. *Canadian Journal of Occupational Therapy, 86*(4), 262–276. https://doi.org/10.1177%2F0008417419832338

Van Niekerk, L., Lorenzo, T., & Mdlokolo, P. (2006). Understanding partnerships in developing disabled entrepreneurs through participatory action research. *Disability and Rehabilitation, 28*(5), 323–331. https://doi.org/10.1080/09638280500166425

Wilding, C., & Whiteford, G. (2008). Language, identity and representation: Occupation and occupational therapy in acute settings. *Australian Occupational Therapy Journal, 55*(3), 180–187. https://doi.org/10.1111/j.1440-1630.2007.00678.x

Additional Resources

Asaba, E., & Suarez-Balcazar, Y. (2018). Participatory research: A promising approach to promote meaningful engagement. *Scandinavian Journal of Occupational Therapy, 25*(5), 309–312. https://doi.org/10.1080/11038128.2018.1541224

Benjamin-Thomas, T. E., Laliberte Rudman, D., Cameron, D., & Batorowicz, B. (2019a). Participatory digital methodologies: Potential of three approaches for advancing transformative occupation-based research with children and youth. *Journal of Occupational Science, 26*(4), 559–574. https://doi.org/10.1080/14427591.2018.1512054

Gubrium, A., & Harper, K. (2013). *Participatory visual and digital methods.* Left Coast Press.

Lunch, N., & Lunch, C. (2006). *Insights into participatory video: A handbook for the field.* InsightShare. Retrieved from https://insightshare.org/resources/insights-into-participatory-video-a-handbook-for-the-field/

Reason, P., & Bradbury, H. (Eds.). (2008). *The SAGE handbook of action research.* SAGE.

12 Visual Arts-Based Methodologies

Laura R. Bowman and Katie Mah

Drawing, painting, sculpting, and coloring are among the most universal and instinctual ways of communicating. From a very young age, children share their experiences of the real and the imagined through creating pictures and sculptures. Throughout society, visual art (painting, sculpture, other created visual representations) are commonplace in homes, buildings, and museums to display the experiences, values, and tone that mark that space. The ubiquity of the use of visuals to communicate experiences in our everyday lives lends to their importance as means of communicating knowledge and experiences in research, despite often being overlooked.

In this chapter, we present how visual arts-based methodologies can be used to drive understandings of human occupations. A 'visual arts-based methodology' does not represent a single methodology but a swell of arts-based methods for data generation, interpretation, and analysis. Such methods have gained traction in occupational science and occupational therapy research due to a need to more deeply and differently explore human engagement and experience (or the multifaceted concept of occupation). One important offering of visual arts-based methodologies is their potential, when deployed reflexively, to destabilize the power differential inherent in the research relationship (further discussed in later sections), by acknowledging the value of participants' first-hand accounts of their health- and disability-related experiences, and inviting participants into the early stages of analysis and interpretation. By illuminating such perspectives through research, the knowledge produced becomes more rich, nuanced, and diverse, as do the practice changes that derive from such an evidence-base.

We will focus specifically on methods of arts-based data generation and visual data analysis. Arts-based research can focus on any number of media—from the visual arts (our area of focus) to the performative (dance, theatre), literary (fiction, story, poetry), musical (songs, sounds) and others. Due to the variation of methodologies across media, this chapter focuses specifically on research that considers the *visual* arts, and marries it with methods of visual analysis, or of what can be seen and interpreted (Pink, 2003; Rose, 2016). We discuss visual arts-based research methodologies as means through which to explore the multiplicity and complexity of human occupation from the perspectives of those who are often excluded from research participation.

We draw on examples from our individual programs of research, both of which center the knowledge and experience of children living with acquired brain injury (ABI). Throughout the chapter, we highlight the similarities and differences of the specific visual arts-based research methods we employed to illustrate why and how they were engaged, as well as their potential implications for research, clinical, and policy outcomes. *"Freaked out" by pediatric concussion: An exploration of drawing and interview data produced by*

DOI: 10.4324/9781003456216-12

children 'at risk' and living with concussion (Mah et al., 2020; henceforth "Katie's study") was a critical qualitative arts-based research project that combined drawing with semi-structured interviewing methods to explore with young people the multiplicity and complexity of childhood concussion as a social phenomenon. *The embodied return to school after ABI* (Bowman et al., in preparation; henceforth "Laura's study") was a body map storytelling project undertaken with elementary school-aged individuals who experienced ABI to explore the embodied journey of returning to school. Both projects used drawing-based methodologies to: (a) explore, with participants, a health-related experience; (b) invite young people into data generation and the early stages of analysis and interpretation; and (c) enable us, as critical qualitative researchers, to explore the effects of contemporary clinical practices on the everyday lives of young people following ABI.

Epistemology, Ontology, Axiology

Research is always and inevitably imbued with assumptions concerning the nature of knowledge and how we know what we know; specifically, what constitutes knowledge, how knowledge is produced, and who is considered knowledgeable in research (Lincoln et al., 2011). Such epistemological assumptions, however, often remain unacknowledged or implicit in published research. In this section we make explicit the epistemological, ontological, and axiological assumptions of visual arts-based methodologies with the goal of increasing the accessibility of such methods to the 'visual-curious' occupational scientist or occupational therapist.

In approaching this section, it is tantamount that we engage in critical reflexivity, acknowledging our own positioning along the continuum of research paradigms, and how this positioning shapes how we have engaged visual arts-based research methods in our respective projects (we return to discuss reflexivity later in this chapter). More specifically, we approach our visual arts-based research studies from the critical social paradigm of inquiry.

While the examples we draw on in this chapter emerge from our critical work, we acknowledge the varied contributions of scholars operating from the constructivist paradigm of inquiry. Both paradigms share an important ontological assumption about the nature of knowledge in relation to visual imagery, including that visual images and objects are never transparent windows into the world (Rose, 2016; Yates, 2010). Indeed, from our critical social stance, we insist that the types of knowledge that are most often accessed through this type of visual arts-based methodology are situated within conflicting social, political, cultural, economic, gender, and identity structures. Additionally, from our axiological perspective, we ourselves (as researchers, practitioners, and holders of many other forms of privilege) bring additional complexity to our research interactions, which must be acknowledged and honored. As such, we and our fellow visual arts-based researchers seek ways to explore and construct knowledge so that we may shift power balances towards equity for groups who are typically marginalized from such acts. As Rose (2016) suggested of visual images and objects, "they interpret the world; they display it in very particular ways; they represent it" (p. 2). That is, rather than offering an objective and self-evident reflection of some supposed 'truth' of the world, visual images and objects are *constructed*; for example, through talk, text, and media. Rose's description highlights the potential of visual images (and the process of their creation) to connect previously disconnected understandings to form new knowledge and promote action.

As researchers operating from a critical social paradigm, we must also attend to the effects of visual materials. Of note, we do not use the term 'effect' to refer to cause and effect, effect size, nor any other concept typically equated with positivist, quantitative research. Instead, we use 'effect' as an English language verb meaning "to cause to come into being" (Cambridge Dictionary, n.d.). From our critical social perspective, we believe visual materials to have their own agency, in that they are not merely put out into the social world to exist 'as is.' Rather, they produce an effect, or *do* something in the social world. As researchers, it is our task to attend to what images do, including the social differences and categories they offer visions of, including those of class, race, gender, age, generation, and able-bodiedness (Rose, 2016). Moreover, as critical researchers, we must attend to the power relations circulating through our research, including through the researcher-participant relationship, and through the visual products of our research (Mah et al., 2020; Rose, 2016). We return to this discussion of power, and to the effects of visual products later in the chapter.

In light of the above understanding of 'the visual,' the visual arts-based methods and methodologies that are the focus of this chapter are discordant with the positivist paradigm of inquiry, which assumes a stable and unchanging reality existing 'out there,' waiting to be found by the objective researcher (Creswell & Poth, 2016). Such an ontology is incompatible with our own assumptions, and with the very nature of visual research which is concerned not with some objective 'truth' of what can be seen, but with the *meaning* attributed to what can be seen (Prosser, 2011). With this understanding of the visual as constructed, visual images and objects cannot be taken at face value in research but must be analyzed and interpreted.

Topics and Questions Best Suited to Visual/Arts-Based Methodologies

As outlined by Mah et al. (2020), when contemplating the adoption of visual arts-based research methodologies appropriate regard must be given to the 'fit' between the method and question being explored:

> As with any method, the potential of the ABR [arts-based research] context must be considered in concert with the research topic and population to posit whether participant and researcher will be able to co-construct knowledge that will be useful and relevant to the research question.
>
> (p. 2973)

Rather than defining a narrow set of criteria for the types of research topics and questions that might be explored using visual arts-based methodologies, we outline a number of common considerations in Tables 12.1 and 12.2. We have constructed these considerations, and 'pause and reflect' prompts, through our own experiences contemplating the uptake of visual arts-based research methods, our interactions with the substantive literature on visual and arts-based methods in research with young people, and our social interactions with visual-curious and novice visual researchers in health and rehabilitation.

Table 12.1 Common reasons for considering a visual arts-based methodology

Consideration	Pause and reflect
My population does not—or prefers not to—communicate verbally	A great thought to consider in both research and clinical practice. Art is *one* other way that people can communicate. We encourage you to stop and consider how your population *does* communicate, or chooses to communicate, which may or may not include through arts-based modes of expression.

(Continued)

Table 12.1 (Continued)

Consideration	Pause and reflect
My topic is really complex	Excellent! Then it is perhaps also a topic that is unexplored, underexplored, or underrepresented in research. Will a visual arts-based medium enable participants to reflect upon and perhaps reconsider their experience, or how best to represent that experience? Will it provide a way to reorganize or re-conceptualize their thoughts? Might an arts-based activity be *part* of your approach to research (an elicitation tool) rather than your sole means of generating data? Will the expectation to produce a visual arts-based representation be overwhelming for your participants?
I want to work with children	Fantastic! Actively engaging children in research that concerns them is an important move toward occupational justice and achieving more equitable representation in research. Children communicate in *a number of* meaningful ways. Take time to consider whether the reflective process of visual arts-based data generation will allow for the shared power and meaning-making needed to co-construct knowledge with your population and on your topic. Consider whether other methods such as observation, document/chart reviews, interviews, story creation or other performative arts-based methods might also be useful.
My population will not want to do 'art'	The visual arts-based products that are co-produced in research are considered and treated as data, not art. That said, if you determine that visual arts-based methods will enable the co-creation of useful and relevant knowledge in relation to your topic, we encourage you to use them. We remind our own participants that the aesthetic of the product (how 'beautiful' or 'neat' or 'creative' it ends up being) is not of concern, and certainly not why we engage such methods. We also remind them that we are researchers, not artists; and as researchers, it is the process of creating the product that is of interest to us. From this perspective, the product becomes a *tool* for connecting with, exploring, and making meaning in relation to the topic of inquiry.
'Art' will be a great way to share our findings	This is a common thought, to which we reply, "yes, and ..." Again, we remind readers that the products of the visual arts-based research process are data (rather than 'art') and must be represented as such. We also recommend discussing data ownership with participants (outlined in the ethics section below). Any plans to share or profit from the products must be considered alongside participants and vetted through an institutional research ethics board (even after the project has closed). We also acknowledge the importance of knowledge dissemination and mobilization. In an ongoing effort to shift knowledge and practice, the findings of research must be accessible to audiences. Tangible ways of connecting to audiences (beyond peer-reviewed publications) can help in that process. With that acknowledgement, we remind readers that producing novel dissemination tools is not reason enough to employ visual arts-based research methodologies. The methodology must first and foremost serve to answer the research question with the given population.

Author created

Table 12.2 Considerations when undertaking visual arts-based methodological inquiry

What type of knowledge?	Are you looking for historical accuracy and fact (veracity) or one's interpretation of their experience (e.g., narrative)? Is this a meaningful way for participants to consider and communicate their experiences?
Who is the target participant?	Consider their preferred mode of communication, interest, and ability to engage with visual arts-based media (e.g., vision, fine motor, fatigue)
What resources are available?	Do team members have the time, materials, and space to facilitate the data generation process? Does the team have expertise (or time and resources to learn/gain expertise) in relation to the philosophical underpinnings, methods of data generation, interpretation, and analysis adopted?
Who are the intended audiences for the constructed knowledge?	Different end-users (e.g., clinicians, policy-makers, advocates) have different information needs. Will the knowledge generated through your research meet the information needs of your target audience?
Is visual arts-based data the primary source of data?	Will you be using visual arts-based methods as the primary means of data generation? Or would the inclusion of visual arts-based methods be helpful as a secondary method of data generation? How might you incorporate visual arts-based data generation, interpretation, and dissemination methods most appropriately for your population, question, epistemological stance, and intended audience?

Author created

In our examples, we chose visual arts-based approaches to explore the experiences of populations who have historically had research conducted on or about them, rather than *with* them. Children living with ABI, who have been described as a 'doubly vulnerable' group by nature of their status as children and cognitive status (Boylan et al., 2009), have largely been excluded from research that concerns them. Their exclusion has been based on concerns of their ability to give historically accurate information, or worries about upsetting them by asking them to discuss a potentially sensitive topic. Such paternalistic exclusion has, however, also led to interventions and policies created without their expert knowledge, which runs the risk of not addressing their actual needs. We approached our respective studies with the following consideration: how might we amplify the voices of so-called vulnerable young people in the literature base, engaging them in research in ways that allow for their meaningful contribution to research that concerns them and produces knowledge regarding their occupational engagement?

Katie's study, which aimed to investigate, challenge, and transform conventional ways of thinking and knowing about concussion and children, invited young people (ages 6–18 years) with and without lived experience of concussion into research as 'knowers.' That is, as experts in their own lives, with the capacity for insight into their health-related experiences, and the competence to recount their experiences through research (Clark & Statham, 2005; Grover, 2004; Kortesluoma et al., 2003; Mah et al., 2021; Morrow, 2008). Participants were invited into data generation and the first stage of data analysis and interpretation. Guided by a Foucauldian-informed conceptual framework (Mah et al., 2020), Katie examined how young people's conceptualizations of concussion were shaped by taken-for-granted assumptions of childhood vulnerability, risk, and responsibility (or what is termed the Pediatric Concussion Discourse) (Mah et al., 2020, 2022).

Laura's team employed a body map storytelling methodology (Solomon, 2007) to explore and highlight the experiences of children (ages 6–13 years) in transitioning from hospital to school following ABI. The co-produced body maps were intended to highlight the children's journeys back to school, and highlight practical aspects of the return-to-school experience that were notably absent from the research-base and school guidelines. Both studies (highlighted in Textbox 12.1) explored children and young people's perceptions of living with ABI, and through the methods, allowed for shared meaning-making in the creative and interview processes.

Textbox 12.1   Example Questions Explored Through Visual Arts-Based Research

In Katie's study, the primary aim was to investigate, challenge, and transform conventional ways of thinking and knowing about concussion and children (Mah et al., 2022). She asked:

1 How does the Pediatric Concussion Discourse (PCD) produce and constrain how children can think and act in relation to pediatric concussion? and
2 How do children 'at risk' of and living with concussion respond to the PCD?

Data were co-produced with participants through drawing (with the option to write) and semi-structured interviewing methods. Drawing was selected to enable participants to actively engage in the co-construction of knowledge while removing the demand of an immediate response as might be expected with words-based methods alone. This provided participants with the temporal space to reflect on a topic they may not have thought about explicitly before (Clark, 2010; Guillemin, 2004; Literat, 2013). Generating drawings in this study allowed for a reflective, meaning-making process that also provided an analyzable product. The inclusion of semi-structured interviews (a words-based method) made it possible for young people to engage in the first stage of analysis and interpretation in situ (i.e., in the research setting), sharing with Katie what their drawings represented, as well as their imagined intended audience.

Beyond the research setting, participant data (drawings, interviews) were additionally analyzed through the Foucauldian-informed theoretical framework guiding the study. This allowed Katie to work toward the broader theoretical aim of the study, accounting for the ways in which young people's conceptualizations of concussion were re/produced by the PCD, as well as how young people negotiated and/or resisted the PCD in their everyday lives. The findings of the study have implications for practice across sectors (e.g., health, education, family, policy).

In Laura's study, the goal was to consider the first-hand accounts of primary and middle school-aged children that were returning to school following an ABI. The questions were:

1 How do children experience the return-to-school journey following an ABI from social, educational, and environmental perspectives? and
2 What are children's experiences of the challenges, barriers, and facilitating factors of their return to community and school following ABI?

Data were co-produced through a body map storytelling process modified from that of Solomon (2007) to suit the topic and participant group. The approach was chosen to allow for reflection, recall, and a common language in the construction of the children's narratives. The strengths-focused methodology aligned with the researcher's and institution's solution-focused practice, and promoted the consideration of factors related to strengths, abilities, and resiliency that were notably absent from the relevant literature on transition to school following ABI for children at the time of the study.

We provide two points of reflection when considering the uptake of visual arts-based methodologies in research with children. The first is not to mistake the common use of visual artistic expression with children as an invitation to use arts-based research to address all research questions with all children. Children learn through play and self-expression, and the arts often play a large part in their occupations as children. Art, however, is not always the most appropriate way to approach a research question, regardless of the population's age or communicative abilities. The second is that visual arts-based research can be resource intensive (time, space, materials, coordination) in relation to data generation, analysis and interpretation, and storage. This intensity should be weighed against what the researcher expects to gain in relation to the production of new knowledge when approaching the research question.

Beyond our own work, visual arts-based approaches are being used to explore human occupation in a number of ways (see Textbox 12.2).

Textbox 12.2   What Is Being Explored in the Occupation-Based Literature?

- In exploring occupational engagement in society, the use of body map storytelling has been used to explore resilience and settlement of refugee youth (Davy et al., 2014) and those of undocumented workers in Canada (Gastaldo et al., 2013).
- Huot et al. (2022) used occupational mapping to explore representations of everyday occupations during long-term unemployment.
- More classically clinical topics also use drawing to explore complex human experiences. In addition to our own work on experiences of ABI, Phillips et al. (2015) explored experiences of chronic pain using drawing and a critical visual analysis methodology.
- Visual arts-based methods are used to explore the practitioner experience as well, such as through the work of Botma and Labuschagne (2019) who used freehand drawings to explore interprofessional education experiences of healthcare trainees.

Recruitment and Sampling

The populations for whom visual arts-based research might be appropriate include those who would benefit from having ways of expressing themselves beyond or in addition to the words-based methods that are so often employed in qualitative health research. We were both intentional in incorporating visual arts-based methods in our respective studies, in addition to words-based methods, to provide an alternate form of expression to a population whose capacity to produce knowledge has often been questioned in research. Children diagnosed with ABI are commonly assumed to be unreliable sources of information, even with respect to their own experiences. They are also often regarded as innately vulnerable within the research relationship (Mah et al., 2020). While we do not discount concerns of vulnerability, we do caution that when such (generally unacknowledged) assumptions are left to circulate through research practices, the perspectives of so-called vulnerable populations remain unexamined. The risk of this practice is that entire bodies of research, clinical practices, and policies may be devoid of the perspectives of those they purport to serve. To avoid perpetuating such exclusionary practices in our own research, we sought research methods that would invite contributions through accessible and familiar modalities (such as drawing and arts) as opportunities for conducting research with (not simply 'about') children diagnosed with ABI.

Considerations for including children with cognitive impairments in research that will impact their care and well-being has its own growing literature base. Visual arts-based methodologies represent one way of engaging children with ABI in research, but authors such as Boylan (2009), Mealings et al. (2012), Teachman and Gibson (2013), and Mah et al. (2021) discuss the wide variety of ways to engage meaningfully with children and youth in research. While the methods of data generation and analysis vary across the studies highlighted in this chapter, both methodologies were deployed in ways that valued the representation of participants and their experiences in meaningful and contextually relevant ways.

When designing the sampling strategy for a visual arts-based research project, the identification of individuals who can provide a deep understanding of the topic at hand is of utmost importance. To avoid perpetuating the exclusion of particular groups from research we recommend seeking their first-hand accounts in research that concerns them, even if this proves difficult. In making this recommendation, we do not suggest that generating knowledge with other sources (e.g., parents, clinicians, educators) might not also be warranted. These groups can be approached to provide contextually-relevant or supplementary knowledge, or when the unit of analysis is the child's social relationship to another. But, when possible, we aim to always engage the population of interest in our research as experts in their own lives (Mah et al., 2022).

When recruiting participants for studies using visual arts-based methods of data generation, creativity in accommodating participants' impairment-related needs (e.g., physical, cognitive, and communicative needs) may be required. For example, when recruiting children with ABI to participate in body map storytelling, Laura's team considered how historical recall, verbal communication, attention span, fatigue, and physical limitation (resulting from or co-occurring with ABI onset) might impact data generation. The research team decided that some impairment-related needs could be accommodated for, some could not, and some impairment-related needs were not 'needs' at all given the study's focus. For example, fatigue could be accommodated by breaking the research into multiple sessions and taking breaks when requested, but an attention span of 20-minute activity blocks was strongly encouraged. The ability to hold/manipulate art supplies (e.g., markers, paint brushes) was not required, and participants could direct others (researcher, parent) to draw/paint what they wanted instead. Functional vision was made a requirement to create and reflect upon the visual body map. Accurate historical recall was not deemed a requirement because participants were being asked to share their experiences rather than the 'facts' of those health-related experiences. After deciding which common ABI-related considerations would impact recruitment, Laura's team connected with participants regarding how they could be involved in the study and provided examples of how the study procedures could and could not be adjusted to accommodate specific needs.

Once recruitment parameters are outlined in alignment with the research topic/questions and the practicalities of research participation, active recruitment can proceed. Laura's study team recruited participants through flyers that were mostly text-based and included a small image to indicate the arts-based nature of the study. Recruitment strategies also included online advertisements on institutional and local association websites, as well as through service providers in the area of pediatric ABI rehabilitation. Katie's study team recruited participants in person at a local science center which was hosting a science exhibit on the human brain. Science center attendees were welcome to participate in a number of studies related to concussion, and Katie's study was among them.

The required number of participants also differed between the two studies. Katie's study delved into a relatively unexplored question, and asked fewer, broad questions. She sought more widespread input from a larger sample to begin to collect experiences and thoughts on the topic so that she might conceptualize a new area of knowledge that can impact practice and policy. Laura's study focused on a topic that has a great deal of research and evidence, and so she sought a few in-depth perspectives to uncover the nuanced experiences from a group of participants from whom such questions had not been asked. As with most qualitative research, there is no power calculation or magic number as to how many participants will allow you to fully address your question. We have found it helpful to think about data generation before number of participants. By this we mean that the researcher should first consider the amount, depth, and quality of the data that will be generated by each participant, and then consider how many participants will be needed to provide the breadth, depth, and diversity of experiences that the research questions require. For Katie, many perspectives on fewer questions were required to give her breadth and understanding of her novel topic. For Laura's question, the existing perspectives on the experiences and procedures of the return-to-school process were well known, so fewer in-depth data sets were most helpful to provide a volume of data on a depth of experience.

Data Generation Methods

In this section, we use the term 'data' rather than 'art' because the creation of the visual representation or output was driven by a research question. When undertaking a visual arts-based research study, the methods for data generation and analysis will vary, but can be considered along some of the parameters outlined below.

What Constitutes Data?

Data are conceptualized as a combination of 'process' and 'product.' The data generation *process* includes the activities, discussions, reflexive moments, and decisions that occur during the creation of the product (see Table 12.3 for examples). The *product* is the resulting visual item that was generated via the process. While one may take for granted that the created visual work (or product) will be considered a source of study data, this is not always the case. The generation of the product may be a mechanism through which meaning is co-constructed, but the product itself may be used solely as an elicitation device and might not be analyzed as data.

The arts-based data generation process may be recorded via video, audio, researcher notes (e.g., ethnographic fieldnotes, analytic memos) all of which should also be considered and treated as data. Additionally, participant reflections (e.g., through dialogue, journaling) may be considered sources of data, contributing important participant-generated insights that may be used to inform analysis and interpretation. Table 12.3 outlines data that can be generated over the course of an arts-based research project.

Table 12.3 Examples of process and product data

Process data	Product data
• Researcher–participant dialogue (recorded and/or transcribed) • The pace of the session • The tone of the session • Decision/choice points (what participants chose to include in their representation, what they chose to exclude) • Mistakes • Revisions • Researcher reflections • Participant reflections	• The visual representation • The aesthetic elements (colors, composition) of the representation • The viewpoint • Use of common imagery (metaphor, representation) and/or words • What is represented • What is not represented (or what is absent)

Author created

The Role of the Researcher

Visual arts-based methodologies, just like other modes of qualitative data inquiry, require the researcher to be 'creatively present' throughout the research process (Eakin & Gladstone, 2020). That is, rather than adopting the removed and objective stance expected of the positivist researcher, the methodologies require the researcher to use themselves as a resource in the analysis and interpretation of visual data produced through arts-based methods (we will return to this later). Said otherwise, the role of the visual arts-based researcher is an *active role*, of acknowledging and accounting for the co-constructive process of data generation, of interpreting and analyzing visual data, and accounting for the social circumstances in which the visual materials are created (e.g., the history, cultural, sociopolitical context) (Guillemin, 2004; Rose, 2016). As Rose (2016) explained, the visual must be understood as "embedded in the social world and only comprehensible when that embedding is taken into account" (xxii). In contrast to the positivist researcher, assumed neutral and objective, the visual researcher who operates from somewhere along the constructivist to critical social continuum is an active co-constructor of knowledge, whose history and values are necessarily imbued in the research process, and thus is inseparable from the knowledge produced (Lincoln et al., 2011; Thorogood & Green, 2009).

Participant Considerations

For populations with clinical involvements (e.g., cognitive, physical, age-related considerations), and in the name of equitable representation in research, it might be necessary to adapt methods. For example, the research team may adapt drawing or body-mapping materials or processes to allow for greater access for those with physical impairments (e.g., decreasing the scale of the project, adding more breaks, providing adapted art materials).

Researchers might also consider adapting the research protocol to allow for the participant to direct another person (researcher, caregiver) to create the visual product, if this is their preference, or if they are unable to access materials. For example, in Laura's study, one participant found it difficult to lower themselves to the floor in order to be traced, and so the paper was taped to the wall; another participant became fatigued and asked to guide the researcher in drawing what they described. These choices were not considered to compromise the integrity of the research process or the data that was generated, and allowed for development of trust and rapport in the research relationship.

Data Generation Procedures

The data generation procedures for visual arts-based projects can vary from a single prompt to a detailed stepwise process depending on the knowledge sought and the amount of direction the researcher has determined participants require. In Katie's study, participants were invited to respond to written prompts, producing a drawing representing their experience with and understanding of concussion (Figure 12.1). Participants who did not self-report a history of concussion were asked to produce a drawing in response to the phrase "When I hear the word concussion, I …". Participants with a self-reported history of concussion were asked to produce two drawings, one in response to the phrase "Before I had my concussion, I …", and a second in response to the phrase "Now, I …" Participants who did not wish to draw were given the option of responding with written text. This approach, wherein few prompts were provided, was chosen to allow for varied responses reflecting the multiplicity of experiences of concussion. For similar reasons, a decision was made not to audio/video record the creative process, allowing participants the time and space to quietly reflect on an abstract topic that they may not have considered before. Following the creation of their drawings, participants were invited to participate in a semi-structured interview to describe their visual (e.g., what was represented, their imagined audience, what they would share about concussion with that audience). During the interview, participants were invited to amend their visual, if desired, as their understanding of the topic changed. The co-constructed meaning-making that occurred during the interview was captured through audio recording, and through alterations made to the visual product. Constraints in the study setting limited researcher–participant interaction to one session. Data generation sessions were thus carefully crafted to enable the generation of rich data in one session only (e.g., in the decision to not record the creation of the visual, in the construction of the semi-structured interview guide).

Laura's study followed a structured body mapping protocol based on the work of Solomon's (2007) *Living with X* project. The protocol included 16 'steps' or prompts that allowed the researcher to walk the participant through their experience of transitioning from care to school following ABI. Examples of steps included tracing their body in a position that represented themselves and how they would like to be seen, representing those people and resources that supported them, identifying sources of power in their bodies, and creating representations of their journey (where they came from and where they imagine themselves going). Figure 12.2 demonstrates the shared participation in the protocol steps. The process facilitates the construction of the story of internal experiences and contextual influences, all mapped out around the individual at the center. Data generation took place over two to three sessions in order to respect the time, attention span, and fatigue of children living with ABI, and to allow for reflection between sessions. The data generation process included an initial interview, the detailed, stepwise body map

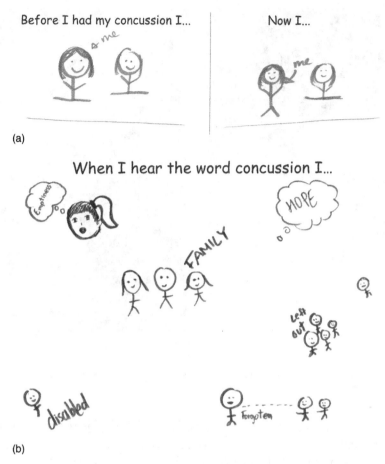

Figure 12.1 (a and b) Sample of visual data generated by Katie's participants. Author created.

storytelling protocol, and a request for the participant's final reflections on the created body map. The process invited ample time for reflection, discussion, and cultivation of a narrative that suited the child.

The body map storytelling process was detailed in the study's letter of information and consent so that potential participants understood what they were agreeing to before starting. Potential participants were asked if they wanted an adult caregiver present in the room at any point (e.g., during the interview for comfort/verification, to help move their body or manipulate materials, to trace their body rather than having the researcher do so). Participants were reminded at the start of each session that they could take breaks at any time or end a session at any point. Regular check-ins and verbal reconsenting were undertaken at the start of each session and throughout sessions.

Data Analysis

Plans for analysis should align with the research team's positioning along the continuum of research paradigms, their standpoint and positionality, the context of the study, as well as its research aims, and the forms of data generated (all outlined in previous sections) in the

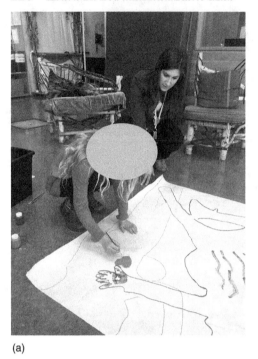

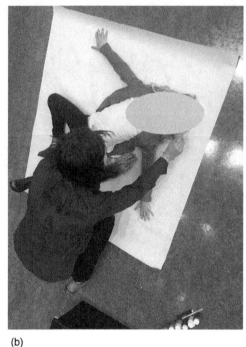

(a) (b)

Figure 12.2 (a and b) Body map storytelling data generation process from Laura's study. Author
created.

interest of achieving coherence throughout the study (Denzin, 2019; Eakin, 2010; Eakin
& Gladstone, 2020). It would be impossible, and even irresponsible, to provide prescriptive rules for the 'how' of analysis in a visual arts-based research project. Such a prescriptive
approach bears the risk of diminishing the role of the 'creatively present' researcher, or the
researcher who is seen not as a source of bias but a source of creativity and insight that is
integral to the research task (Eakin & Gladstone, 2020). As Eakin and Gladstone (2020)
explained:

> The notion of "value-adding" draws on the idea that the data do not speak for them-
> selves, and that it is the researcher who adds value to the research by interpreting data
> (assigning them meaning), by conceptualizing them (seeing them as instances of or
> types of more general or abstract concepts), and by "theorizing" them (linking, explain-
> ing and accounting for data and concepts). That is, researchers read, organize, and
> assign meaning to data, and produce "findings."
>
> (p. 3)

This notion of 'value-adding' analysis is fruitful when working with all forms of data (i.e.,
visual and otherwise). We highlight it in this chapter because we have both fielded questions from diverse audiences that lead us to wonder if visual data is somehow more likely
to be taken at 'face value' or as a window onto some supposed 'truth' of the phenomenon
than other forms of data (e.g., words-based data including interview transcripts, ethnographic fieldnotes) (Yates, 2010). The products of visual arts-based research must be

subject to the same rigorous analysis and interpretation as their forms of data. Just because this data may be 'seen' differently does not mean that what is seen should be taken as 'fact.' Moreover, visual data must be considered reflexively. As Rose (2016) noted, researchers need to consider where they 'see' from, acknowledging that ways of seeing are always historically, geographically, culturally, and socially specific (i.e., there is no view from nowhere).

An in-depth accounting of practices for the deep and contextualized analysis that is a marker of quality qualitative analysis is beyond the scope of the chapter (for helpful resources see Becker, 1998; Coffey & Atkinson, 1996; Eakin & Gladstone, 2020; Jackson & Mazzei, 2013; MacFarlane & O'Reilly-de Brún, 2012). Instead, we walk the reader through how we applied a number of "analytic devices" in our respective studies (Eakin & Gladstone, 2020, p. 3). Of note, the analysis presented below is not confined to a distinct analysis stage but is a *process* that is ongoing and iterative, beginning at the time of study conceptualization and the formation of the research question, through to the co-construction of data with participants and the deployment of specific analytic procedures within and across the data (Johnny & Mitchell, 2006).

In both of our studies, participants were invited into the first stage of analysis and interpretation when they were asked to describe what they created, and why they chose to represent their experiences as they did. Participants shared the intended meaning of the visual product, the intended audience for the product, and what they would like their imagined audiences to understand about their experience upon encountering and interacting with their visual product (Guillemin & Gillam, 2004; Johnny & Mitchell, 2006; Mah et al., 2022; Mah et al., 2020; Rose, 2016). While the studies shared some analytic practices, we describe each study in turn below.

Katie's study generated a large amount of data, which needed to be made more manageable for analysis. A number of techniques were used: interviews were transcribed, drawing data were digitized, and a summary of each participant's drawing and interview data was created in an Excel spreadsheet. We include these techniques here, under a discussion of analysis, because these were *conceptual acts*. For example, in summarizing each participant's data, deciding what words to use to describe the images, or what aspects of the image to comment on, required Katie to think about the data in new ways. To gain deep familiarity with the data, Katie engaged in multiple readings of the data (i.e., the drawing or written response data, interview data and data summaries), extensive reflexive memo writing, and generative coding (Birks et al., 2008; Coffey & Atkinson, 1996; Eakin & Gladstone, 2020; Miles & Huberman, 1994). Analysis was guided by the study's Foucauldian framework (Foucault, 1971, 1980, 1982a, 1982b) and oriented by interrogative questioning with regard to the production, content, and intended audience for the data (Eakin & Gladstone, 2020; Guillemin, 2004; Guillemin & Gillam, 2004; Rose, 2016). Questions asked of the data included: *what is represented in this drawing/interview? What discourses were in operation for this participant to experience and represent concussion in this way? What alternative discourses are offered?* In asking these questions of the data, Katie became able to account for the role of discourse in shaping how young people experienced concussion, moving her understanding of the topic beyond the self-evident meanings of the data to re-conceptualize what is known about concussion. The practical contribution of her research is an expanded understanding of concussion, a way of considering concussion not only as a biomedical injury but also as a social phenomenon that young people come to know and make sense of through discourse.

In Laura's study, the data that were analyzed included the constructed body maps (product) along with transcripts from the data generation sessions and researcher notes and reflections (process). Team members first analyzed the body maps one at a time, and then considered them as a collective. The product was analyzed first to allow for fresher eyes without pre-constructed codes based on deep engagement with the process data. Each body map was explored for its general impression and elements (what stood out, the colors and tone, size and relation of elements), and then considered alongside each question in the body mapping protocol (Figure 12.3). The same process was undertaken across the entire sample of body maps. Key words and phrases were recorded as early codes as well as research team reflections. Transcripts of the body mapping sessions were then reviewed by two researchers who provided early impression and initial codes, using participants' own language whenever possible, integrating the codes derived from the body maps themselves. Discussion of the early codes from the entire data set were considered collectively by the broader research team, and a codebook was created to be applied to the full data set (visuals and transcripts). Codes were brought back to the team along with the visuals and sample transcript quotes to collectively identify themes to be presented through different dissemination channels (publications, presentations, community events). Findings were shared with participants and their families and feedback was considered by the team and integrated into the code set as applicable. Digital pictures of the body maps and the individual elements of each map were taken, and the original maps were offered back to

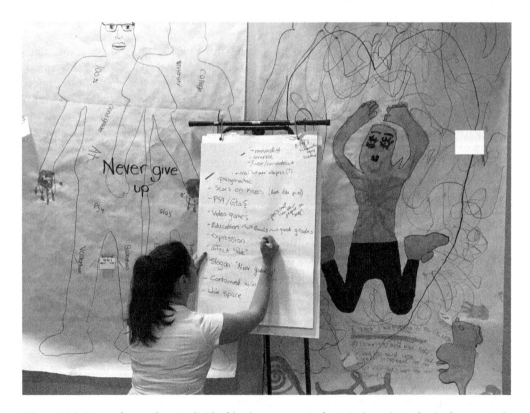

Figure 12.3 Researcher analyses individual body maps as products in Laura's study. Author created.

participants. For those who did not want their body maps back, the body maps were stored in a secure location within the research office (storage for up to seven years), as per ethics review board guidelines.

Rigor and Ethics

In tandem with the proliferation of arts-based research in the health and social sciences, there has been an expansion in the availability of ethical guidelines pertaining to such methods. Here, we outline some key considerations. Examples of additional criteria are available in the works of Boydell et al. (2012), Rose (2016), and Cox et al. (2014a).

In arts-based research, we suggest adopting an 'ethics-as-process' approach, wherein participants are informed prior to study participation, and reminded throughout study participation, that they can stop the process of data generation, refuse to answer a question or produce a visual, or withdraw from the study at any time (Ramcharan & Cutcliffe, 2001). From a procedural perspective, informed consent/assent should account for the emergent nature of the research and the notion that a participant cannot provide informed consent for a visual product that they have not yet produced. We both used a two-step consent procedure (Gladstone & Stasiulis, 2019) including: (1) the participant providing informed consent for study participation and the production of data; and (2) re-visiting the informed consent discussion following the production of data. This second-step involves providing informed consent for the public display and use of the visual product for knowledge dissemination purposes (e.g., publications, conference presentations).

Along with the discussion of the public display of the visual product comes the more nuanced consideration of product ownership. In most research, the product of data generation may be assumed to be owned by the research team and shared in ways outlined in a research protocol (e.g., publication, presentations). With the creation of a visual product, additional consideration must be given to who owns the original or digital copies of the data, when the visual data can be shared, and how. This nuanced discussion becomes more complex when considering whether data can be shared on personal social media, if it requires re-consenting each time it is shared, how many ways it can be presented, and by whom. For example, in Laura's study, participants were allowed to take photos of their body maps if they wished at any point, but were asked not to share them on social media because of their status as in-progress data. Once the data were preliminarily analyzed by the research team and photos were taken of all body maps, participants were offered the choice to keep their original body maps, as the owners and creators, and were informed that same-size prints would be made for dissemination purposes.

Adhering to a model of 'ethics in practice' or the "day-to-day ethical issues that arise in the doing of research" (Guillemin & Gillam, 2004, p. 264) was particularly useful in attending to ethically important moments that might arise in the 'doing' of arts-based research. For example, during Katie's study, a participant produced a particularly vivid drawing of himself experiencing violence that resulted in concussion. When speaking about how he sustained his injury, this participant became withdrawn, preferring to focus instead on the details of his recovery. While Katie initially probed around the violent nature of the injury, she soon recognized his attempts to shift the conversation back to his recovery as a protective instinct. She followed his lead despite her curiosity and made a choice, in the moment, to prioritize the emotional safety of the participant and the integrity of the research relationship over the depth of the data. In the thick of this ethically important moment, Katie chose to interact with this participant in a non-exploitative and humane way, upholding her ethical obligation to the participant. This is one example of the ways in which visual methods can create forms of harm that are unforeseen, or beyond the harmful experiences that might normally be considered by ethics review boards (Cox et al., 2014a), but that can be accounted for in our care and safety plans (e.g., through the inclusion of local emergency numbers, locations of mental health emergency walk-in clinics).

Addressing questions of rigor, or of how to establish the quality of a visual arts-based research project, will differ depending on the project being undertaken. Similar to Eakin and Mykhalovskiy (2003), we support the notion that qualitative research requires quality criteria that differ from conventional criteria for judging quantitative research, and even from parallel criteria for judging qualitative research from within the post-positivist paradigm (Lincoln et al., 2011; Morrow, 2005). Instead, we propose a substantive approach to establishing the quality of a visual arts-based research study, wherein the focus is on the analysis put forward and on the relationship between the research practices adopted and that analysis (Eakin & Mykhalovskiy, 2003). Within this substantive approach, research practices are used as resources—for engaging with the topic of inquiry, interpreting and analyzing the data, and producing a convincing and meaningful account of the data (Eakin & Mykhalovskiy, 2003).

Critiquing Visual Arts Research

While we cannot provide a blanket response to the question of how to establish quality in visual arts-based research (because this answer will be epistemology and project dependent), we have outlined a number of overarching questions to consider when evaluating the quality of studies claiming a visual or arts-based research methodology (see Textbox 12.1). Importantly, when referring to Textbox 12.3, the answers to the overarching questions will likely not be readily available but will require the reader to read between the lines of published research reports. For example, word limits might constrain the research team from outlining how they engaged reflexively with their methodology. Accordingly, we have provided a number of interrogative prompts to help readers think through the larger overarching questions.

Application to Occupational Science

Beyond illuminating the tacit through re-conceptualizing it in the form of visuals, visual and arts-based methodologies have allowed us to challenge current understandings *about* children with ABI that are primarily created *without* them. For our studies and others that seek to explore the nuanced experiences of occupational marginalization, deprivation, and disruption, creating safer and shared means of expression and reflection have been essential. As an interdisciplinary science that contributes understanding of the study of human occupation to many fields, the inclusion of visual arts-based research methods (along with other participant-driven, creative, and reflective ways of engaging) will allow for deeper and more diverse insight into issues of occupational justice. Outcomes of such research in the field of occupational science can illuminate the potential impact of marginalization on the eventual care, services, and opportunities made available to children diagnosed with ABI, as an example.

Textbox 12.3   Critiquing Visual Arts-Based Research – Questions to Ask

Is there *'fit' across the project*?

Is the philosophical orientation (i.e., ontology and epistemology) of the visual arts-based research project expressed, either implicitly or explicitly?

Is there coherence (i.e., fit) between how the visual arts-based methodology has been theorized and how it has been taken up?

Has the research team expressed why they used this methodology with this population? Does the methodology seem to 'fit' the needs and preferences of the population?

Has the research team *engaged reflexively* with the methodology?

Why was a visual arts-based methodology adopted in approaching this particular research question? Does the methodology 'fit' the question?

What does a visual arts-based methodology add to the study beyond the benefits of qualitative inquiry more generally?

Has the research team provided rationale beyond 'innovation' for engaging a visual arts-based methodology?

Has *appropriate regard* been given to the products of the visual arts-based methodology (e.g., photographs, drawings, body maps)?

Have the products of the visual arts-based methodology been regarded as data, subject to the same rigorous analysis and interpretation as other forms of data (e.g., interview transcripts, ethnographic fieldnotes)?

Have the methods of visual analysis and interpretation been adequately described?

Has the analysis and interpretation of the visual product been illustrated? For example, has the research team *described* their interpretation of the visual data and *illustrated* their interpretation through sharing examples of that data?

Adapted from Boydell et al. (2012) and Mah et al. (2020)

Note: these questions and considerations apply to the outputs of visual or arts-based research, whether in the form of published articles, web-based content, and/or public art/research installations.

Application to Occupational Therapy

Occupational therapy has deep roots in 'doing.' Meaningful engagement is at the heart of exploring, understanding, and intervening in human occupations (Townsend & Polatajko, 2007). From the profession's earliest days, the potential of crafting to promote motor skills, reflection, mastery, and healing has been recognized (Friedland, 2011). Even in the current evidence- and outcomes-driven health care systems, occupational therapy has moved increasingly towards co-creating approaches, going beyond the standard of client-centered care to a more inclusive approach (ACOTRO et al., 2021). Visual arts-based practices in therapeutic and research contexts provide processes for co-creating meaning and goals with clients/participants. Research that situates knowledge in a way that aligns with the practice philosophy of occupational therapy (i.e., co-creation approaches) has the potential to yield meaningful evidence to inform the development of practices and programs better suited to client and family needs.

Authors' Reflections

We have each worked clinically and in research with young people with ABI. As we dug deeper into the evidence base that supported and drove our work, we became increasingly aware of the stark absence of children's perspectives regarding their own experiences. As clinicians and researchers based in a clinical organization, we recognized the power that formal evidence has in our health and social care systems. We found ourselves at a crossroads of adhering to the language and constraints of biomedical investigation which limited the ways we could engage children in research, and engaging in child-oriented ways that risked removing ourselves from the realm of 'valued' evidence. In the end, we were each drawn to visual and arts-based methodologies as a different way of thinking about, engaging with, and representing the health- and disability-related experiences of our participants/clients. We quickly became convinced of the potential of visual and arts-based research to bring participants/clients into the co-creation of knowledge in more equitable ways, using methods that suited the abstract topics we sought to explore. However, even with the increasing presence and systematization of visual and arts-based methods, we continue to face questions of legitimacy, with the value of our research and results minimized when compared to those produced through other paradigms or research traditions. We persist because we believe in a more just and equitable research enterprise, are committed to amplifying the voices of groups whose participation in research has been limited by assumptions of vulnerability or inability, and know the importance of knowledge and evidence that is driven by experience.

Conclusions

By the very nature of considering occupations, occupational scientists and occupational therapists address both the highly complex and contextualized and the very abstract and tacit. When deployed reflexively, visual and arts-based methodologies provide opportunity to explore topics, experiences, and contexts that are not commonly studied due to their complexity (e.g., occupational marginalization) or tacit nature (e.g., occupational disruption). Moreover, such methods can enable the co-creation of knowledge with groups of participants that have long been underrepresented in research. In addition to enabling the production of new knowledge from oft overlooked groups, researchers employing visual and arts-based methods can leverage the power of the visual to disseminate findings to broad audiences with impact in an effort to influence change.

References

ACOTRO, ACOTUP, & CAOT. (2021). *Competencies for occupational therapists in Canada/ Référentiel de Compétences pour les Ergothérapeutes au Canada.* https://acotro-acore.org/sites/default/files/uploads/ot_competency_document_en_hires.pdf

Becker, H. S. (1998). *Tricks of the trade: How to think about your research while you're doing it.* University of Chicago Press.

Birks, M., Chapman, Y., & Francis, K. (2008). Memoing in qualitative research: Probing data and processes. *Journal of Research in Nursing*, *13*(1), 68–75. https://doi.org/10.1177/1744987107081254

Botma, Y., & Labuschagne, M. (2019). Students' perceptions of interprofessional education and collaborative practice: Analysis of freehand drawings. *Journal of Interprofessional Care*, *33*(3), 321–327. https://doi.org/10.1080/13561820.2019.1605981

Bowman, L. R., Rowland, E., Crossman, S., & King, G. (in preparation). Children's experiences of transitions back to school following acquired brain injury: A body map storytelling study.

Boydell, K. M., Volpe, T., Cox, S., Katz, A., Dow, R., Brunger, F., Parsons, J., Belliveau, G., Gladstone, B., & Zlotnik-Shaul, R. (2012). Ethical challenges in arts-based health research. *International Journal of the Creative Arts in Interdisciplinary Practice*, *11*(1), 1–17.

Boylan, A.-M., Linden, M., & Alderdice, F. (2009). Interviewing children with acquired brain injury (ABI). *Journal of Early Childhood Research*, *7*(3), 264–282. https://doi.org/10.1177/1476718X09336970

Cambridge Dictionary. (n.d.). *Effect*. https://dictionary.cambridge.org/dictionary/english/effect

Clark, A. (2010). Young children as protagonists and the role of participatory, visual methods in engaging multiple perspectives. *American Journal of Community Psychology*, *46*(1), 115–123. https://doi.org/10.1007/s10464-010-9332-y

Clark, A., & Statham, J. (2005). Listening to young children: Experts in their own lives. *Adoption & Fostering*, *29*(1), 45–56. https://doi.org/10.1177/030857590502900106

Coffey, A., & Atkinson, P. (1996). *Making sense of qualitative data: Complementary research strategies*. SAGE.

Cox, S., Drew, S., Guillemin, M., Howell, C., Warr, D., & Waycott, J. (2014a). *Guidelines for ethical visual research methods*. Visual Research Collaboratory Parkville.

Creswell, J. W., & Poth, C. N. (2016). *Qualitative inquiry and research design: Choosing among five approaches*. SAGE.

Davy, C., Magalhães, L. V., Mandich, A., & Galheigo, S. M. (2014). Aspects of the resilience and settlement of refugee youth: A narrative study using body maps. *Cadernos Brasileiros de Terapia Ocupacional*, *22*(2), 231–241. http://dx.doi.org/10.4322/cto.2014.045

Denzin, N. K. (2019). The death of data in neoliberal times. *Qualitative Inquiry*, *25*(8), 721–724. https://doi.org/10.1177/1077800419847501

Eakin, J. (2010). Towards a 'standpoint' perspective: Health and safety in small workplaces from the perspective of the workers. *Policy and Practice in Health and Safety*, *8*(2), 113–127. https://doi.org/10.1080/14774003.2010.11667751

Eakin, J. M., & Gladstone, B. (2020). "Value-adding" analysis: Doing more with qualitative data. *International Journal of Qualitative Methods*, *19*, 1–13. https://doi.org/10.1177/1609406920949333

Eakin, J. M., & Mykhalovskiy, E. (2003). Reframing the evaluation of qualitative health research: Reflections on a review of appraisal guidelines in the health sciences. *Journal of Evaluation in Clinical Practice*, *9*(2), 187–194. https://doi.org/10.1046/j.1365-2753.2003.00392.x

Foucault, M. (1971). Orders of discourse. *Social Science Information*, *10*(2), 7–30. https://doi.org/10.1177/053901847101000201

Foucault, M. (1980). *Power/knowledge*. Vintage Books.

Foucault, M. (1982a). *The archaeology of knowledge*. Pantheon Books.

Foucault, M. (1982b). The subject and power. In H. L. Dreyfus & P. Rabinow (Eds.), *Michel Foucault: Beyond structuralism and hermeneutics* (pp. 208–226). University of Chicago Press.

Friedland, J. (2011). *Restoring the spirit: The beginnings of occupational therapy in Canada, 1890–1930*. McGill-Queen's Press-MQUP.

Gastaldo, D., Carrasco, C., & Magalhães, L. (2013). The creation of a mobile workforce: Latin American undocumented workers in the Greater Toronto Area. *Encounters*, *1*(1), 18–32.

Gladstone, B. M., & Stasiulis, E. (2019). Digital storytelling method. In P. Liamputtong (Ed.), *Handbook of research methods in health social sciences* (pp. 1303–1319). Springer Singapore.

Grover, S. (2004). Participating in social research why won't they listen to us? On giving power and voice to children. *Childhood, 11*(1), 81–93. https://doi.org/10.1177/0907568204040186

Guillemin, M. (2004). Understanding illness: Using drawings as a research method. *Qualitative Health Research, 14*(2), 272–289. https://doi.org/10.1177/1049732303260445

Guillemin, M., & Gillam, L. (2004). Ethics, reflexivity, and "ethically important moments" in research. *Qualitative Inquiry, 10*(2), 261–280. https://doi.org/10.1177/1077800403262360

Huot, S., Aldrich, R. M., Rudman, D. L., & Stone, M. (2022). Picturing precarity through occupational mapping: Making the (im)mobilities of long-term unemployment visible. *Journal of Occupational Science, 29*(4), 529–544. https://doi.org.10.1080/14427591.2020.1821244

Jackson, A. Y., & Mazzei, L. A. (2013). Plugging one text into another: Thinking with theory in qualitative research. *Qualitative Inquiry, 19*(4), 261–271. https://doi.org/10.1177/1077800412471510

Johnny, L., & Mitchell, C. (2006). "Live and let live": An analysis of HIV/AIDS-related stigma and discrimination in international campaign posters. *Journal of Health Communication, 11*(8), 755–767. https://doi.org/10.1080/10810730600934708

Kortesluoma, R. L., Hentinen, M., & Nikkonen, M. (2003). Conducting a qualitative child interview: Methodological considerations. *Journal of Advanced Nursing, 42*(5), 434–441. https://doi.org/10.1046/j.1365-2648.2003.02643.x

Lincoln, Y. S., Lynham, S. A., & Guba, E. G. (2011). Paradigmatic controversies, contradictions, and emerging confluences, revisited. In N. K. Denzin & Y. S. Lincoln (Eds.), *SAGE handbook of qualitative research* (4th ed., pp. 97–128). SAGE.

Literat, I. (2013). "A pencil for your thoughts": Participatory drawing as a visual research method with children and youth. *International Journal of Qualitative Methods, 12*(1), 84–98. https://doi.org/10.1177/160940691301200143

MacFarlane, A., & O'Reilly-de Brún, M. (2012). Using a theory-driven conceptual framework in qualitative health research. *Qualitative Health Research, 22*(5), 607–618. https://doi.org/10.1177/1049732311431898

Mah, K., Gladstone, B., Cameron, D., & Reed, N. (2021). Re/producing the Pediatric Concussion Discourse in clinical rehabilitation practice. *Disability and Rehabilitation*, 1–11. https://doi.org/10.1080/09638288.2021.1996645

Mah, K., Gladstone, B., Cameron, D., & Reed, N. (2022). Thinking otherwise: Bringing young people into pediatric concussion clinical and research practice. *Brain Impairment, 23*(1), 104–117. https://doi.org/10.1017/BrImp.2021.28

Mah, K., Gladstone, B., King, G., Reed, N., & Hartman, L. R. (2020). Researching experiences of childhood brain injury: Co-constructing knowledge with children through arts-based research methods. *Disability and Rehabilitation, 42*(20), 2967–2976. https://doi.org/10.1080/09638288.2019.1574916

Mealings, M., Douglas, J., & Olver, J. (2012). Considering the student perspective in returning to school after TBI: A literature review. *Brain Injury, 26*(10), 1165–1176. https://doi.org/10.3109/02699052.2012.672785

Miles, M. B., & Huberman, A. M. (1994). *Qualitative data analysis: An expanded sourcebook.* SAGE.

Morrow, S. L. (2005). Quality and trustworthiness in qualitative research in counseling psychology. *Journal of Counseling Psychology, 52*(2), 250–260. https://doi.org/10.1037/0022-0167.52.2.250

Morrow, V. (2008). Ethical dilemmas in research with children and young people about their social environments. *Children's Geographies, 6*(1), 49–61. https://doi.org/10.1080/14733280701791918

Phillips, J., Ogden, J., & Copland, C. (2015). Using drawings of pain-related images to understand the experience of chronic pain: A qualitative study. *British Journal of Occupational Therapy, 78*(7), 404–411. https://doi.org/10.1177/0308022614562791

Pink, S. (2003). Interdisciplinary agendas in visual research: Re-situating visual anthropology. *Visual Studies, 18*(2), 179–192. https://doi.org/10.1080/14725860310001632029

Prosser, J. (2011). Visual methodology: Toward a more seeing research. In N. K. Denzin & Y. S. Lincoln (Eds.), *The Sage handbook of qualitative research* (4th ed., pp. 479–498). SAGE.

Ramcharan, P., & Cutcliffe, J. R. (2001). Judging the ethics of qualitative research: Considering the 'ethics as process' model. *Health & Social Care in the Community, 9*(6), 358–366. https://doi.org/10.1046/j.1365-2524.2001.00323.x

Rose, G. (2016). *Visual methodologies: An introduction to researching with visual materials.* SAGE.

Solomon, J. (2007). *"Living with X": A body mapping journey in the time of HIV and AIDS. Facilitators guide.* Regional Psychosocial Support Initiative (REPSSI).

Teachman, G., & Gibson, B. E. (2013). Children and youth with disabilities: Innovative methods for single qualitative interviews. *Qualitative Health Research, 23*(2), 264–274. https://doi.org/10.1177/1049732312468063

Thorogood, N., & Green, J. (2009). *Qualitative methods for health research.* SAGE.

Townsend, E. A., & Polatajko, H. J. (2007). *Enabling occupation II: Advancing an occupational therapy vision for health, Well-being.* Canadian Association of Occupational Therapists.

Yates, L. (2010). The story they want to tell, and the visual story as evidence: Young people, research authority and research purposes in the education and health domains. *Visual Studies, 25*(3), 280–291. https://doi.org/10.1080/1472586X.2010.523281

Additional Resources

Caldairou-Bessette, P., Nadeau, L., & Mitchell, C. (2020). Overcoming "you can ask my mom": Clinical arts-based perspectives to include children under 12 in mental health research. *International Journal of Qualitative Methods, 19,* 1609406920958959. https://doi.org/10.1177/1609406920958959

Cox, S., Drew, S., Guillemin, M., Howell, C., Warr, D., & Waycott, J. (2014b). *Guidelines for ethical visual research methods.* The University of Melbourne. https://edisciplinas.usp.br/pluginfile.php/4434501/mod_resource/content/1/Ethical%20guidelines%20for%20visual%20ethnography.pdf

Gastaldo, D., Magalhães, L., Carrasco, C., & Davy, C. (2012). *Body-map storytelling as research: Methodological considerations for telling the stories of undocumented workers through body mapping.* www.migrationhealth.ca/sites/default/files/Body-map_storytelling_as_reseach_HQ.pdf

Hartman, L. R., Mandich, A., Magalhães, L., & Orchard, T. (2011). How do we 'see' occupations? An examination of visual research methodologies in the study of human occupation. *Journal of Occupational Science, 18*(4), 292–305. https://doi.org/10.1080/14427591.2011.610776

13 Visual Methodologies

Photovoice in Focus

Eric Asaba, Melissa Park, Margarita Mondaca and Debbie Laliberte Rudman

Visual images evoke elements of human consciousness that words alone cannot; images evoke both more information and different kinds of information (Harper, 2002). Not surprisingly, images are being utilized in research to access meaning, as well as deepen critical understanding of how individuals and social groups are situated within, and 'read' the contexts in, which their lives are negotiated (Coemans et al., 2019). Visual research methods encompass systematic ways in which visual materials are gathered or generated to understand, explain, or express phenomena—a process that is in constant development (Pink, 2012). For example, visual methods can draw upon pre-existing photos or videos or alternatively generate photos and videos during the research process. Moreover, these visual materials can be drawn upon, gathered, or generated by researchers, informants, and/or in collaboration (Prosser & Schwartz, 1998).

Visual methods can be used for varying purposes such as documenting observations, capturing processes as they occur, facilitating dialogue, and constructing counter-stories (Goessling, 2018; Prosser, 2011; Prosser et al., 2008; Prosser & Schwartz, 1998; Wang & Burris, 1997). The nomenclature for visual methods in health and social sciences have developed over the years to include photo elicitation, photo tour, video diaries, photo story, body mapping, film elicitation, photo novella, and photovoice. All these terms can be taken to reflect a set of assumptions about visual literacy—that visual artifacts can be 'read' as a text (Catalani & Minkler, 2009; Elkins, 2008; Hartman et al., 2011; Lal et al., 2012; van Nes et al., 2012).

Although the possibilities for using visual images are plentiful, assumptions around literacy, particularly in the context of research, can come with risk. For example, there is a need to consider who has the power in photography, as well as the various ways in which the social positions of the photographer and subject come into play when a photograph is taken during photo elicitation (Harper, 2002). The shift away from a realist assumption that images 'speak' for themselves places a greater demand on researchers to contextualize and interpret images and attend to positionality (Prosser, 2011). More recently, it has been argued that visual research, itself, continues to fail to "sufficiently theorize power in relation to ethics" (Harley & Langdon, 2018, p. 188). We contend that it is particularly important to be reflexive regarding how the 'visual' is understood, constructed, and interpreted within any study (Banks, 2007; Prosser & Schwartz, 1998). In his introduction to *Visual Literacy*, James Elkins (2008), an art historian, wrote:

> Since the 1980s the rhetoric of images has become far more pervasive, so that it is now commonplace in the media to hear that we live in a visual culture and get our information through images. It is time, I think, to take those claims seriously.
>
> (p. 4)

DOI: 10.4324/9781003456216-13

Yet, Elkins also argued that scholars too often assume a certain literacy of visual images; this literacy needs to be learned. Greater attention needs to be given to how epistemologies or ways of knowing largely determine 'ways of seeing' (Berger, 1972/2002), including how the relatively easy production and reproduction of images with the advent of film and photography also politicized them (Benjamin, 1935/1986).

Epistemology, Ontology, Axiology

Much like the aperture on a camera, epistemologies determine what is foregrounded or backgrounded and, thus, what becomes the focus of inquiry and interpretive processes. Hence, the researchers' epistemologies also directly shape the results as well as how they are represented and disseminated. For example, within a transformative paradigm that draws upon critical social theories (e.g., Freire, 1973), the focus is on how visual images can facilitate dialogue and conscientization to empower persons or a community that they represent to identify and explore topics considered relevant by them for them (Wang & Burris, 1994; Wang et al., 1996), or how visual images as a symbolic representation of political or historical situations can stimulate dialogue in the public realm for education, debate, and/or policy changes (Carlson et al., 2006). In comparison, within an interpretive paradigm that draws upon critical phenomenological theories, an 'imagistic approach'— textual, verbal, pictorial, or other form—can provoke reflection on social structures from a first-person, experience-near perspective (Mattingly & Gron, 2022). This can 'defrost' or question established conceptual categories (Mattingly, 2019). This type of imagistic approach can also provide metaphors to engage people in communication about experiences that are difficult to grasp, which can facilitate understanding and empathy (Woodgate et al., 2021).

Occupational science is, arguably, a pluralistic epistemic community in which researchers effectively draw upon a range of epistemologies (cf. Kinsella, 2012), dependent upon the aim or purpose of the project. Although rarely made explicit, reflexivity on and articulation of epistemologies *prior to* beginning a photovoice project has both scholarly and practical implications. Understanding the situatedness of photovoice research requires attending to epistemological positioning and inter-related ontological and axiological assumptions. Epistemologies are guided by ontologies, or assumptions about what constitutes knowledge or world views. Further, ontologies have related axiologies or values, "Ontology and epistemology provide insight into what the researcher believes to be the nature of truth, the nature of the world, and ways of being in that world; together they describe the world view or the researcher" (Beryman, 2019, p. 272). The stances taken are also moral or ethical ones, which guide choices about the 'good' of certain types of questions (i.e., whether for information, meaning, or critique), the quality of collaborative relations developed and enacted, and the ways in which images are used and contextualized.

Although we have utilized a variety of visual methods (e.g., video/film, drawing, photography), this chapter will focus on photovoice, both because it allows us to draw from our experiences with projects that span three countries, and because photovoice has received attention from scholars within occupational science and occupational therapy. It can be worth noting that literature within occupational science and occupational therapy in which photovoice is used only emerged substantially in the discipline and practice literature after 2010 (Lal et al., 2012), with rapid expansion during the past decade. Since that time, photovoice has been used with a diversity of epistemologies, either explicitly or, more often, implicitly. Depending upon these epistemologies, this body of research has focused on understanding (e.g., interpretive) or interrogating (e.g., critical) a range of occupations and occupational inequities to, often, redress them with a variety of participants and or co-researchers. Work within a critical paradigm begins with the ontological assumption of the tentative and power-laden nature of what has come to be taken as 'real,' pointing to the potential for transformation. Moreover, such work is often explicitly informed by particular values, thus embracing an axiological stance in which research and community values are central to project aims and on-going reflexivity (Goessling, 2018; Liebenberg, 2018).

The ambition in this chapter is to use illustrations and reflections from our own projects, aligned by their epistemological stances, in order to provide key examples of how theoretical frameworks can be used to guide planning, conducting, analyzing, and presenting findings in photovoice research (see Table 13.1). Moreover, we will examine how epistemological orientations guided choices in the field; specifically, approach to ethics; relationships with those who were engaged in the photovoice projects; and how data were generated, analyzed, interpreted, and disseminated.

Background: Photovoice History and Methodology

Photovoice, initially referred to as photo novella, was coined by Wang and colleagues in a project focusing on maternal and child health in rural China (Wang & Burris, 1994, 1997; Wang et al., 1996). As Wang and colleagues have purported, photovoice as a participatory methodology involves a group of people producing, sharing, and discussing photos that pertain to shared experiences in order to enable the group to identify and build on community strengths, engage with each other through dialogue, and potentially reach diverse community stakeholders and policy makers through media and methods not otherwise accessible. Photovoice challenges the traditional hierarchies between *researchers* and *researched* (Carlson et al., 2006). A more detailed and retrospective account of the history and reflections around the development of photovoice has been shared by one of the founders, and can be useful for the reader to explore (Wang, 2022).

There are three major theoretical influences on the development of photovoice as a methodology. First, photovoice incorporates Freire's approach to critical education in that it emphasizes "people's sharing and speaking from their own experience" (Wang & Pies, 2008, p. 184), the need for people to identify "the historical and social patterns that bind their individual lives together" (Wang & Pies, 2008, p. 184), and the capacity of people to generate collective solutions for enacting change (Freire, 1973, 1993; Wang & Burris, 1994; Wang & Pies, 2008). Freire (1973) emphasized reflexive discussions of everyday struggles within communities in order to evoke social transformation. Second, photovoice has also been influenced by critical feminist theory, particularly emphasizing voice and a platform for vantage points expressed by those who have or are experiencing forms of oppression (Wang & Pies, 2008). In application, this means asking whose knowledge is valued. Following from this, attention is also given to where and how knowledge is obtained, by whom, from, and for whom and what purposes (Brinkmann, 2018). These questions and opportunities for reflection are relevant to participatory approaches, which directly concern active work with populations experiencing oppressive and constraining life conditions to enact social change. Third, theoretical underpinnings commonly associated with documentary photography are seen as particularly relevant with regard to how the camera functions as a tool in a process of consciousness raising, capacity building and moving to action (Castleden et al., 2008).

Table 13.1 Authors' photovoice projects drawn upon for this chapter

Project (participants)	Research aim	Stated methodology and theoretical frameworks	Visual methods	Dissemination
Creating Inclusive Communities (2010–2012) Adults 60+ who had internationally migrated to Sweden during adult life, and adults 60+ who had internationally migrated to Japan during adult life. Photovoice groups were held in Stockholm, Sweden, and Kobe, Japan, respectively.	To explore experiences of aging among older adults who had migrated	Ethnography Photovoice	Participant observation, share occupations in community settings, photos, objects used in show and tell.	Public community exhibition, academic conferences, website, and published works. Johansson et al. (2013)
Everyday Life with Spina Bifida (2017–2020) Adults with spina bifida including cognitive and/or physical disabilities.	To explore the meaning of dialogue and action as methodologically pivotal for the relevance of photovoice as community-based participatory research (CBPR)	Community-based participatory Photovoice Critical dialogue Narrative	Digital photos using a camera or mobile telephone. Photos served as data, support in discussions, and as a tool in analyzing materials together in the PV group.	Photo exhibition with panel debate and politician involvement, travelling exhibition at sites such as public library, disability conferences, universities among more. Social media. Gabrielsson et al. (2020) Gabrielsson et al. (2022)

(Continued)

Table 13.1 (Continued)

Project (participants)	Research aim	Stated methodology and theoretical frameworks	Visual methods	Dissemination
Sens.és Making (2014–2021) Children with autism, autistic youth, and adult mentors, family members who participated as co-researchers.	To understand sensory barriers to, and create actions for, socio-spatial inclusion in local communities	Mixed methodology (Visual ethnography, Participatory, Photovoice) Conceptual frameworks: Narrative and Aesthetics; Narrative Phenomenology and Critical phenomenology 2.0; Critical dialogue	Photographs and mini-video clips using box cameras and mobile telephone by children, youth, parents. Photos and video clips served as data to support sharing of experiences in group meetings using collective narratives (e.g., see Mattingly, 2010 for description of *Collective Narratives*)	Academic and autism conferences, educational brochures for distribution in local community, including health care sites, policy makers at federal and provincial levels, website, and social media. Clement et al. (2022) www.connectednarratives.org/project/sense-making/
Vision Quest (2008–2012)	To increase understandings of the a) strengths, assets and needs of First Nations youth in relation to performance study experiences and visions of success, and b) supports and barriers encountered by First Nations youth in local context	Photovoice Critical Indigenous scholarship Critical dialogue Critical occupational science	Digital photos taken with cameras Individual qualitative interview with each youth regarding photos about educational journey; focus group dialogue (all youth, elder, 2 researchers; each youth shared 3 photos)	Photo-exhibit at local Indigenous friendship center involving youths' invited guests, educational admin and policy makers, and related community-based organizations; local media coverage; academic conferences; and integration into Faculty of Health Sciences Task force addressing Indigenous education. Laliberte Rudman et al. (in press)

Author created

The theoretical influences behind photovoice are conceptually important for three reasons. First, persons who engage in photovoice research projects are often considered in public discourses to have access to fewer resources; yet their unique experiences can critique social structures, while contributing new knowledge that lead to the development of new or the transformation of old practices. Photovoice research advertly shifts focus from vulnerability as individual or collective weakness to conscientization about vulnerability created by structural conditions (Freire, 1973, 1993) as a common platform from where structural mechanisms can be redressed. From this perspective, it can be possible to pursue different understandings and different actions. Second, photovoice research challenges the extractivist view of persons as only participants or source of information; and, instead, resituates persons as co-researchers in defining what questions, information, and even concerns are of relevance within a particular context that can substantially reframe research inquiries. Third, photovoice can be a way to connect with or engage community members, particularly when projects are enacted in ways that attend to how power is shared and trust is built, the level of commitment to capacity building and responsiveness to the worldviews and resources of those involved (Carlson et al., 2006).

Photovoice groups capture a dimension of events, contexts, or stories using photographs, which serve as a representation of daily socio-political realities experienced by the individual or group (Wang & Burris, 1997). Photos, and the dialogue they ignite, can serve as a catalyst for further narrative exploration and transformed understandings or consciousness regarding broader social and political forces shaping possibilities for being and doing (Wang & Burris, 1994, 1997; Wang et al., 1996). Thus, photovoice can be conceptualized as situated methodologically between narrative and participatory approaches, while centralizing visual elements (refer to Chapters 8, 11, and 12 for exploration of narrative and participatory approaches).

Linking to Examples

Photovoice has been widely used within community-based research projects to address issues of injustices, disparities, marginalization to name a few (Castleden et al., 2008; Coemans et al., 2019; Goessling, 2018; Haque & Eng, 2011; Novek et al., 2012; Wang & Pies, 2008). Along with a common focus on groups who are viewed or socially positioned as marginalized or vulnerable, there is a commitment with photovoice as originally presented to collectively identify socially and politically produced barriers faced by such groups and how these continue to be perpetuated, and bring to light the strengths, capacities, resources, and contributions of people. For instance, in one study addressing high school dropout, the authors shifted away from examining negative student and family characteristics to attending to broader economic, political, and social factors; and also shifted the focus "towards adolescents' strengths and factors that they perceive as supporting school attendance" (Lieblein et al., 2018, p. 3) as a means to generate new solutions to support school belonginess.

Examples that have more explicitly integrated occupational perspectives include aging and place among international migrant groups (Asaba et al., 2010); exploration of participation and everyday life among children and adults with intellectual and development disabilities (Gabrielsson et al., 2022; Gabrielsson et al., 2020; Heffron et al., 2018; St John et al., 2021); everyday life with a rare disease (Mälstam et al., 2018); understanding barriers and possibilities in the return to work process among adults with spinal cord injuries (Holmlund et al., 2018); religion and spirituality (Eyres et al., 2019); and advocacy messages with caregivers of children with disabilities (Rabaey et al., 2021).

From the perspective of being inclusive, photovoice can be useful in that it taps into modes of expression beyond oratory or literary skills (Wang & Pies, 2008). Prosser and Schwartz (1998) wrote:

> Photographs may not provide us with unbiased, objective documentation of the social and material world, but they can show characteristics and attributes of people, objects and events that often elude even the most skilled wordsmiths.

(p. 335)

Hence, one of the advantages of photovoice is its accessibility to and for participants whose perspectives might otherwise be excluded from research. Photovoice can be useful in understanding questions related to occupation and its negotiation in everyday life with power relations, contending that the sense of immediacy and accessibility of visual images can provide a potent vehicle for knowledge mobilization, community dialogue, exchange, and informing social change.

Topics and Questions Best Suited for Photo Voice Studies

Broadly, research questions are often framed as having to do with addressing a knowledge gap, either in finding new knowledge or exploring new ways to understand phenomena. In photovoice, research questions ideally develop during collaboration with co-researchers (i.e., all participants in a project who are part of the social setting and/or group being studied). Through such collaboration, research questions evolve to reflect issues of relevance to a setting or group, and in this way contribute to defining the knowledge gap or the problematic to be addressed. For example, in one of our early photovoice projects (Asaba et al., 2010), the question originally posed was, "What characterizes possibilities and barriers to feeling included in society among older adults whom have experienced international migration?" However, at the first meeting, the participants of the photovoice group posed questions such as, "Why are we portrayed so poorly in media?" and "Why don't people see the resources we bring?" Each session, the group discussed potential questions with which to work and finally agreed on a question with which to move forward for that week. This was repeated each week during the duration of the project, providing an opportunity to return to. as well as address, several questions.

Recruitment

Wang and Burris (1997) asserted that "the ideal 'who' or 'where' for using photovoice is a community or group in which people are involved in all major phases of selecting and planning the process" (p. 377). In photovoice, recruitment is not about selecting a representative sample of people; rather, it is about collaborating to define what parameters to apply in looking for partners (partnering). A simple visual overview of phases from recruitment to exhibition based on our experiences is provided (see Figure 13.1). An important aspect for consideration is how we define the 'people' in 'all' major phases, something that is a contentious point. In most research projects within occupational science and occupational therapy, the academic partner is responsible for funding and the initial alignment between concepts and methods. Thus, the collaborative research endeavor in this case often commences after recruitment has been completed. Although not as common, there are also cases in which partnering occurs either in preparation for the grant application or is initiated and directed by the community partner.

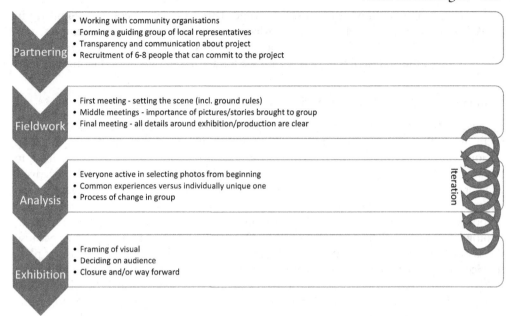

Figure 13.1 Overview of the photovoice process. Author created.

For instance, in Vision Quests (Laliberte Rudman et al., 2023) a mixture of personnel from local reserve communities whose positions address work and/or health, the Director of Indigenous Services at the local university, and a First Nations undergraduate student, among more, were invited to initial discussions for a project, with seed funding from a provincial ministry focused on work and education. Building upon this engagement process, potential research foci and methods were discussed as well as ethical issues and principles of research outlined by both Indigenous and research organizations in Canada to guide the conduct of research with Indigenous peoples. Everyone was invited to be part of a subsequent grant proposal, thereby involved from the onset of planning a photovoice project that had a focus on First Nations youth transitions from secondary to post-secondary education.

In another example, the Disabled Refugees Welcome (DRW) project based in Sweden incorporated photovoice as one of their projects funded by Allmana Arvsfonden (www.arvsfonden.se/). The grant application, funding, recruitment, and running of the project was conducted solely by the community organization Independent Living Institute in Stockholm, Sweden. After the project was completed, the community organization and participants of the photovoice group contacted members of the academic community to explore possibilities for secondary analyses of data. In the case of DRW, partnering was initiated by the community organization and ethics approval (EPM Dnr#2020-04100) was sought by the academic partner in a collaborative manner with DRW.

Close collaboration in partnering can thus unfold in different ways, and it can be a benefit that the research design closely reflects the community's local knowledge, for instance as in Vision Quests to: (a) include elders in the research process to ensure cultural safety and guidance for the youth; (b) provide a space for the youth to individually talk about their photos before bringing them to a group; and (c) ensure youth had multiple decision points regarding what photos they would share and in what contexts. Similarly, in DRW it was important to reflect local knowledge about terminology and discourses such as: (a) persons with disability versus disabled persons, (b) unique challenges nestled between migration and disability, and (c) a need for a sense of safety and belonging.

Data Gathering and Data Generation

Because of the nature in which photovoice groups work with data, we suggest that it is useful to think in terms of generating data rather than gathering data. Although group sessions and discussions are often recorded using audio or video and later transcribed, in this way similar to many other qualitative data gathering methods, data are collaboratively generated through the selection of photos brought to sessions and dialogue regarding the images. Wang and Burris (1997) described the challenge of offering guidelines that open up possibilities and build on community strengths rather than using language and methodological structures that limit or "pathologize" (p. 378) people. This is important because the distinction between facilitating and leading a group is subtle, and in the case of photovoice a risk is that the facilitator's voice becomes too dominant; thereby detracting from ideals of empowerment and participation. The number of sessions held, the duration of data generation, or the number of participants appropriate for a group all depend on the context and questions characterizing the project. We have found that fewer than five participants can at times feel like too few, especially if someone is ill or needs to miss a meeting; conversely more than eight participants in a group can lead to limitations in time for each person to share. The precise instructions for running a photovoice group will thus vary greatly depending on circumstances. Here we put forth seven reflections that can guide a process of planning data generation.

Lessons From the Field 1: Setting the Scene

At the first meeting with a photovoice group it is relevant to describe the project and overall aims, do a round of introductions, discuss and establish ground rules for the group, as well as decide on times to meet. It is important that participants feel safe and that everyone can participate on equal terms. Although a photovoice group might be homogenous in relation to a particular identity 'marker,' such as belonging to an ethnic minority, experiencing homelessness, or being a migrant worker, photovoice participants might see each other as diverse in terms of values, customs, and in relation to other intersecting identities. For this reason, we have found it appropriate to allocate time during the first session to let each person share about themselves and talk about ground rules. Ground rules can consist of things such as: being on time, calling if late, being respectful of other participants' perspectives, and not answering a mobile telephone during group time. It is important that the group jointly agrees on the processes. Deciding on a time frame and schedule allows everyone to commit to and plan their presence and participation. We have found this structure instrumental in ensuring continuity. However, it has also been important to remain flexible to changes proposed by the group. For instance, in one of our projects, the group initially agreed to only meet for two hours per week during an eight-week period. However, at the second session participants communicated that two hours was not enough time and subsequent sessions were extended to three hours. At week six, participants agreed that more time was needed in order to complete their work, thus the duration for the group was extended another four weeks. In this way the group decided the amount of time spent conducting group work. Certain cultural rituals were also acknowledged; for example, fika in Sweden (Swedish custom of sharing coffee/tea and something to eat between a day's main meals).

Lessons From the Field 2: Technological Development, and to Instruct or Not?

Much has developed in terms of technology since 2010 when some of the initial projects were conducted. At the time, some type of simple camera (digital or with film) was preferred by participants of photovoice groups. Over the years, we have found that participants of photovoice groups more often want to use their own smartphone instead of carrying an extra gadget. The freedom for each participant of a photovoice group to use their own camera can be beneficial in many ways; however, there are some challenges that can be noted. First, when sharing or downloading pictures there is a risk that there are several different operating systems and software products that need to be synchronized. Second, picture quality can vary depending on the device. Third, there is a risk that photos are shared via cloud services and other social media despite the group agreeing not to do so.

In early photovoice work, perspectives differed about whether facilitators/researchers should provide instruction in *how* to take a picture. On the one hand, aesthetically pleasing photographs with particular attention to focus, framing, depth, or color can be desirable; while on the other hand, a focus on such elements can be detrimental to the metaphoric qualities or in-the-moment experiences of the photographer. If much time is spent on how-to instruction pertaining to photography, people are likely to produce photographs in keeping with a style in which they received instruction. Focusing on how-to can also lead to feeling pressured to produce a particular type of picture or a certain quality which, at times, can stifle creativity or a freedom to express something that is not yet well understood for oneself. By not providing instruction, people are less likely to be steered in a particular direction about how to take a picture, although there can be frustration with feeling a lack of skill or later feeling that a picture does not aesthetically measure up to a desired quality for an exhibition. However, these latter concerns can be dealt with more readily in a photovoice project through discussion and group processes as well as captions or written texts during exhibitions.

Lessons From the Field 3: Groupwork with Pictures

In many photovoice projects, sharing stories about pictures with others in a group serves as an important part of generating data. Castleden et al. (2008), in working with First Nations youth, raised concerns regarding the risks of participation in focus groups as well as the cultural appropriateness. Utilizing 'Sharing Circles,' something recognized and grounded in a local community practice, in which each person is given space to talk if they so choose, could be an effective way for youth to share their thoughts and experiences with each other. Generating data can thus vary broadly between projects depending on the aim, research question, and community ways of doing.

Lessons From the Field 4: Frequency of Meetings

A benefit of not meeting frequently is that there is more room for freedom in scheduling and less time is required from already busy lives. Conversely, the continuity of meeting and sharing on a regular basis can provide a sense of belonging and the possibility to change direction in relation to emerging topics. Whatever the interval of gathering visual material, an important aspect of photovoice research is that participants have an opportunity to explore what the picture represents for each person and what the picture can communicate about individual as well as shared experiences.

Lessons From the Field 5: Storing and Selecting Photos

It is worth considering the participatory processes with extensive amounts of photographic material. The longer a project runs, the more pictures are likely to be produced. In this sense it is also relevant to consider how pictures are stored. A systematic way of storing and retrieving pictures will be particularly helpful when planning the final exhibition. In one of our projects where we had more than 700 photos, the group decided that each participant/photographer would choose three pictures from each session that they wanted to put in an archive. By doing this, the group was able to begin with approximately 80 pictures instead of 700 when discussing which pictures to include and how to frame the exhibition.

Lessons From the Field 6: Dialogue Is Critical

Dialogue is a powerful tool and an important quality to attend to within a photovoice project. When a safe space for individual narratives to emerge and for agreement/disagreement to unfold are fostered, dialogue between participants of the group becomes possible. From Freire's (1993) perspective, dialogue was a requisite for communication which, in turn, was necessary to foster a sort of critical stance to the status quo in a group in which issues of injustice were being worked with. The reason why this is important to be aware of is because one of the common adaptations to photovoice studies is to trim aspects of the study such that dialogue is no longer part of the group process, in turn, leading to missed opportunities to generate knowledge through this important process. In order to facilitate a participatory and collaborative process with participants of a photovoice group, dialogue will be an instrumental part to refine and integrate (Gabrielsson et al., 2022).

Lessons From the Field 7: Visual Images and Embodied Experiences

Arguably, video methods provide opportunities to study occupation in all its complexity and, specifically, the multi-modal sensory qualities linked to occupational identity within particular and unfolding contexts of everyday life (Bailliard, 2015) as well as the creation of intersubjective moments of connection and transformation in clinical contexts (Park, 2010). Yet, photographs also provide valuable and viable access to multi-modal sensory experiences. By capturing a moment or an experience to be shared, viewer reflections on a singular image taken at one point in time and space also evoke related sensations as well as emotions. For example, in the *Inclusive Communities* project the participants discussed the meaning of food that included smell and taste. As participants in the photovoice groups discussed, they raised the issue of how the sensory dimensions of the meal experience were lost in the photos and were not done justice by telling a story about how it was. The referral to embodied experiences then shaped the photo exhibition, as the participants wanted viewers to actually be able to open a jar of spices and smell it (Asaba et al., 2010). In the *Sens.és Making* project, when the youth shared their photographs of the sensory challenges in public spaces, everyone started to share both their embodied emotional and social experiences, which were inextricable from their multi-sensory experiences (Clement et al., 2022). Often sensory experiences are invoked in the viewer, through image alone, as in an image of flames and smoke in the *Vision Quest* project that can evoke the embodied smells of a fire.

Data Analysis

In photovoice research, analysis starts when participants begin sharing ideas about the meanings of pictures. The sharing of pictures is, therefore, not merely an event of viewing the 'generated data,' but a collaborative event of sharing experiences and beginning to interpret the visual and experiential information.

> Photovoice is not intended to produce a body of visual data for exhaustive analysis in the social science sense … In contrast, photovoice offers a new framework and paradigm in which participants drive the analysis – from selecting photographs that they feel are most important or simply like best to the 'decoding' or descriptive interpretation of the images.
>
> (Wang & Pies, 2008, p. 192)

It is rare that pictures are analyzed for content, since photographs are used as catalysts for discussion and as representations for something that someone in a group wants to highlight. The methodological plasticity of photovoice means that participants can shape and tailor both the information gathered as well as the way in which this information is analyzed. This is important because in cases where participants in a project have experienced social exclusion or alienation from participation in local activities, it is likely that new ideas come up spontaneously during group work. For example, in the *Vision Quest* project, a participant presented photographs in a storied form (Isaac, 2012), which influenced the group to adopt a photo-narrative approach to presenting stories through pictures. This provided a presentation of experiences across time and context as well as thematically presenting common experiences among participants. In this way, analysis was performed through group discussions and engagement in a process of writing detailed descriptions relating to concrete or symbolic aspects of each photo (Van Leeuwen, 2001).

It is also possible that certain experiences of relevance that have been dormant can come to be expressed because of the empowerment felt through a group where several people share similar experiences. For example, in one of our projects a participant brought a picture of a dandelion, which had been taken during late autumn when dandelions typically are not in bloom. For the person who took the photograph, the dandelion first represented beauty and strength in later life, the ability to bloom even during late autumn days; but through the group's discussion, it also came to represent national policies around immigration (dandelion as undesired weed or as a burden in a garden), and the inevitable fact of modern migration (even if the dandelion is weeded it will keep returning, metaphorically migration will continue to occur even in light of barriers and challenges). Discussions can be captured in different ways such as through audio recording or video recording photovoice sessions as well as taking fieldnotes. Moreover, groupwork during photovoice sessions that results in artefacts such as writings on a whiteboard or post-it notes can also be included as recorded data.

Dissemination

In some cases, participants of the photovoice group might want to invite an artist to provide advice on framing and displaying the photographs such as in the *Inclusive Communities* project or *Everyday Life with Spina Bifida* (Asaba et al., 2010; Gabrielsson et al., 2020). An artistic consultation can be structured to include a first meeting to listen to stories from the group (i.e., what the group wants to express, and the types of spaces in which the pictures would be displayed). In a second meeting, the artist can provide concrete examples and feedback to the group about alternatives for the visual presentation of the pictures depending on color schemes, size, framing, height from ground, and symmetry versus asymmetry, among more. Feedback through this type of consultation can be helpful for the group to make decisions about how well the emerging display of pictures is in fact communicating that which the group intends or wishes to express. Whether this level of work with aesthetics is required or whether it is positive can be debated. Not every project in which we have worked has devoted this amount of time and detail to issues of presentation. We have found the contribution of an artist to be valuable in making the exhibition's message come across clearly, and in raising a sense of pride and dignity to the group's work. This was not something that was planned, rather something that grew from the group processes.

The outcome of analyses in a photovoice project can vary. In most cases the outcome is at least a photographic exhibition where a community/audience is invited to the visual (and often textual via captions) expression of experiences as well as a dialogue with the group. However, a photo production can also be online (https://disabledref ugeeswelcome.se/wp-content/uploads/2020/11/PhotovoiceBroschy-En.pdf) or via a printed pamphlet (Mälstam et al., 2018). Within photovoice projects underpinned by a critical epistemology, and thus aiming to mobilize knowledge into action, there is a need to consider how the dissemination process, including exhibitions, can be organized in ways that reach audiences that include 'power brokers' whose zone of influence relates to desired change (Liebenberg, 2018). Achieving social change or impacting directly upon the community in which the project is conducted is a central tenet in photovoice. However, it should also be noted that the measure of social change is a debated concept. In all instances, there is a need for transparency regarding a researcher's commitment to working with communities towards desired social change, and a need to avoid the pitfall of raising consciousness regarding situations of oppression and marginalization without also facilitating exploration of meaningful ways forward to address such situations (Johnston, 2016; Liebenberg, 2018). In many cases, researchers involved in a project also have academic career interests or grant obligations where scientific publication is an outcome. Authorship and co-authorship can be negotiated as in any group where a joint work is produced, and efforts can be made to publish in ways that raise consciousness of diverse audiences, such as academics, policy professionals, and health care professionals.

Rigor and Ethics

Ethical aspects of conducting photovoice research are of critical importance. This section has both an instrumental aspect related to informed consent and the use of visual material, as well as a reflective aspect related to challenges that we have come across in conducting our projects.

Photovoice entails additional ethical challenges when compared to other qualitative or participatory methods because photos are used (Wang & Redwood-Jones, 2001); for example, the act of taking pictures in a community is a political act, that both discloses that which is photographed and hides what is not. Photography can be intrusive and lead to unintended consequences (Castleden et al., 2008). Dealing with anonymity and confidentiality is also challenging, although strategies such as addressing ethics in photovoice training sessions, using informed consent forms (from those photographed), transcription verification (allowing participants to delete any potentially harmful photos and transcripts), and photo release forms (ensure understanding of what photos would be used for and where photographs would be published) can be used. Photovoice projects often involve people who experience conditions creating vulnerability or marginalization; it is thus critical to emphasize that no picture is worth taking if it brings the photographer or subject of the photograph harm (see Table 13.2 for potential risks).

Photovoice research projects need to be anchored in a local context and in struggles experienced by the participants, otherwise there is a risk of it being used as an instrumental approach to gathering photos as a complement to group interviews. If there is a lack of participatory elements that are central within an epistemology of photovoice research, then projects that do not involve group discussion, stakeholder consultation, or identification of action strategies do not meet the rigor of being participatory (Gabrielsson et al., 2022). Lal et al. (2012) argued that sole reliance on individual interviews regarding photos, as opposed to group discussions, significantly detracts from the positive effects that arise from enactment of participatory principles and a transformative group context. It has been argued that if the methodology does not contain an action component where photos and discussions do not come from community participants, then it should not be labeled as photovoice (Hartman et al., 2011). As with many methods, adaptations to the photovoice method have been observed; the most common adaption observed in disability research was to replace the dialogue that unfolds through discussions in a group with individual interviews (Shumba & Moodley, 2018). We argue that dialogue is a crucial dimension that cannot be methodologically justified if removed from photovoice (Gabrielsson et al., 2022).

Table 13.2 Potential risks and strategies for working with risks

Potential risks	*Strategies*
Taking pictures that portray community, group, or individuals in a negative light.	Discussing risks and ensuring match between participant resources and aim of project.
Pointing out a group/community as 'marginalized,' 'oppressed,' and 'vulnerable' can contribute to stigmatization and further marginalization of group.	Being attentive to language use, discussion around risks associated with presentations, and having representative reference groups.
Photography can be interpreted as intrusive.	Discussion about informed consent and forms needed when taking pictures of people.
People in pictures are no longer anonymous.	Discussion of informed consent and possible risks of being identified in a photo.
Excluding people who might be seen as limited in taking pictures due to physical, sensory, or cognitive barriers.	Working with reference groups in order to find adaptive strategies to make project inclusive or consider how techniques can be adapted.

Author created

Another aspect is the need for redefinition of power positions and relationships; experts are the participants themselves whereas researchers are often acknowledged as resources that can facilitate the negotiated and sanctioned agendas pertaining to the identified social issues. A perpetual challenge in photovoice projects is future sustainability of social actions in line with the social issues identified by the group. In particular, when underpinned by critical epistemology, the ethical imperative of researchers involves not only ensuring that "the ways we engage in research with communities honor their wisdom and expertise" (Liebenberg, 2018), but also ensuring that there is a commitment to converging action and research to meaningfully address highlighted issues and support social transformation. This aim for social transformation aligns with directions in occupational science and occupational therapy to mobilize occupation as a means to address social and occupational injustices (Schiller et al., 2022). Enacting this ethical imperative requires that resources and capacity are in place to support meaningful community collaboration in knowledge generation, identification of ways forward in addressing community concerns, and dissemination to relevant power brokers. It is also crucial to avoid downloading the responsibility for enacting social transformation solely onto participants and communities facing marginalization and enduring resource inequalities; thus, requiring that attention is paid to building and mobilizing partnerships within actions directed towards social and policy change (Johnston, 2016; Liebenberg, 2018).

There are limits to what is observable and what can be photographed—both for practical and ethical reasons (Castleden et al., 2008); while we found participants to be incredibly creative in how they used photos to comment on non-tangible items or issues, we also found that combining photos with individual interviews opened space for discussion regarding the issues that participants could not photograph. For example, in the *Sens.és Making* project the youth co-researchers understood that they needed to get the consent of anybody who was caught in the frame of their photographs. Thus, this ethical aspect of taking photographs in public venues took away from their ability to capture many of the sensory-social aspects of their everyday environments that the youth felt oppressive (e.g., crowded metros, smoking at bus stops, lines at amusement parks, etc.). Similarly in the *Inclusive Communities* project (Asaba et al., 2010), participants at times felt uncomfortable asking for consent to include strangers in their photos. In the *Inclusive Communities* project, the dilemma became most clear when the group wanted to use a particular picture for which the photographer had not solicited informed consent from all persons in the picture. After long deliberation around possibilities, the group ended up printing only a portion of the picture in which the feet of a dancing couple could be identified but no persons. The group reasoned that the picture communicated what it needed to communicate without showing the persons or broader space in which the occupations were unfolding.

The democratic ideal of an equal partnership emphasizes the unique strengths, expertise, and shared responsibility of all partners who are engaged in a joint process, and involves all partners' input into all phases of a project. However, achieving equal participation can be challenging for various reasons; for example, in one project, two of the executive directors who were part of the project group left their organizational positions in the later phases of the project, and the project focus was negotiated with the mandate of a funding source. Three partnering organizations wanted to have input in shaping the research questions and being part of community presentation of findings where potential action strategies were discussed, but at the same time indicated they did not have time or interest to participate in the photovoice process or in analysis.

This raises questions about what counts as 'participatory.' Similarly, participants in another one of our projects expressed that they did not want to spend time in the latter parts of the analytic process through creating an exhibition. Rather, they suggested that the researchers make a suggestion to which they could make revisions. Cargo and Mercer (2008) have raised a distinction between equal and equitable partnership, which we find useful here; an equitable partnership enables the contribution of each partner to be negotiated, rather than expected, and to align with each partner's resources and strengths.

Finally, how to handle social interactions and dynamics between group participants within the research processes can be challenging. One woman in the *Inclusive Communities* project in Sweden became very invested in the ideas of being part of the group and making a change. She consistently came with pictures that she had taken and expected a platform to share these ideas at length. At times this led to conflict. In retrospect, and after some reflection, it is interesting to think about what it was that got this person so invested in the questions and the process. Her passion and commitment was, in many ways, an expression and affirmation of the 'empowerment' upon which the method in part rests. Her role in the group also led to 'conflicts' and 'making up,' which in part also led to discussion around issues that allowed for the group to reach deeper insights about 'participation' and investment in a process. She was also a person from our project who explicitly expressed how she would integrate new activities in her everyday life that were made possible through a sense of confidence that she had gained through her involvement in the photovoice groups. In her case, it meant volunteering to show and share her migration experiences grounded in a historical perspective using a collection of personal artifacts as portable exhibition.

Critiquing Photovoice Studies

In Textbox 13.1, we offer some questions that readers of photovoice studies might ask to ascertain the quality of the methodology and the overall study.

Textbox 13.1   Questions to Ask in Critique Photovoice Studies

1 To what degree is the problem/challenge *grounded in a local context*?
2 To what degree is the *data-generating process* participatory?
3 How does the interpretive process provide space for *collective discussion and analysis*?
4 How is *authorship* of the generated data addressed in the project?
5 Are the authors transparent regarding how *ethical guidelines* for photo taking and exhibition were established?
6 To what degree are *findings presented* within the community? In which forms? Is it collaborative and who constitutes the audience?
7 What are the *epistemologies* underlying not only the research question but those that guide the various researchers' and participants' on the team?
8 How are *sustainability issues* addressed with the community/local context?
9 How is the project *transformative of the societal challenge* addressed?

Implications for Occupational Science

Drawing on photovoice to examine barriers and constraints to occupational engagement for groups experiencing marginalization or socially positioned as being marginalized has potential to enhance understanding of the ways in which various layers and elements of contexts influence the occupations in which individuals and collectives engage. For instance, photovoice can be a useful approach in projects where occupational deprivation (Wilcock, 1993, 1998) is in focus and where locally rooted change is of interest. In keeping with Hartman et al. (2011), photovoice can advance the study of occupation through enabling researchers to gain access to tacit and commonplace elements of occupation that may be difficult to verbally describe or not immediately available to conscious reflection, such as experiences linked to spirituality (Eyres et al., 2019), structural inequity (Gabrielsson et al., 2020; Holmlund et al., 2018; St. John et al., 2021), or even how structural inequity is linked to multi-modal and embodied experiences (Clement et al., 2022). The use of visual methods can also bring to light cultural elements of occupation (Agaronov et al., 2019; Berinstein & Magalhaes, 2009), such as the ways in which curriculums exclude Indigenous ways of knowing and doing and thereby limit occupational possibilities (Laliberte Rudman et al., 2010/2011) or how the experiences of aging among international migrants are strengthened through the integration of their culture of origin into everyday life practices (Asaba et al., 2010). Photovoice methods can also speak to the broader health care and social practices relevant to occupation as well as advance transformative occupation-based research (Benjamin-Thomas et al., 2019; Benjamin-Thomas et al., 2022). Finally, photovoice is inherently occupational in the sense that engagement in the project means that people will plan things, do things, reflect on their plans and engagements, share in other people's experiences, as well as communicate all this visually, textually, and/or verbally. We also advocate for reflecting on the epistemologies guiding the projects. Not only is this part of our shared task of articulating our epistemic communities (Kinsella, 2012) but it foregrounds or backgrounds the degree of focus on transformation, and how that plays out at various levels.

Implications for Occupational Therapy

There are many examples of how photovoice has been used to involve communities in health promotion initiatives and to inform health policies, systems, and programs (Wang & Pies, 2008). Given that the focus on participation and collaboration aligns well with client-centered approaches in occupational therapy practice, as does the use of activity and group work (Lal et al., 2012), photovoice can be mobilized to inform occupational therapy, in terms of managing and living with chronic illness (Mälstam et al., 2018); understanding health disparities (St. John et al., 2021); in-patient environments (Birken & Bryant, 2019); child-directed assessment (Greco et al., 2017); community participation (Heffron et al., 2018); and empowering caregivers (Rabaey et al., 2021). Photovoice can be used to address many types of research aims relevant for informing occupational therapy practice and advocacy, such as raising awareness around environmental barriers to participation, engaging in a group process aimed at changing aspects of peoples' daily lives, or raising awareness of the social and political production of marginalization to key stakeholder groups (Lal et al., 2012).

Authors' Reflections

Our personal reflections are integrated throughout this chapter hermeneutically in order to maintain connections between the what, why, and how in our project endeavors. What is intriguing about photovoice—and particularly appealing to us—was the ambition of collaborating with people in a process that would contribute to building knowledge in an academic sense and have a potentially immediate impact on communities/organizations with whom the work was being carried out. In these participatory processes, the use of visual materials provided a wealth of information, a depth of understanding of the meaning of images from both individual and group perspectives, and the opportunity to better communicate and thus collaboratively build knowledge and transformational actions strategies guided by those with whom we worked through relationship building and dialogue. The most challenging part for novice researchers using photovoice could be the shift in power relationships between the researchers and participants, and the unexpected directions the projects can take because of exercising democratic dialogue in research.

Conclusion

Photovoice research requires a comfort with the unknown, a readiness to embrace the unexpected, a willingness to de-center the 'power' of the researcher, and the patience to let the group process unravel in organic ways. For occupational scientists and occupational therapists, the theoretical underpinnings of photovoice and our examples drawn from four projects, can be used to focus attention on how the methodology of photovoice aligns with underlying assumptions in the practice of occupational therapy and/or applications or research practices within occupational science; that is, how engaging occupations can contribute to participation in society and how the potential of visual images can support learning, engaging together, communication, and a personal to social transformation. We hope that a focus on epistemologies sheds light on implications for rigor in the continued development of research about human occupation.

References

Agaronov, A., Entwistle, T., & Leung, M. M. (2019). From the lunch table, to the family table: A grounded theory approach to understanding urban adolescents' experiences of food culture mismatch between school and home environments. *Ecology of Food and Nutrition, 58*(1), 23–44. https://doi.org/10.1080/03670244.2018.1554566

Asaba, E., Laliberte-Rudman, D., Park, M., Borell, L., Kottorp, A., Josephsson, S., & Luborsky, M. (2010). *Creating inclusive communities: Challenging the status quo through a multi-national innovative integration of ethnography and photovoice among elder migrants* (D10-R-0076) [Grant].

Bailliard, A. L. (2015). Video methodologies in research: Unlocking the complexities of occupation. *Canadian Journal of Occupational herapy, 82*(1), 35–43. https://doi.org/10.1177/0008 417414556883

Banks, M. (2007). *Using visual data in qualitative research.* SAGE.

Benjamin, W. (1935/1986). The work of art in the age of mechanical reproduction (H. Zorn, Trans.). In J. G. Hanhardt (Ed.), *Video culture: A critical investigation* (pp. 27–51). Peregrine Smith Books in association with Visual Studies Workshop Press.

Benjamin-Thomas, T. E., Rudman, D. L., Cameron, D., & Batorowicz, B. (2019). Participatory digital methodologies: Potential of three approaches for advancing transformative occupation-based research with children and youth. *Journal of Occupational Science, 26*(4), 559–574. https://doi.org/10.1080/14427591.2018.1512054

Benjamin-Thomas, T. E., Rudman, D. L., McGrath, C., Cameron, D., Abraham, V. J., Gunaseelan, J., & Vinothkumar, S. P. (2022). Situating occupational injustices experienced by children with disabilities in rural India within sociocultural, economic, and systemic conditions. *Journal of Occupational Science, 29*(1), 97–114. https://doi.org/10.1080/14427591.2021.1899038

Berger, J. (1972/2002). *Ways of seeing.* British Broadcasting Corporation and Penguin Books.

Berinstein, S., & Magalhaes, L. (2009). A study of the essence of play experience to children living in Zanzibar, Tanzania. *Occupational Therapy International, 16*(2), 89–106. https://doi.org/10.1002/oti.270

Beryman, D. (2019). Epistemology, Ontology, methodology, and methods: Information for librarian researchers. *Medical References Services Quarterly, 38*(3), 271–279. https://doi.org/10.1080/02763869.2019.1623614

Birken, M., & Bryant, W. (2019). A photovoice study of user experiences of an occupational therapy department within an acute inpatient mental health setting. *British Journal of Occupational Therapy, 82*(9), 532–543. https://doi.org/10.1177/0308022619836954

Brinkmann, S. (2018). The interview. In N. K. Denzin & Y. S. Lincoln (Eds.), *The SAGE handbook of qualitative research* (5th ed., pp. 576–599). SAGE.

Cargo, M., & Mercer, S. L. (2008). The value and challenges of participatory research: Strengthening its practice. *Annual Review of Public Health, 29*, 325–350. https://doi.org/10.1146/annurev.publhealth.29.091307.083824

Carlson, E. D., Engebretson, J., & Chamberlain, R. M. (2006). Photovoice as a social process of critical consciousness. *Qualitative Health Research, 16*(6), 836–852. https://doi.org/10.1177/1049732306287525

Castleden, H., Garvin, T., & Nation, H.-A.-A. F. (2008). Modifying photovoice for community-based participatory indiginous research. *Social Science & Medicine, 66*(6), 1393–1405. https://doi.org/10.1016/j.socscimed.2007.11.030

Catalani, C., & Minkler, M. (2009). Photovoice: A review of the literature in health and public health. *Health Education & Behaviour, 37*(3), 424–452. https://doi.org/10.1177/1090198109342084

Clement, M.-A., Lee, K., Park, M., Sinn, A., & Miyake, N. (2022). The need for sensory-friendly "zones": Learning from youth on the Autism spectrum, their families, and Autistic mentors using a participatory approach. *Frontiers Psychology – Perception Science.* https://doi.org/10.3389/fpsyg.2022.883331

Coemans, S., Raymakers, A. L., Vandenabeele, J., & Hannes, K. (2019). Evaluating the extent to which social researchers apply feminist empowerment frameworks in photovoice studies with female participants: A literature review. *Qualitative Social Work, 18*(1), 37–59. https://doi.org/10.1177/1473325011769263

Elkins, J. (Ed.). (2008). *Visual literacy.* Routledge.

Eyres, P., Bannigan, K., & Letherby, G. (2019). An understanding of religious doing: A photovoice study. *Religions, 10*(4), 269. https://doi.org/10.3390/rel10040269

Freire, P. (1973). *Education for critical consciousness.* The Continuum Publishing Company.

Freire, P. (1993). *Pedagogy of the oppressed.* Penguin Classics.

Gabrielsson, H., Cronqvist, A., & Asaba, E. (2022). Photovoice revisited: Dialogue and action as pivotal. *Qualitative Health Research, 32*(5), 814–822. https://doi.org/10.1177/10497323221077300

Gabrielsson, H., Hultling, C., Cronqvist, A., & Asaba, E. (2020). Views on everyday life among adults with spina bifida: An exploration through photovoice. *International Journal of Qualitative Studies on Health and Well-being, 15*(1). https://doi.org/10.1080/17482631.2020.1830702

Goessling, K. P. (2018). Increasing the depth of the field. Critical race theory and photovoice as counter storytelling praxis. *The Urban Review, 50*, 648–674. https://doi.org/10.1007/s11256-018-0460-2

Greco, V., Lambert, H. C., & Park, M. (2017). Being visible: Photovoice as assessment for children in a school-based psychiatric setting. *Scandinavian Journal of Occupational Therapy*, 24(3), 222–232. https://doi.org/10.1080/11038128.2016.1234642

Haque, N., & Eng, B. (2011). Tackling inequity through a photovoice project on the social determinants of health. Translating photovoice evidence to community action. *Global Health Promotion*, 18(1), 16–19. https://doi.org/10.1177/1757975910393165

Harley, A., & Langdon, J. (2018). Ethics and power in visual research methods. In R. Iphofen & M. Tolich (Eds.), *The Sage handbook of qualitative research ethics* (pp. 188–202). SAGE. https://doi.org/10.4135/9781526435446.n13

Harper, D. (2002). Talking about pictures: A case for photo elicitation. *Visual Studies*, 17(1), 12–36. https://doi.org/10.1080/14725860220137345

Hartman, L. R., Mandich, A., Magalhaes, L., & Orchard, T. (2011). How do we 'see' occupations? An examination of visual research methodologies in the study of human occupation. *Journal of Occupational Science*, 18(4), 292–305. https://doi.org/10.1080/14427591.2011.610776

Heffron, J. L., Spassiani, N. A., Angell, A. M., & Hammel, J. (2018). Using photovoice as a participatory method to identify and strategize community participation with people with intellectual and developmental disabilities. *Scandinavian Journal of Occupational Therapy*, 25(5), 382–395. https://doi.org/10.1080/11038128.2018.1502350

Holmlund, L., Hultling, C., & Asaba, E. (2018). Mapping out one's own paths towards work - Focus on experiences of return to work after spinal cord injury. *Qualitative Health Research*, 28(13), 2020–2032. https://doi.org/10.1177/1049732318782706

Isaac, A. (2012). *Educational vision quests: Using photovoice to explore the perspectives of First Nations youth during their transition of post-secondary education* [Doctoral thesis, University of Western Ontario]. London, Ontario, Canada.

Johansson, K., Rudman, D., Mondaca, M., Park, M., Josephsson, S., Luborsky, M., Asaba, E. (2013). Moving beyond 'aging in place' to understand migration and aging: Place making and the centrality of occupation. *Journal of Occupational Science*, 20(2), 108–119. https://doi.org/10.1080/14427591.2012.735613

Johnston, G. (2016). Champions for social change: Photovoice ethics in practice and 'false hopes for policy and social change. *Global Public Health*, 11(5–6), 799–811. https://doi.org/10.1090/17441692.2016.1170176

Kinsella, E. A. (2012). Knowledge paradigms in occupational science: Pluralistic perspectives. In G. E. Whiteford & C. Hocking (Eds.), *Occupational science: Society, inclusion, participation* (Chapt. 6, pp. 67–85). Wiley-Blackwell.

Lal, S., Jarus, T., & Suto, M. J. (2012). A scoping review of the photovoice method: Implications for occupational therapy research. *Canadian Journal of Occupational Therapy*, 79(3), 181–190. https://doi.org/10.2182/cjot.2012.79.3.8

Laliberte Rudman, D., Richmond, C., Huot, S., Klinger, L., Maghalaes, L., Mandich, A., Orchard, T., Shaw, L., Thomas, D., & White, J. (2010/2011). *Learning with First Nations youth: A photovoice study addressing visions of education and work success (in partnership with Indigenous Services at Western N'Amerind Friendship Centre and Southwestern Ontario Aboriginal Health Access Centre)* [Grant].

Laliberte Rudman, D., Richmond, C., Orchard, T., & Isaac, D. (2023). Educational Vision Quests of Canadian First Nation Youth: A photovoice exploration. In H. V. Bruggen, S. Kantartzis, & N. Pollard (Eds.), *And a seed was planted…Occupation based approaches for social inclusion* (Vol. 3). Whiting & Birch.

Liebenberg, L. (2018). Thinking critically about photovoice: Achieving empowerment and social change. *International Journal of Qualitative Methods*, 17(1). https://doi.org/10.1177/1609406918757631

Lieblein, V. S. D., Warne, M., Huot, S., Rudman, D. L., & Raanaas, R. K. (2018). A photovoice study of school belongingness among high school students in Norway. *International Journal of Circumpolar Health*, 77(1). https://doi.org/10.1080/22423982.2017.1421369

Mälstam, E., Bensing, S., & Asaba, E. (2018). Everyday managing and living with autoimmune Addison's disease: Exploring experiences using photovoice methods. *Scandinavian Journal of Occupational Therapy, 25*(5), 358–370. https://doi.org/10.1080/11038128.2018.1502351

Mattingly, C. (2019). Defrosting concepts, destabilizing doxa: Critical phenomenology and the perplexingparticular. *AnthropologicalTheory,19*(4),415–439.https://doi.org/10.1177/1463499619828568

Mattingly, C., & Gron, L. (2022). Imagistic inquiries: Old age, intimate others, and care. In C. Mattingly & L. Grøn (Eds.), *Imagistic care: Growing old in a precarious world* (pp. 1–30). Fordham University Press.

Novek, S., Morris-Oswald, T., & Menec, V. (2012). Using photovoice with older adults: Some methodological strengths and issues. *Aging and Society, 32*(3), 451–470. https://doi.org/10.1017/S0144686X11000377

Park, M. (2010). Beyond calculus: Apple-Apple-Apple-Ike and other embodied pleasures for a child diagnosed with Autism in a sensory integration based clinic. *Disability Studies Quarterly: Special Topic: Autism and Neurodiversity, 30*(1). Retrieved from https://dsq-sds.org/article/view/1066/1232

Pink, S. (Ed.). (2012). *Advances in visual methodology*. SAGE.

Prosser, J. (2011). Visual methodology: Toward a more seeing research. In N. K. Denzin & Y. S. Lincoln (Eds.), *The SAGE handbook of qualitative research* (4th ed., pp. 479–496). SAGE.

Prosser, J., Clark, A., & Wiles, R. (2008). *Visual research ethics at the crossroads*. NCRM Reality Working Paper.

Prosser, J., & Schwartz, D. (1998). Photographs within the sociological research process. In J. Prosser (Ed.), *Image-based research: A sourcebook for qualitative researchers* (pp. 101–115). Falmer Press.

Rabaey, P. A., Hepperlen, R., Manley, H., & Ament-Lemke, A. (2021). Empowering caregivers of children with disabilities in Zambia: A photovoice study. *American Journal of Occupational Therapy, 75*(4), 7504180030. https://doi.org/10.5014/ajot.2021.045526

Schiller, S., van Bruggen, H., Kantartzis, S., Laliberte Rudman, D., Lavalley, R., & Pollard, N. (2022). 'Making change by shared doing': An examination of occupation in processes of social transformation in five case studies. *Scandivanian Journal of Occupational Therapy*. https://doi.org/10.1080/11038128.2022.2046153

Shumba, T. W., & Moodley, I. (2018). Part 1: A review of using photovoice as a disability research method: Implications for eliciting the experiences of persons with disabilities on the Community Based Rehabilitation programme in Namibia. *African Journal of Disability, 70*, 418. https://doi.org/10.4102/ajod.v7i0.418

St. John, B., Gray, M., Malzacher, A., Hladik, L., Lurie, S., & Ausderau, K. (2021). Using photovoice with people with intellectual disability to illuminate definitions of health and factors influencing participation in health promotion. *Journal of Applied Research in Intellectual Disability, 34*, 866–876. https://doi.org/10.1111/jar.12868

Van Leeuwen, T. (2001). Semiotics and iconography. In T. Van Leeuwen & C. Jewitt (Eds.), *Handbook of visual analysis* (pp. 92–118). SAGE.

van Nes, F., Jonsson, H., Hirschier, S., Abma, T., & Deeg, D. (2012). Meanings created in co-occupation: Construction of a late-life couple's photo story. *Journal of Occupational Science, 19*(4), 341–357. https://doi.org/10.1080/14427591.2012.679604

Wang, C., & Burris, M. A. (1994). Empowerment through photo novella: Portraits of participation. *Health Education Quarterly, 21*(2), 171–186. www.ncbi.nlm.nih.gov/entrez/query.fcgi?cmd=Retrieve&db=PubMed&dopt=Citation&list_uids=8021146

Wang, C., & Burris, M. A. (1997). Photovoice: Concept, methodology, and use for participatory needs assessment. *Health Education Behaviour, 24*(3), 369–387. www.ncbi.nlm.nih.gov/entrez/query.fcgi?cmd=Retrieve&db=PubMed&dopt=Citation&list_uids=9158980

Wang, C., Burris, M. A., & Ping, X. Y. (1996). Chinese village women as visual anthropologists: A participatory approach to reaching policymakers. *Social Science & Medicine, 42*(10), 1391–1400. https://doi.org/0277953695002871

Wang, C., & Pies, C. (2008). Local knowledge, local power, and collective action. In P. Liamputtong (Ed.), *Performing qualitative cross-cultural research* (pp. 186–211). Cambridge University Press.

Wang, C., & Redwood-Jones, Y. A. (2001). Photovoice ethics: Perspectives from flint photovoice. *Health Education & Behavior, 28*(5), 560–572. https://doi.org/10.1177/109019810102800504

Wang, C. C. (2022). The Tai Qi of photovoice. *Health Promotion Practice, 23*(2), 205–210. https://doi.org/10.1177/15248399211069905

Wilcock, A. (1993). A theory of the human need for occupation. *Journal of Occupational Science, 1*(1), 17–24. https://doi.org/10.1080/14427591.1993.9686375

Wilcock, A. (1998). *An occupational perspective of health.* SLACK.

Woodgate, R. L., Tennent, P., & Legras, N. (2021). Understanding youth's lived experience of anxiety through metaphors: A qualitative, arts-based study. *International Journal of Environmental Research & Public Health, 18*(4315). https://doi.org/10.3390/ijerph18084315

Additional Resources

Photovoice related websites that can be of interest: https://photovoice.org

14 Community-Based Research

Roshan Galvaan and Pam Gretschel

Community-based research is an orientation to inquiry (Boyd, 2020) that has its broadest goal as a "just, equitable and sustainable society" (Stutts, 2004, p. 69). It has a broad history that varies across geographical locations and disciplines. Paolo Freire's popular education, proposing a more humanist approach to education and inquiry, had a marked influence on community-based research. Freire's impact is evident in the value given to community participation and the transformative potential of ordinary people's subjective experiences in community-based research (Munck, 2014). The broad and diverse historical roots of community-based research are closely aligned with types of inquiry that have progressed into research designs with different emphases (Strand et al., 2003). For instance, action research and participatory research designs (Johnson, 2017a; Strand et al., 2003) evolved in line with varying priorities at particular historical moments, leading to distinctions between the designs and the scope of the political nature of the research. These distinctions are noticeable in the extent of community participation in the research process.

In this chapter, we begin by detailing how perspectives of what a community is and who constitutes it are reflected in the distinguishing features of community-based research. We discuss the approach to generating data in community-based research and describe key considerations for working with communities. We identify possible tensions that researchers must navigate during the research process. We share two practice examples of community-based research conducted in South Africa: one with a community of schools to address challenges relating to education, and one with a group of occupational therapists designing a new intervention for caregivers of children who are HIV positive. Our examples elucidate varied constitutions of communities, providing a glimpse of the nuances of applying the research processes and the lessons learnt following engagement in community-based research. We conclude by describing the alignment of community-based research with the discipline of occupational science and the profession of occupational therapy, and our reflections on what has drawn us to this research orientation and our experiences of engaging in this research.

Distinguishing Features of Community-Based Research

A community-based research orientation to inquiry requires partnerships with communities and expects people's lived and experiential knowledge to guide the research processes (Coghlan & Brydon-Miller, 2014). Selected research across disciplines such as education, social sciences, and health sciences seeks to uncover multiple, diverse community perspectives and, in partnership with communities, produce meaningful responses and solutions to particular concerns (Johnson, 2017a). What constitutes a community is not taken for

DOI: 10.4324/9781003456216-14

granted. The assumption that communities are diverse positions the troubling of the notions of community as an integral part of a community-based research project. The distinguishing features of community-based research are summarized in Table 14.1 and discussed below.

In community-based research, a community is defined as a group of people with shared experience and may include a variety of stakeholders. The boundaries of communities are demarcated using markers of shared geographies and place, sharing social meaning, or shared purposes (Le Dantec & Fox, 2015). For example, a community may be a group of people with the shared experience of using a service or a community may be those with experience of doing a certain kind of work, or a group of people who frequent a particular place. One of the first responsibilities of a community-based researcher is to connect with the community and, in partnership with them, develop an understanding of how the community defines themselves. One of the aims of building this understanding of how the community constitutes and defines themselves, is to identify how the community could be authentically represented in a study.

A community-based research orientation appreciates the diversity of knowledges and experiences present in and emerging from communities, and seeks to understand how this relates to and is influenced by broader political influences that contribute to experiences of oppression and privilege by members of the community. In this wider social and political context, multiple role-players and stakeholders are people associated with or connected to the community and may include policy and decision-makers and service providers. In occupational science and occupational therapy research, there is often a focus on a particular situation or phenomena that a community may have experienced, and stakeholders are connected to the phenomena or problem. Such stakeholders could be part of an inquiry as they are vested in the phenomena studied, and their views may enhance the inquiry. Stakeholders could contribute by sharing their links to and experiences of the phenomena, the actions they might have taken, and the outcomes. They might also suggest connections with different stakeholders linked to the phenomenon and, in this way, deepen the inquiry. For a study to be community-based, communities must have a significant say in the research (Johnson, 2017a). Ideally, communities would actively work with researchers and may even, at times, take the lead in the research process

Table 14.1 Characteristics of community-based research

Distinguishing features of community-based research	*Description*
Collaboratively delineating the community	The community has a say in defining itself and this informs how they are represented and what is represented in the research.
Values diversity of knowledges and experiences	The range and types of knowledge and experiences that communities hold are viewed as worthy for the research.
Relates to the community's social issues	The research phenomenon is located in relation to an interest driven by the needs as expressed by the community.
Respecting the power and self-determination of communities	The right of the community to exercise its agency and make decisions is valued.

Author created

to address the social issues they have raised. This framing emphasizes the value of communities as owners of knowledge and wisdom, recognizing that gaining insight from communities about respective situations of success and concern, facilitates producing knowledge relevant to and meeting their needs.

Since community-based research is collaborative in its approach and encourages a critical stance and a transformative agenda (Johnson, 2017a), researchers must negotiate their power with communities. Power refers to the extent of control over the research process, from conceptualization to dissemination, and occurs in the differential knowledge, resources, and interpersonal dynamics between those involved in the research. Power differentials and existing hierarchies must be considered so that the research process advances equitable participation for everyone involved. Such equitable participation is shaped during the research process and reflects how interpersonal, institutional, and organizational power are negotiated. The scope of community participation at various stages of the research may also vary based on the design and the way of dealing with power within the research. Communities could contribute to conceptualizing the research, formulating the research questions, recruiting participants, and analyzing and disseminating findings to varying extents. The intention here is not to oversimplify the interpretation of power; instead, we wish to draw attention to the pragmatic and conceptual influence on how power is conceived and navigated during community-based research.

A Decolonial Lens on Community-Based Research

A decolonial lens draws from a large body of theory which opposes the ongoing domination of Eurocentered and Western supremacy on political, social, and cultural life (Quijano, 2007). Decolonial perspectives value the often dismissed and invisibilized ways of being, doing, and knowing of Indigenous and minority groups (Quijano, 2007). Disrupting coloniality challenges researchers to break with hegemonies of knowledge that reproduces narratives of inferiority. Applying a decolonial praxis to community-based research can counter the often-invasive nature of research. To do this, Tuck and Yang (2014) proposed "refusal" (p. 812) as a mode of doing research that prevents researchers from objectifying participants and exploiting their knowledge for the benefit of academia. As community-based researchers we refuse to engage in research which objectifies communities by describing them in disenfranchizing ways. Instead, applying decolonial perspectives in community-based research demonstrably respects communities' agency, personhood, authority, and sacred knowledge and power as a way of countering ongoing colonial influences in people's lives. Showing this respect occurs through intentionally discussing and, where needed, negotiating aspects of the research.

Root (2007) advocated that community-based research combines research, activism, and education opportunities. In occupational science and occupational therapy, community-based research offers insights into the occupational engagement of communities while prioritizing their concerns and needs. Prioritizing communities' voices ensures that research is socially responsive. Thus, community-based research has the potential to actively involve communities by working on matters guided by the community in ways that resonate with them. The data generated from community-based research can inform advocacy and lobbying activities that could advance change aligned with a community's needs. The participatory research process and the data generated create opportunities to raise awareness and opportunities for learning for everyone involved. However, tangible change takes time, and communities may not experience immediate benefits.

These intentions to contribute to long-term change or the slow pace of immediate change may lead to communities becoming disgruntled with the research. A study's immediate, visible gains to those in the academy (i.e., a student graduating or a journal article publication) may be more than the immediate gains and outcomes felt by the community. This tension has to be managed so that the research contributes or supports shorter term changes where possible. The research process involves examining and questioning existing theories and concepts against data generated with communities to reveal opportunities for change. Researchers have to take responsibility for contributing to and drawing the community's attention to the possibility of gradual and incremental changes, which may be possible as changing theory influences social systems. The incremental and longer-term changes that may come about through advocacy and scholarship promoting transformation require that researchers apply research findings to shift practices and policies that affect the community.

We participated in a community-based action research project to improve education through changing school-based policies and practices in a low resource setting in South Africa. Bringing about change in this education system was a long-term project. This project formed part of the University of Cape Town Schools Improvement Initiative (SII), a university-school-community partnership between the University of Cape Town, the Department of Education, and schools in Khayelitsha in Cape Town (South Africa). Some of the challenges in education for schools in Khayelitsha, a historically black township, include a long history of systemic underinvestment, poor infrastructure and overcrowded classrooms, and low levels of literacy and numeracy. The curriculum in Khayelitsha schools inadequately prepares learners for further education in numerous ways. A key concern is that the medium of instruction does not accommodate most learners who speak English as an additional language. The schoolteachers and principals were keen to find new ways to involve parents and community members in the efforts to improve the school as a learning environment. Shortly after the SII's launch, we were part of a group that initiated a research project with a community-based orientation and action research design to work with the schools to explore possible strategies for improving the education system through sustaining partnerships and implementing strategies with the school and surrounding community (Silbert et al., 2018). In the work of the SII, the community included all teachers, learners, family members, and residents associated with the eight schools and the university staff members affiliated with the SII. Drawing on our knowledge of occupational science and occupational therapy, this project focused on the occupation of learning in context, asking: How is the occupation of learning in the SII partner schools best understood? (Galvaan et al., 2015a, 2015b). The community-based orientation of the research was a natural fit for the SII initiative, given the research team's interests in creating mutual opportunities for learning.

Epistemology, Ontology, Axiology

The paradigmatic stance (i.e., worldviews) underpinning community-based research are discussed below, drawing on the notions of axiology, epistemology, ontology, and theory. Axiology refers to the values of the researcher and what they believe should be researched. These values influence the research process. Community-based researchers value research which is anchored in developing partnerships to pursue actions which meet their individual and collective wants and needs of communities. Research is not undertaken for research sake. There is a deliberate intent to purposefully understand and effect changes while partnering with communities. This positioning reflects the strong alignment of community-based research with emancipatory paradigms (Guba & Lincoln, 1994) and participatory research designs (Peralta, 2017).

Ontology considers what is there to know; that is, the nature of knowledge. Community-based researchers recognize and search for epistemic pluralism. This ontological stance extends beyond a positivist paradigm in which an objective researcher searches for a singular reality. Community-based researchers value alternate forms of *evidence* and prioritize "local knowledge over universal knowledge" and value "experiential over abstract knowledge" (Munck, 2014, p. 18). In practice, this means that community-based researchers seek to discover knowledge located in the experiences and realities of communities, and develop an interpretation of this knowledge reciprocally with communities. Communities are considered to be intellectual spaces with rich and authentic knowledge linked to their contextually situated experiences (Johnson, 2017a). In the SII project, we believed that the opportunities for learning provided through education could make a difference in improving access to quality education for learners at the SII schools. We envisaged that improving education would increase opportunities for access to further education and decent work, reducing unemployment and the prevalence of social inequality in South Africa. However, we also recognized that through partnering with the schools in the community we could leverage our collective knowledge to support change together. This mode of partnering fitted with the ontology of community-based research.

Epistemology refers to the process by which the researcher will engage in the research with communities. Epistemologically, the community-based researcher considers themselves to be a collaborator who partners with communities to understand the issues they wish to bring to the fore. Partnering to collaborate with a community departs from traditional research and changes the relationships between what is researched and researchers. People in communities are owners of knowledge, skills, and expertise and are viewed as co-researchers. Democratizing knowledge generation by recognizing ownership differs from decolonizing processes in community-based research, where the roots of knowing are part of social movements and Indigenous ideologies (Fernández, 2021).

Theoretically, community-based research is primarily positioned within an interpretivist approach. An interpretivist approach is one in which the researcher/s and community aim to gain a fuller understanding of the community assets and needs, and the community is actively involved in developing a co-constructed understanding. Researchers may wish to frame their use of collaboration within a critical stance to advance social change. Adopting a critical stance shifts from understanding a community to a more transformative plan in which the community and the researcher partner seek to address relevant social, economic, and moral injustices. In the SII study, an occupational justice approach to occupational therapy and speech therapy student practice placements positioned these as critical service learning placements (Abrahams et al., 2018; Galvaan & Silbert, 2018). Our students' contributions to change formed part of the community-based research. Community-based research positioned in transformative approaches aligns with the work of Freire (1970) in its intent to raise critical consciousness and engage in actions which have the potential to advance change (Johnson, 2017a).

Community-based research does not impose solutions or rescue people from situations of marginality. It recognizes that the contributions that communities bring and the value of their diverse ways of knowing resists the powerful dominance of euro-centric knowledge. Foregrounding the knowledge and the concerns that communities bring, offers the change for research to be framed as praxis (theory and practice). This appreciation of scholarship as praxis can facilitate change in academic institutions holding power to legitimize knowledge (Fernández, 2021; Kessi, 2017).

Communities are heterogenous, with people possessing diverse societal power living alongside each other. There are layers of representations of power within the community that the researcher has to consider during the research. Researchers, communities, and participants must negotiate their power when forming relationships as it impacts the initiation, development, and maintenance of relationships. The negotiations are complex due to the multiple representations of power in a community.

Through enacting refusal (Tuck & Yang, 2014), researchers mindfully and consistently think through the complexities of power as they come to know the intricacies of a community, ensuring that the rituals of a community are respected. The researcher navigates power cautiously to ensure to not exert superiority and dominance over communities involved. Kessi (2017) described the re-inscription of dominance as examples where the research "links Black people with violence, women with irrationality, the poor with ignorance, or young people with deviance" (p. 507). Community-based research resists re-inscription of inferiority and instead seeks to use research to understand how experiences of and resistance to marginalization and oppression can inform liberatory goals and systemic change. Using a reflective map, in which elements of power within the research process are shared, aids in describing how the research field is developed and how instances of power and coloniality are accounted for during the research. During the SII study, a colloquium was hosted with community partners and used as an opportunity for everyone involved to map our reflections on power as a collective. This dialogue shaped the research process.

In her research example presented in more detail later in the chapter, Gretschel describes how she generated a reflexive statement when developing her research protocol which she gradually added throughout the research process to describe and reflect on her own positionality and the impact of this on her interactions with the community. This personal statement also presented other possible intersections of power in line with the differing positionalities of the members of the community.

Topics and Questions Best Suited for Community-Based Research Studies

Community-based research may be conducted for the purposes of seeking possibilities for change and discovering how and why experiences and efforts have been shaped and sustained, in some cases. Questions focused on during inquiry may include:

1 How is a particular phenomenon of human behavior shaped by both personal and external and systemic influences?
2 How could collaborative action address key issues and create shifts in policies and practices?
3 What are the opportunities for raising consciousness about entrenched and limiting actions and practices in a community?
4 What possible actions, strategies and approaches could be adopted or implemented to resist forms of coloniality in a specific setting?

Other examples of community-based research in occupational science and occupational therapy can be seen in Textbox 14.1.

Textbox 14.1   Examples of Community-Based Research

Community-Based Participatory Research Remodelling Occupational Therapy to Foster Older Adults Participation (Turcotte et al., 2019)
   This study explored the factors that affect social participation in community occupational therapy services in Canada, with the aim of service improvement. A steering committee consisting of academics and an array of 12 stakeholders who were knowledge users, came together to engage in the research. The research question posed was: "Which factors have the potential to affect the integration of social participation interventions in community occupational therapy with older adults based on the perspectives of potential knowledge users?" (Turcotte et al., 2019, p. 264).

Social Occupational Therapy, Impoverished Youth, and Everyday Urban Mobility (Gonçalves & Malfitano, 2021)
   This study explored the daily movements of youth within urban socio-cultural settings where marginalization is prevalent in Brazil. It aimed to describe how practices in social occupational therapy could address concerns related to everyday urban movements of young favela dwellers who have minimal social participation.

The detailed questions cannot be fully developed in advance; rather, they emerge as shaped by an agenda which should be set mainly by and with the direction from the community. The approach to crafting the research question with the community recognizes the value of the community's everyday realities (Lather, 1986).

In the SII research project, developing the overall research question emerged through an eight-month period in which the practice partnership was established. The broad research question was shaped through dialogues with community stakeholders about concerns related to learning and our practice contributions during this period. The overall research question was finally agreed upon through building consensus with the school management teams, the education district managers, and parents involved in programs at the school. The broad research question was framed as: What are the implications of a university–school partnership for capacity building of the schools (principals, teachers and senior management teams, the learners, the university students, and staff members) and the Education District (circuit managers, subject advisors, and other officials)? Specific sub-questions were crafted with different groups, such as learners, parents, and teachers who were part of practice projects. These sub-questions reflected the concerns related to each sub-group. For example, occupational therapy students together with their clinical education supervisor partnered with teachers to explore how they could support the learners' development of their handwriting through classroom-based interventions.

Recruitment of Community and Participants

Researchers have to invest in building relationships with a community before the selection of participants. The intentional choice of a community is guided by the phenomenon to be studied, and access is most often negotiated with key 'inside' community members. Negotiating permission to conduct research with communities takes time and community processes should not be bypassed by privileging academic timelines. Waiting and working at the community's pace may lead to significant amounts of time spent waiting. Time taken to wait for data collection, seen as a process of waiting inherent to community-based research, allows an opportunity for reflexivity on the research and self-reflection in such a way that knowledge emerges from the immersion (Palmer et al., 2018). The concept of what will be sufficient time (i.e., for selecting participants), needs to be open to allow communities to shape the selection. Research processes, thus, have to adjust to the community's time frames.

After initial partnering, the researcher and community must choose who will participate in the various research activities. Inclusion criteria to select participants could be co-designed with communities to identify whole collectives or selected participants for purposive recruitment. Often researchers work through key community decision-makers or establish a reference group to facilitate meaningful collaboration with communities. However, researchers must remember that communities are diverse and fluid in their composition. Thus, researchers must remain open to the participation of various people at various parts of the research process. Snowball sampling may well become one of the vital sampling strategies, with the researcher steered by the perspectives of the community who will guide who should participate and contribute to the research activities.

The community engages as co-researchers who adopt distinct roles to address issues in the research process. The more active involvement of the community as engaged researchers may be a challenging shift for researchers accustomed to more traditional forms of research, as they renegotiate their role not as leaders but supporters of their co-researchers' extended roles in the research process. Our approach to establishing the SII practice involvement in Khayelitsha was to negotiate formal permission to work at schools through entering into negotiations and agreements with the education district and the Khayelitsha Development Community Forum prior to entering the schools. Since the research emerged from this practice contribution, the recruitment of participants could occur by inviting those who were already part of practice programs to contribute to the research. When researchers explicate the research process, it provides a context for understanding the study (Le Dantec & Fox, 2015). Researchers must detail how they facilitate the partnership, who represents the community, how research and recruitment choices are made, and how initial research questions may change as the partnership develops. These explanations support researchers' efforts toward refusal and epistemic justice (Tuck & Yang, 2014).

In the SII research, the key school representatives and participants actively participating in SII projects (such as the learners, the library assistants, and parent volunteers at the schools) were the community partners for the research project. One of the co-researchers had worked as an educator in Khayelitsha before joining the university as a staff member. Thus, he was already well known in the Khayelitsha community. The rest of the participants who became stakeholders in the research were involved at different stages of the research process. These participants were organically selected to participate in the research based on their active participation in practice projects from which the research emanated. Their participation was thus reflective of the time they were actively involved with projects at the school. For example, school library assistants working to establish a reading program with occupational therapy students were involved for shorter periods during the practice projects but continued to work at the school and contributed to the community-based research project. The challenge of negotiating and including different participants at different stages in an equitable way reflected the challenges of working at different levels of partnership with communities. The number of participants recruited depended on how many people participated in the project. Most project participants contributed to the research and were accommodated through various logistical arrangements. Since the aim of this project was not to generalize the findings or find a universal truth, the number of participants included were also managed based on what was practically possible in data collection in relation to the ongoing contributions to practice involvements. Practice involvements were prioritized over the research. This meant that not all volunteers were necessarily included in the study but that diversity of people and views were sought and, once it appeared that this was reached, then, through consensus with our community partners, we stopped inviting participants to sign up. This was managed by allocating specific periods for data collection. This approach ensured that the research did not become burdensome for community members.

The researcher and interested community may have to navigate many barriers to meaningful community participation in community-based research. Sometimes, based on prior experiences, a lack of trust in the researcher and the purpose of the research may exist. Researchers should be clear about the strengths and limitations of the research focus and process, and how this could contribute to meeting a community's priorities. The researcher's task is to build a trusting rapport with the community and to transparently articulate and shape the research with communities so that any potential contributions of the research that may emerge are apparent. This shaping may involve dialogue with communities about underlying assumptions about the research or the phenomena to be researched; exchanging ideas and expectations about which language is used to communicate and how language is used in the research. Investing in such dialogue contributes to building trust and showing respect to communities.

Where differences in priorities and perspectives exist between the community and the research, researchers may need to find creative means of mediating toward a consensus. This may include extending available social networks and resources to leverage access to the resources necessary to facilitate change. Opportunities to access education and training through research, increase the visibility of community needs in the media, or advance local advocacy agendas are contributions that communities may find beneficial and valuable. Similarly, using languages and vocabularies that resonate with communities communicates respect for ways of thinking in communities. Given perceptions of different positionalities between the academics involved in the SII research and the community partners, we engaged reflectively and created consistent efforts for dialogue throughout the research. In dialogues with teachers, occupational therapy students, and supervisors, we created regular reflective spaces to talk through our experiences of the interventions. Through doing this frequently we built trust to be able to share authentically with each other. An occupational justice perspective to the overall research framed the research purpose as providing equitable opportunities for learning through recognizing how systemic factors contributed to everyday life.

Data Collection

A challenging aspect of conducting community-based research is the developmental nature of the research inquiry. Just as the questions are shaped and directed by the community involved, so too must researchers and the community work collaboratively to agree on the data collection methods. Community-based research is mainly rooted in qualitative designs but could include quantitative data and adopt a mixed methods design. Methods commonly used are qualitative in-depth interviews and participatory methodologies such as photovoice, digital storytelling, focus groups or inquiry meetings, and photo-elicitation interviews. These methods facilitate conversations rather than fixed responses and allow for exploring uncharted areas with which communities may wish to engage. In addition, they create opportunities for rich engagement in the issues which arise and problem-solving to find relevant responses and solutions. Survey data may quantify the extent of a problem or describe a concern in a way that is directly useful to the community. Such data can help support service development or lobbying for change.

Relationality between the researcher and community is exceptionally important in community-based research, with priority given to what matters to the community. The process of generating data must reflect, for example, respect for different cultural and social ideologies and expectations in a community. This relational aspect of data collection requires that researchers engage in reflexivity. Reflexivity refers to the researcher actively examining their assumptions, beliefs, and actions and how these might influence the research process. (Kinsella, 2005; Kinsella & Whiteford, 2009) This active examination involves a critical awareness of the researcher's privileges associated with their positionality. Practically, this means the researchers need to be conscious of how the community may view them and how the knowledge they value and have access to might differ from the knowledge communities' value. The steps they will take to continue to privilege the knowledge emerging from communities over that of researchers should be explicit. In the SII research example, the community were provided with several informal opportunities to share their perspectives, and challenge ideas introduced by the researchers. The influence and progress of the research was also tabled for discussion during frequent meetings where the practice partnership was monitored. Finally, a forum was created near the end of the research process in which representatives from the community shared their experiences of the outcomes and their learning in the research process.

Peer debriefing is a strategy which researchers use to ensure their reflexivity (Morrow & Smith, 2000). For example, researchers may use research journals and critical conversations with peers as mechanisms to ensure that they remain reflexive. Through peer debriefing, researchers may seek guidance regarding the theoretical and practical aspects of conducting the research. The reflexivity associated with debriefing can ensure that communities' voices and decision-making are honored during data generation and analysis.

As members of the SII, we were acutely aware of the power that came from being associated with the academy and the limitations of the scope of improvement that was possible in a system that, structurally, was just inadequate. This critique informed ongoing practice at the schools and ensured continuous vigilance about using power. An ideal and consistent research partnership was challenging to attain. Instead, the reality became a model for awareness of how we, especially the university and school representatives, used our power. This became a pivotal part of where we focused our inquiry. Being able to embrace the evolution of participation as a reality and reflecting on our power as a mode of doing our research was well aligned with a community-based research orientation.

Data collection involved semi-structured interviews with teachers, interviews with learners, reflexive accounts of photovoice practice projects, and document reviews. The data collection was devolved to practitioner–researchers who practiced in the schools and thus could discern and apply the necessary relational ethics to understand and reasonably include and represent the voices of those involved. The project group met regularly, generating data as a focus group to reflect on and critique ourselves and as people. Acknowledging that many aspects of power were far from equal, the negotiation of power between university academics and key representatives and stakeholders, such as parents and educators, was reflected in different gains from the research. This included widening access to services, such as access to rehabilitation screening for learners, and facilitated sessions where teachers discussed the hidden curriculum and identified changes they could implement. Another gain was principals from across schools demonstrating how they can form supportive coaching communities of practice that challenge the assumptions about limited parent involvement in schools.

Data Analysis

It is a complex task to organize, analyze, and interpret these multiple data sources. It is best practice for data to be stored electronically in folders which clearly label the date and nature of the engagement on a secure platform which is accessible to all involved in the analysis and write up of the research findings. The chronological organization of data allows for a detailed overview of the data collection process across the duration of the research process.

The relationality in community-based design is complex given that data may be generated and analyzed across various sites, and the plurality of communities and constraints of structures have to be contended with in the research (Le Dantec & Fox, 2015). Doing data analysis can occur as part of being in the research field and after all the data have been collected. Applying reflexive thematic analysis (Braun et al., 2019), the researcher codes the qualitative data to identify patterns that can be grouped into themes (see Table 14.2 for an example of coding and themes). Thematically analyzing high school learners' interviews on their experiences of mentoring primary school learners as part of a homework program yielded the following codes, sub-themes, and theme:

Table 14.2 Example of grouping codes into themes

Codes	Sub-theme	Theme
Inspiring change "Patience and understanding and I know how to motivate them. Like when someone doesn't believe more in themselves, I am able to make them believe more and more in themselves"—Mbuyi, high school learner	Making a difference	Wanting to give back to the community
Contribution to community change "what informed my decision to join the homework program was to like share my knowledge with other kids to help them improve with their school marks. Seeing that like my school is at a better level compared to some other schools in Khayelitsha, so I was like motivated to bring about change in my community"—Noma, high school learner and "To me at first it was all about to put something on my CV. But now it's all about helping."		
Feeling stuck "The other support that I need is to be helped as to how to let the student who just looks in the eyes and be like: so what, what are you going to do. And I just don't know what to do with them."	Facing the challenges	
Resources needed "I had to like take out my own calculator to help another kid. And I also had to take out my own eraser. also I had to take out my own pen. They're all—like some of them just like I don't have a pen."		

Author created

This analysis can be conducted with or presented to community members to guide the analysis process (Johnson, 2017b). The above theme was discussed with the teachers and learners, leading to practical responses within the homework program. Similarly, the findings from the data analyses throughout the process can be synthesized by identifying assertions. Assertions are statements that capture interpretations of the data in relation to the study's focus (Johnson, 2017b). Through developing and confirming the assertions with the community the what, how, and why of community actions can be considered. The community can contribute to developing the assertions or the researcher can present preliminary assertions to the community.

In the SII project, we generated high volumes of data through the involvement of diverse stakeholders, multiple data collection methods, and the prolonged nature of engagement. The researchers and community partners involved in each project thematically analyzed the data and then team sessions were held where the data analysis was discussed in order to develop assertions. Examples of assertions related to the homework program are presented below (Textbox 14.2).

Textbox 14.2 Examples of Homework Program Assertions

1 The opportunity to inspire primary school learners through contributing to the homework program leaves high school learners feeling that they are making a difference in their community.
2 Facing resource challenges can be frustrating, but high school learners are earning to contribute what they can and use their resources to strengthen our context

---

This continuous and sequential approach to data analysis informed the ongoing actions and aligned with the action based approach often adopted in community-based research. Analysis is complete when there is consensus between the researchers and community that the findings, in this case the themes, fully and accurately represent the data essence of the data.

Findings

Using a community-based research orientation in the SII study revealed the challenges with education experienced in the community and the difficulties in professional practice that are navigated. The project created a more participatory mode of engagement between teachers and learners; and produced innovative programs to support learning in the school. Lastly, it established an openness within the district and with the teachers and managers to crafting new opportunities for learning. In terms of scholarship, the project illustrated the potential of community-based practice for speech and language therapy as a way of shifting professional identity and extended how occupational therapy positioned its contributions in schools. Disciplinary and professional boundaries restricted students and academics from being able to formulate responses that matched the contextual demands. This led to opportunities for further theorizing and revising interpretations of what was deemed possible for practice. It became apparent, for example, that some of the practitioners with firmly established traditional, individualistic practices became agitated and affronted with the critique offered through community-based research. It took patience and openness from all involved to acknowledge possible shifts to consider.

Overall, the limitations of current conceptualizations and theories were exposed, and the research brought academics closer to the real struggles of the education system. Solutions were, of course, not to be found within a single project. What the project did, was elucidate some of the strengths and limitations of a university–school–community partnership aiming to improve the quality of education.

Some of the questions that we are left with following the study are:

a Are the small shifts and changes enough? How could we have used advocacy more to advance sustainable change?
b What is a sufficiently accountable amount of change that a community-based research project can show when the changes needed are systemic?

These remaining questions inform the continuing practice at the SII and in similar school settings, providing impetus to continue to use opportunities for lobbying and advocating for change. Situating community-based research in relation to existing community practices promotes accountability and contributes to sustainable change.

Rigor

In community-based research, the social-constructivist nature of engagement between the researcher(s) and community can facilitate rigor by encouraging a collective commitment to ensuring that the research is being done well (Kingsley & Chapman, 2013). Specific attention must fall on the subjectivity and reflexivity of the researchers and community; the sufficiency of, and immersion in all the data collected; the adequacy of data; and issues related to how the data are interpreted and presented (Morrow & Smith, 2000). The researcher(s) must describe in sufficient detail the community context to ensure that readers can apply their interpretation of the data to their contexts (Creswell, 2007). Communities will play a key role in shaping this description of their context. It is the responsibility of the community-based researcher to not only document and share their subjectivity; that is, their intentions and expectations about the research process with the community, but also to create spaces for the community to share their subjectivity. In the SII this was possible given that the researchers were also practitioners and thus the community members were familiar with who they were and had close experiences with how they worked and what was valued. Also, in designing the research, the opportunity to collect multiple sets of data and reveal different perspectives allowed for a fuller view in response to the research question. This approach to creating and supporting data collection enhances the rigor of community-based research (Morrow & Smith, 2000). Lastly, communities have to be given multiple opportunities to share their views of the findings and have the opportunity to weigh in on representations of data which do not align with their lived realities.

Ethical Research with Communities

Sound and ethical research in community-based research should be nested in the relational ethics framework rather than fixed expectations of absolutes of what can and cannot be done. Relational ethics is a framework developed to help researchers negotiate ethical considerations in complex environments. The researcher's responsibility to their participants and themselves is central to relational ethics (Pollard, 2015). Relational ethics resonates with experiences expressed by Indigenous people and communities who appreciate the ongoing considerations of ethical practice concerning issues that may arise during the research process. It requires that ethics is applied not only as a formula or procedures to be followed but that there is a continuous investment in working out what is ethical in the context of communities' ways, agendas, and needs. Relational ethics suggests a continual consideration of and, in practice, respect for ethics throughout the research activities. In practice this is linked to the following actions:

1 Placing continual emphasis on the value of the collective spaces of research engagement, highlighting that the information shared in the space must not be unduly shared.
2 Continually checking in with each other to make sure that being part of the research process is largely beneficial and not arduous.
3 Creating and facilitating access to sources of support or changing the research as necessary, should engagement in the research process cause distress for any participants.

Ensuring ethical practice in the research process cannot take place without consideration of possible factors which may influence the establishment of a relationship between the researcher and communities and impact the processes used to generate and interpret the data emanating from the study. Since knowledge emanating from marginalized groups (e.g., persons with disabilities and Indigenous groups) have historically been denied within academia, privileging the ways of knowing and being of these groups is essential in community-based research. The influence of possible factors on this relationship becomes even more important when it is recognized that there are various mechanisms of dominance that have historically oppressed communities that are still at play.

When health professionals engage in community-based research, the power associated with their professional identity creates an implicit hierarchy that may add to the quite established views of deference to the expertise of researchers. Here the researcher needs to be conscious of how communities may view them and plan approaches to mitigate against this view, and demonstrate actions which foster collaborative partnerships instead. These actions and approaches could include abandoning the use of professional titles and emphasizing the value of each person's contributions, continuing to intentionally create spaces for all to have the opportunity to share their views when they wish to, and foregrounding the requests of the community in the research process.

Educators in the SII project required encouragement to voice both their experiences and their suggestions for change, given that they had frequently found themselves as the recipients of instructions placed on them by statutory and regulatory educational bodies. Researchers contributed as active listeners to facilitate optimal participation of all stakeholders. This allowed for open sharing and novel ideas to be shared.

Hacker (2013) suggested careful consideration of the following questions when planning and engaging in community-based research: How and in what ways is the research project acceptable to the community? Have all relevant community leaders played a part in determining the acceptability of the research project? Have they been asked to suggest who should be involved in the project and in what ways? Have they been encouraged to highlight any potential issues which the researchers should be attentive to when entering into and engaging with the community? Are community leaders actively and continuously involved in steps relating to the research process?

Practice Example of Community-Based Research

The two practice examples shared above (SII) and below (Gretschel et al., 2017) describe our work with communities as researchers. We explain how notions of power surfaced in partnering with communities, highlighting concepts of negotiating the influences of power in line with the intended aims of our research projects. In both examples, as the researchers, we adopted stances which drove efforts to critically review and transform the practices of higher education institutions and health professionals, practices which are still anchored in colonial roots. To do this, we could not shy away from exploring moral and social justice issues linked to our intersectional identities relating to race, gender, ethnicity, class, and sexual orientation and how these might marginalize certain groups.

Research Example: Community-Based Research Within a Co-Operative Inquiry

In this second example, we describe a research partnership between Pam, an occupational therapy researcher, and a group of six occupational therapists working for a non-profit organization (NPO) providing services to HIV-positive children living in low-income conditions in South Africa (Gretschel et al., 2017). This research is shared to provide an example of community-based research with a community who were similarly positioned to the researcher.

Nolu, a senior academic at the place where Pam worked, had a strong association with the NPO, volunteering there and then serving on the board. Nolu tasked the group with designing a new occupational therapy intervention which focused more on the caregivers of the children, empowering them to draw on the constructs of play and playfulness to promote the development of their children and the engagement of their children in play and learning. Nolu invited Pam into the NPO as a possible research and practice space, given her past work experiences with children and their caregivers. The community of six occupational therapists was an accessible sample, representative of occupational therapists working in the area of early child development, and the researcher was familiar with the group. The researcher was drawn to understanding how a group of professionals empowered with education and experience would take the opportunity to reflect on and revise their current practices.

Considering that the profession of occupational therapy is linked to understanding occupation and how it is shaped by the interchange of both personal and contextual factors, the researcher identified that engagement in designing a new intervention as a collective was an occupation. Specifically, she was interested in exploring how occupational therapists' values, professional identities, the broader influences of their profession, and tangible contextual factors during engagement influenced their individual and collective action. She approached the group with this intent, and they responded positively, indicating that given the collective and novel nature of designing the intervention, they welcomed the opportunity to join the researcher as co-researchers.

The co-researchers agreed to a process of reflection and then reflection on action as they designed their new intervention. Pam partnered with the group within the ambit of a co-operative inquiry to document their process of creating the intervention (Heron & Reason, 2001). This methodology recognizes the similarities between the researchers and participants and, because of the seemingly comparable backgrounds, abandons the traditional role of a researcher who researches others, instead positioning participants as co-researchers who can decide how and in what ways the research process should unfold. The group welcomed this approach and contributed, offering suggestions on how they could engage with each other to design the intervention and vocalizing aspects they were not happy with. They also requested that Pam not only observe but also join in on the practical tasks of designing intervention elements. Despite these positive aspects, careful negotiation of power influenced the development of their work as a community of practice. Pam often had to encourage the co-researchers to vocalize their contributions to the research process (Gretschel et al., 2017). This emphasizes the continued effort of researchers to encourage co-researchers to share their contributions.

In addition to being aware of how power contributed to shaping the research, the study also raised awareness about the multiple contributions of diverse stakeholders across the research process, which were not necessarily anticipated during the development of the study proposal. At different stages of the research, various stakeholders requested to enter the space and contribute to designing the intervention. The group then wanted to invite other people to join the study. Here, Pam had to remain open to different people's contributions and ensure that informed consent was gained from all contributors. This example flags possible considerations for researchers as they plan community-based research projects.

A chronological sequencing of the data collection took place to organize the data, which were then analyzed using thematic analysis (Braun & Clarke, 2006; Clarke & Braun, 2017). Pam and co-researchers made use of multiple data collection methods such as researcher journaling, participant reflective pieces, individual interviews, participant observation of the intervention design meetings, and document and artefact review. These methods drove the co-operative inquiry and encouraged us as a group to reflect during and after our actions in designing the intervention over a period of 30 months.

Cultural historical activity theory, derived by Vygotsky, from German philosophy and Russian social science theory, was drawn on to describe and understand the activity of this community; that is, their process of designing the intervention (Gretschel et al., 2017). The multi-faceted focus of this theory allowed for a recognition of the many factors and interplay of these factors on individual and collective human action. In reviewing the analyzed data, cultural historical activity theory facilitated a discussion of how the actions of this specific community were shaped by their cultural views and resources, recognizing the inseparable influence of history on thinking and actions.

In summary, this example draws attention to a group of professionals who formed the community as a community of practice with whom the researcher partnered to engage in an agreed project. This example highlighted that even though the diversity in the positionalities of the group members was not extensive, given the homogenous composition, navigation of perceived power differences took place.

Application to Occupational Science

Community-based research shares strong links with critical theoretical perspectives in occupational science, which describe the value of being in dialogue with communities while building partnerships that embrace diverse knowledges and opportunities for dealing with systemic challenges (Mondaca, 2021). The common interest in addressing people's vulnerabilities and marginality collaboratively in contexts brings the orientation to research offered by community-based research into alignment with occupational science. It has the potential for enhancing how knowledge is generated in occupational science, what knowledge is generated, and extends on traditional notions of who is involved. It allows occupational scientists to consider the political context of knowledge generation, bringing theory into conversation with local realities.

Application to Occupational Therapy

Qualitative research is widely recognized as an invaluable tool to gain insights into the experiences, perspectives, and external influences on collective human action (Frank & Polkinghorne, 2010). Community-based research extends these aims in its intent to understand how communities are influenced by factors in their contexts; and how they are, in turn, influencing their contexts. Considering its focus on the praxis of communities (Johnson, 2017a), community-based research aligns with the goal of occupational therapy to promote participation in everyday life that resonate with communities. Insights generated through community-based research can thus strengthen occupational therapy services by ensuring greater coherence with community's experiences of human occupation in everyday life.

Critiquing Literature

The characteristic focus of community-based research in working collaboratively with communities, advancing socially transformative goals, and advocating for change provides a starting point for reviewing the use of community-based research. In Table 14.3 we present Johnson's (2017a, pp. 4–5) suggested questions linked to each characteristic and extend with questions (inserted in italics) which we propose should be asked to assess the quality of a community-based research project. Studies claiming to be community-based research can be critiqued using these questions as prompts.

Table 14.3 Questions for critiquing literature

Characteristic of community-based research	*Questions to explore evidence of elements of the foci*
Collaborative	What was the partnership? *How well are the strengths and weaknesses of the partnership described?* How was partnership initiated? How was partnership sustained? *Who was selected to partner and who was left out? And what was the reasoning for selecting partners? How were decisions made about including and selecting stakeholders? Has reflexivity been applied in how power was navigated within the study?*
Transformative	What social injustices were identified, by whom and why? *To what extent were communities' voices prioritized in agenda setting?* What changes were affected? What impact did they have? *What were the barriers to sustainable change?*
Advocacy	How is action taken and supported to advance change? Who is involved? How are they involved? *Who benefits from the advocacy initiatives and in what ways? What opportunities for education emerged and how were these harnessed?*

Author created

Authors' Reflections

We share the attraction to the possibilities that community-based research brings for knowing the world anew and the openness that it allows. The openness allows for creativity in the research process and, in our view, allows for more equitable ways of making decisions. Thus, it allows us to think about and conduct research in ways that do not over-emphasize technical and procedural correctness over community common sense and justice-based perspectives. There are many opportunities to grow—personally, spiritually, and professionally—for individuals and collectives involved in this research; and thus, we work together as humans bringing different capacities. The possibilities for equity in a world filled with injustices is appealing. The process of engaging in this type of research created awareness of the challenges and continual effort that needs to be invested in ensuring that the researcher does not slip into the traditional researcher role and take over ownership of the research process. Community-based research demands that the researcher abandons the notion that the research endeavor is theirs alone. This is done by creating and sustaining an environment in which community members are encouraged and feel free to contribute to, and lead, the direction of the research inquiry. The voluminous and intertwined nature of community-based research requires that researchers plan how they will document the process in an authentic and detailed manner which is reflective of the voices of all involved in the research. The realness and messiness of this type of research and opportunity to present multiple, shifting, and static perspectives is rewarding. The potential (not always achieved) of this methodology to create critical consciousness and effect change fuels the possibilities to ensure that scholarship serves the struggles of those who are marginalized.

Conclusion

Community-based research requires varying layers of commitment on the part of the researcher. To begin with, researchers need to invest time in building a relationship with communities, appreciating that they will need to connect with different and diverse stakeholders as guided by key members in the community. They need to relinquish their need to have a 'control' over the research process, remaining true to the collaborative intent of this research design and honoring the issues which communities wish to work on. The process is complex and dense, employing varied sources of data which must be carefully organized and analyzed to develop a complete picture of the research activities and outcomes. We have argued in this chapter that despite the intensity of these commitments, the alignment of community-based research with the values of occupational therapy, supports it continued and more extended use in occupation-focused research.

References

Abrahams, K., Kathard, H., Mostert, L., Walters, F., & Galvaan, R. (2018). Facilitating social inclusion through communication: How do speech- and language therapy students negotiate their transition into community practice? In P. Silbert, R. Galvaan, & J. Clarke (Eds.), *Partnerships in action: University-school-community* (pp. 181–197). HSRC Press.

Boyd, M. R. (2020). Community-based research: A grass-roots and social justice orientation to inquiry. In P. Leavy (Ed.), *The Oxford handbook of qualitative research* (2nd ed., pp. 741–771). Oxford University Press.

Braun, V., & Clarke, V. (2006) Using thematic analysis in psychology. *Qualitative Research in Psychology, 3*(2), 77–101. https://doi.org/10.1191/1478088706qp063oa

Braun, V., Clarke, V., Hayfield, N., & Terry, G. (2019). Thematic analysis. In P. Liamputtong (Ed.), *Handbook of research methods* (pp. 843–860). Springer Singapore. https://doi.org/10.1007/978-981-10-5251-4_103

Clarke, V., & Braun, V. (2017). Thematic analysis. *The Journal of Positive Psychology*, *12*, 297–298. https://doi.org/10.1080/17439760.2016.1262613

Coghlan, D., & Brydon-Miller, M. (2014). *The Sage encyclopedia of action research*. SAGE.

Creswell, J. W. (2007). *Qualitative inquiry & research: Choosing among five approaches* (2nd ed.). SAGE.

Fernández, J. S. (2021). Decolonising participatory action research in community psychology. In S. Kessi, S. Suffla, & M. Seedat (Eds.), *Decolonial enactments in community psychology* (pp. 29–51). Springer. https://doi.org/10.1007/978-3-030-75201-9_3

Frank, G., & Polkinghorne, D. (2010). Qualitative research in occupational therapy: From the first to the second generation. *OTJR: Occupational Therapy Journal of Research*, *30*(2), 51–57. https://doi.org/10.3928/15394492-20100325-02

Freire, P. (1970). *Pedagogy of the oppressed*. Seabury Press.

Galvaan, R., & Silbert, P. (2018). New possibilities or supporting homework practices through a university-school partnership. In P. Silbert, R. Galvaan, & J. Clarke (Eds.), *Partnerships in action: University-school-community* (pp. 167–180). HSRC Press.

Galvaan, R., Peters, L., & Gretschel, P. (2015a). Embracing an 'occupational' perspective to promoting learning in context. *South African Journal of Higher Education*, *29*(3), 281–293. https://doi.org/10.20853/29-3-498

Galvaan, R., Gretschel, P., & Peters, L. (2015b). Occupational therapy in the school context: An occupational perspective. In S. Moonsamy & H. Kathard (Eds.), *Speech pathology and audiology within an educational context: Principles and practices* (pp. 261–274). Van Schaik.

Gonçalves, M. V., & Malfitano, A. P. (2021). Social occupational therapy, impoverished youth, and everyday urban mobility. *South African Journal of Occupational Therapy*, *51*(4), 32–40. https://doi.org/10.17159/2310-3833/2021/vol51n4a5

Gretschel, P., Ramugondo, E. L., & Galvaan, R. (2017). *A case study on designing an occupational therapy intervention for caregivers of children on ART living in low-income conditions in South Africa*. [Unpublished Doctoral thesis, University of Cape Town].

Guba, E. G., & Lincoln, Y. S. (1994). Competing paradigms in qualitative research. In N. K. Denzin & Y. S. Lincoln (Eds.), *Handbook of qualitative research* (pp. 105–117). SAGE.

Hacker, K. (2013). *Ethical considerations in CBPR*. SAGE. https://doi.org/10.4135/9781452244181

Heron, J., & Reason, P. (2001). The practice of co-operative inquiry: Research with rather than on people. In P. Reason & H. Bradbury (Eds.), *Handbook of action research: Participative inquiry and practice* (pp. 179–188). SAGE.

Johnson, L. R. (2017a). *Community-based qualitative research: Approaches for education and the social sciences*. SAGE.

Johnson, L. R. (2017b). *Analysis of data in community-based qualitative research*. SAGE. https://doi.org/10.4135/9781071802809

Kessi, S. (2017). Community social psychologies for decoloniality: An African perspective on epistemic justice in higher education. *South African Journal of Psychology*, *47*(4), 506–516. https://doi.org/10.1177/0081246317737917

Kingsley, B. C., & Chapman, S. A. (2013). Questioning the meaningfulness of rigour in community-based research: Navigating a dilemma. *International Journal of Qualitative Methods*, *12*(1), 551–569. https://doi.org/10.1177/160940691301200129

Kinsella, E. A. (2005). Constructions of self: Ethical overtones in surprising locations. *Journal of Medical Ethics: Medical Humanities*, *31*(2), 67–71. https://doi.org/10.1136/jmh.2005.000201

Kinsella, E. A., & Whiteford, G. E. (2009). Knowledge generation and utilisation in occupational therapy: Towards epistemic reflexivity. *Australian Occupational Therapy Journal*, *56*(4), 249–258. https://doi.org/10.1111/j.1440-1630.2007.00726.x

Lather, P. (1986). Research as praxis. *Harvard Educational Review*, *56*(3), 257–277. https://doi.org/10.17763/haer.56.3.bj2h231877069482

Le Dantec, C. A., & Fox, S. (2015, February 28). *Strangers at the gate. Proceedings of the 18th ACM Conference on Computer Supported Cooperative Work & Social Computing.* Vancouver, Canada. https://doi.org/10.1145/2675133.2675147

Mondaca, M. (2021). "Doing hope" as a possible way towards a responsive occupational science. *Journal of Occupational Science, 28,* 19–28. https://doi.org/10.1080/14427591.2020.1797858

Morrow, S. L., & Smith, M. L. (2000). Qualitative research for counseling psychology. In S. D. Brown & R. W. Lent (Eds.), *Handbook of counseling psychology* (3rd ed., pp. 199–230). Wiley.

Munck, R. (2014). Community-based research: Genealogy and prospects. In R. Munck, L. McIlrath, B. Hall, & R. Tandon (Eds.), *Higher education and community-based research: Creating a global vision* (Chapt 2.). Palgrave MacMillan.

Palmer, J., Pocock, C., & Burton, L. (2018). Waiting, power and time in ethnographic and community-based research. *Qualitative Research, 18*(4), 416–432. https://doi.org/10.1177/1468794117728413

Peralta, K. J. (2017). Toward a deeper appreciation of participatory epistemology in community-based participatory research. *PRISM: A Journal of Regional Engagement, 6*(1). Retrieved from https://encompass.eku.edu/prism/vol6/iss1/4

Pollard, C. L. (2015). What is the right thing to do: Use of a relational ethic framework to guide clinical decision-making. *International Journal of Caring Sciences, 8,* 362–368.

Quijano, A. (2007). Coloniality and modernity/rationality. *Cultural Studies, 21*(2–3), 168–178. https://doi.org/10.1080/09502380601164353

Root, M. (2007). Community-based research. In W. Outhwaite & S. Turner (Eds.), *The SAGE handbook of social science methodology* (pp. 565–577). SAGE. https://doi.org/10.4135/9781848607958

Silbert, P., Galvaan, R., & Clark, J. (2018). *Partnerships in action.* HSRC Press.

Strand, K., Marullo, S., Cutforth, N., Stoecker, R., & Donohue, P. (2003). *Community-based research and higher education: principles and practices.* Jossey-Bass.

Stutts, N. B. (2004). Review essay of community-based research and higher education by Kerry Strand, Sam Marullo, Nick Cutforth, Randy Stoecker, and Patrick Donahu. *Michigan Journal of Community Service Learning, 10*(2), 69–72. http://hdl.handle.net/2027/spo.3239521.0010.206

Tuck, E., & Yang, K. W. (2014). Unbecoming claims: Pedagogies of refusal in qualitative research. *Qualitative Inquiry, 20*(6), 811–818. https://doi.org/10.1177/1077800414530265

Turcotte, P.-L., Carrier, A., & Levasseur, M. (2019). Community-based participatory research remodelling occupational therapy to foster older adults' social participation. *Canadian Journal of Occupational Therapy, 86*(4), 262–276. https://doi.org/10.1177/0008417419832338

Additional Resources

PAN. (2023). *Methods in community-based research.* https://paninbc.ca/resources-2/cbr-toolkitresources/methods-in-community-based-research/

Pilkerton, E. L. (2021). Community-based occupational therapy: Promoting family centered care. *Occupational Therapy Capstone Presentations, 53.* https://red.library.usd.edu/ot-capstone/53

SAGE Publications. (2023). *Laura Ruth Johnson defines community-based qualitative research.* https://methods.sagepub.com/video/laura-ruth-johnson-defines-community-based-qualitative-research

15 Qualitative Evidence Synthesis

Carolyn Murray, Katie Robinson and Mandy Stanley

Qualitative studies provide rich insightful findings that can contribute to knowledge about occupation and inform occupational therapy practice. Qualitative evidence synthesis is an umbrella term for systematic reviews which allows findings from multiple original qualitative studies to be synthesized, thereby allowing richer interpretation of a phenomenon or an experience than individual qualitative studies could achieve (Flemming & Noyes, 2021). Since the publication of the first edition of this book, there has been continued qualitative evidence synthesis methodological development. Different terms have been used to describe the process of synthesizing qualitative research and the lack of consensus persists across health and social science disciplines. For the purposes of this chapter, we will use the broad umbrella term 'qualitative evidence synthesis.' The term refers to the different approaches to qualitative synthesis and is the preferred term of the Cochrane Qualitative and Implementation Methods Group (Booth et al., 2016).

Over 30 different approaches to the synthesis of qualitative research have been identified including meta-ethnography, grounded theory, thematic synthesis, textual narrative synthesis, meta-study, meta-narrative, critical interpretative synthesis, ecological triangulation, framework synthesis, and meta-aggregation (Barnett-Page & Thomas, 2009; Flemming & Noyes, 2021; Lockwood et al., 2015). Among these approaches, there is now growing recognition of the value of qualitative evidence synthesis with an increasing number of such studies being conducted. In this chapter, we draw on our collective experiences of using qualitative evidence synthesis to inform our research in occupational science and occupational therapy across the fields of aged care, neurological and musculoskeletal rehabilitation, developmental coordination disorder, the neonatal intensive care unit, and in teaching and learning. Specifically, in this chapter, we draw extensively on a qualitative synthesis of the perspectives of people with a spinal cord injury co-authored by Carolyn, Mandy and colleagues (Murray et al., 2019) to illustrate the process of qualitative evidence synthesis.

Background

The meta-ethnography approach was the original qualitative evidence synthesis approach derived by Noblit and Hare (1988) within the discipline of anthropology. With this approach, results of included studies identified through systematic searches (including concepts and themes) are extracted from the papers and re-analyzed using an interpretative, inductive process whereby the studies are synthesized to arrive at 'a new line of argument' in the form of higher order analytical theories or themes (France et al., 2019a; Liamputtong, 2013; Sattar et al., 2021). Using our example (Murray et al., 2019), the interpretative

DOI: 10.4324/9781003456216-15

approach with data from 801 participants arrived at two new analytic themes with sub-themes that explained choice and control following spinal cord injury (experiencing vulnerability and security and adapting to bounded abilities). Other examples using meta-ethnography include theorizing challenges in occupational therapy practice (Murray et al., 2015), explaining experiences of pain and function after total knee replacement (Taylor et al., 2022), and exploring why allied health professionals are not using stroke clinical guidelines (Halls et al., 2021). As can be seen from these examples, there is potential within occupational science and occupational therapy to use meta-ethnography to maximize the contribution of numerous published small-scale qualitative studies. Meta-ethnography can enable generation of theory, development of enriched understandings of people's experiences, and can inform intervention development and evaluation (France et al., 2015).

Meta-aggregation is another approach to qualitative evidence synthesis and occurs when existing findings of studies are synthesized into narrative statements and descriptive recommendations (Korhonen et al., 2013). Using this type of qualitative evidence synthesis, extracted data from studies are analyzed and findings are reported under descriptive themes (or headings). A meta-aggregation may occur where the topic is specific and pragmatic outcomes are sought (Lockwood et al., 2015). In contrast to meta-ethnography, meta-aggregation data are presented without re-interpretation by the synthesis authors. The findings of meta-aggregation are statements that stay close to the findings of the included studies rather than generation of new theory as occurs in meta-ethnography (Lockwood et al., 2015). A recent systematic review and meta-aggregation of qualitative research by occupational science and occupational therapy researchers aimed to capture the scope and quality of literature about the occupational experiences of homeless persons in high income countries and aggregate the findings of these studies with at least 335 participants (Marshall et al., 2020). The review included disciplines outside of occupational science and occupational therapy which the authors note enriched the review. Similar to many other review methods, qualitative evidence synthesis allows researchers to map the evidence on a topic and identify where further studies may be redundant or where gaps exist.

Epistemology, Ontology, Axiology

Synthesis of qualitative research has parallels with synthesis of quantitative research; however, it is important to acknowledge the differing epistemological and ontological positions underpinning these two approaches to evidence synthesis. Those completing qualitative evidence synthesis need to remain interpretative and open to multiple viewpoints and diversity in their review, rather than seeking to uncover a single objective reality (Malterud, 2019c). Given these differing positions and the focus of qualitative research on the ideographic rather than the nomothetic, it is worth considering whether synthesis is even compatible with the qualitative approach. As such, qualitative researchers have warned against the unquestioned adoption of methods for synthesis developed to suit quantitative research (Downe, 2008; Malterud, 2019c). For example, when conducting a systematic review of randomized controlled trials to determine the effectiveness of an intervention, it is critically important to include all studies that meet the inclusion criteria. Whereas in qualitative evidence synthesis it is acceptable to use purposive and theoretical approaches to sampling included studies (described below). Another example is that critical appraisal is a crucial part of the review process in quantitative evidence synthesis, but the purpose and helpfulness of critical appraisal in qualitative evidence synthesis is questionable (also discussed further below). Toye et al. (2014) raised the question of whether synthesis of qualitative research moves researchers too far from the unique contextual experience of participants in the original studies. They concluded that synthesis *is* compatible with a qualitative approach, if qualitative synthesis methods ensure interpretations are grounded in the primary qualitative studies included in the synthesis. This practice requires there be explicit consideration of the epistemology at the outset of a synthesis.

The RETREAT framework offers a criterion-based approach to help researchers select the most appropriate approach to qualitative evidence synthesis (Booth et al., 2018). This framework with seven domains—review question, epistemology, time/timescale, resource, expertise, audience, and purpose—can help researchers ensure congruence between the aims of the synthesis and the selected qualitative evidence synthesis approach. Epistemology, one of the aforementioned seven domains, is defined in the framework as, "the assumptions on the nature of knowledge that underpin the synthesis method and the extent to which these permit the review team to achieve their purpose" (Booth et al., 2018, p. 44). Epistemological positions can be organized along a spectrum from idealism to realism. The different approaches to qualitative evidence synthesis can be broadly mapped along this spectrum. Approaches such as critical interpretative synthesis reflect a 'subjective idealist' approach to knowledge; whereas approaches such as framework synthesis are informed by realist worldviews.

Review authors should also consider their own axiological perspectives during the qualitative evidence synthesis alongside the axiological perspectives of the studies they include. This consideration involves making explicit the intrinsic values inherent in the research questions guiding the synthesis and included studies. Analysis by Kelly et al. (2018) indicates that in at least one field of research (health professions education research) the axiological dimensions of included sources in qualitative evidence synthesis are rarely considered let alone accommodated in synthesis techniques.

Articulating the Review Question

Some approaches to synthesizing qualitative evidence favor establishing a question at the outset, while other approaches acknowledge that the review question may be shaped by emergent findings. When establishing an a priori question, it is often tightly articulated such as, "What are the perspectives of allied health professionals about the variability in the use of evidence-based clinical guidelines in stroke rehabilitation?" (Halls et al., 2021, p. 2). Frameworks are commonly used to support development of an appropriate question for a qualitative evidence synthesis with three examples provided in Table 15.1: SPIDER (Sample, Phenomenon of Interest, Design, Evaluation, Research type) (Cooke et al., 2012); SPICE (Setting, Perspective, Intervention or Phenomenon of Interest, Comparison, Evaluation) (Booth, 2006); and PerSPecTiF (Perspective, Setting, Phenomenon of Interest/Problem, Environment, Comparison (optional), Time Timing, Findings) (Booth et al., 2019). As well as assisting in developing the research question, these frameworks can support identification of search terms for electronic database searches to identify potential studies for inclusion in the qualitative evidence synthesis.

In our work we have always set out the question beforehand. One benefit of articulating the research question before beginning a qualitative evidence synthesis is that you can publish a protocol paper in a journal or register the review on the protocol registration platform Prospero (International Prospective Register of Systematic Reviews) (www.crd. york.ac.uk/prospero/). A qualitative evidence synthesis protocol defines the parameters of

Table 15.1 Examples of qualitative evidence synthesis questions framed using the SPIDER, SPICE, and PerSPecTiF frameworks

SPIDER	SPICE	PerSPecTiF
Example question: What are the activity related experiences and beliefs of older adults living in nursing homes/residential care settings?	Example question: What are the views and experiences of adolescents and young people with spina bifida, their families and health care providers of transition to employment from education?	Example question: How do the experiences of people in the first three months after stroke of early supported discharge in high income countries (with established community services for people with stroke), compare with the experiences of people after stroke who receive hospital based or rehabilitation unit-based rehabilitation?
S: Older adults living in nursing home/residential care settings	S: Community based	P: From the perspective of people after stroke
P: Participation in activity in nursing home settings	P: Adolescents and young people with spina bifida, family members of adolescents/young people with spina bifida, Healthcare practitioners working with adolescents/young people with spina bifida	S: Living in community settings
D: Qualitative research designs	I: Transition from education to employment	P: The experience of early supported discharge
E: Views, experiences, and beliefs	C: By implication only, compared to those who do not transition to employment	E: Within high income countries with established community services for people with stroke
R: Qualitative or mixed methods studies	E: Views and experiences	C: (optional) Compared with experiences of hospital-based rehabilitation
		Ti: In the first three months after stroke
		F: in relation to the views and experiences of people after stroke

Author created

the review and enables development of the case for the importance of the review (Flemming & Noyes, 2021). Publishing the protocol reduces research waste by preventing duplication. One of the first steps in the qualitative evidence synthesis process is to check the registration platforms to find the extent and scope of qualitative evidence synthesis related to your topic currently in progress.

Drawing on disability rights and related literature, Carolyn, Mandy, and colleagues developed an argument for the need to focus on how choice and control are conceptualized by people with spinal cord injuries. They used a PICo framework (population, interest, context) to refine their review question to "What are the views of people with spinal cord injury on their ability to exercise choice and control in their daily lives?" Carolyn and

Mandy registered their review about the views of people with spinal cord injury on choice and control on PROSPERO in May 2016 (available at: www.crd.york.ac.uk/prospero/display_record.php?RecordID=38682) and their PROSPERO registration gave full details on their proposed search strategy, approach to data extraction, and analysis plans (Murray et al., 2019).

Study Inclusion

Sampling processes will depend largely on the review question/topic framework and the resulting inclusion and exclusion criteria for papers. Inclusion and exclusion criteria are usually established a priori based on the question, target population, and scope of the review. These criteria are then applied as the reviewers screen the studies that were exported from the databases with the intent to exhaustively include all papers that are eligible based on these criteria. However, there are questions raised in methodological discourse about the positivist nature of this approach and whether 'all inclusive' is appropriate for the interpretive and exploratory nature of qualitative epistemologies (Downe, 2008; Malterud, 2019c; Thorne, 2022). Is there value from a qualitative perspective in synthesizing data from a raft of homogenous papers that all have similar focus and findings? How many papers are enough? Is there a point where saturation has been reached and more papers are no longer adding value to the meta-synthesis (Downe, 2008; France et al., 2019a; Suri, 2011)?

Alternatively, there are suggestions that broader review questions and a more strategic approach (as opposed to exhaustive) to study selection may present findings that set out to include similar as well as refutational data (Downe, 2008; Liamputtong, 2013). This process would take a purposive and theoretical sampling approach to study selection rather than wholly criterion based (Malterud, 2019a). For example, purposive sampling could involve only selecting papers that are conceptually information-rich and of the highest methodological quality (Sattar et al., 2021; Suri, 2011). To create heterogeneity in included papers, there may also be scope for maximum variation sampling or extreme/deviant sampling, whereby selected papers are included if they address the review question from diverse perspectives (Patton, 2002; Suri, 2011). This approach could then include theoretical sampling where papers are sought based on gaps identified by the researchers in the developing theory with the intent of achieving theoretical saturation (Suri, 2011). From a pragmatic perspective, a strategic approach may suit the current climate of plentiful and rapidly expanding information available, which leads to reviews with high numbers of papers that makes analysis and reporting unwieldy. A worked example of the use of purposive sampling in qualitative evidence synthesis can be found in Ames et al. (2019) who adopted this approach due to a high volume of papers about their topic (parental perceptions of vaccine communication). The team used a three-step framework to sample studies from among those eligible for inclusion. The framework allowed them to prioritize studies from low- and middle-income countries, studies that scored high for data richness, and studies that most closely matched the synthesis objectives. As with rigor in any qualitative study, if this approach were taken, researchers would still need to justify their process, explain how they managed bias in study sampling, and provide an auditable outcome (Thorne, 2022).

Given the apparent tensions between the fit of qualitative evidence synthesis with the positivist origins of systemic reviews, there is scope for further guidance from the field in these interpretive approaches to study selection and sampling (Malterud, 2019b). The approach of being strategic rather than exhaustive aligns closely with the qualitative ontology of 'quality of data over quantity' but requires experienced researchers in qualitative sampling and analysis (Malterud, 2019a; Thorne, 2022). It is possible that an attractive aspect of the traditional guides to screening and study selection in qualitative evidence synthesis is the opportunity to work with qualitative research in a way that is systematic and guided. For this reason, qualitative evidence synthesis may provide some occupational scientists and occupational therapists a good entry point to learning about qualitative research, but they must ensure all relevant data are extracted and analyzed with curiosity (avoiding confirmation bias while also managing other biases).

Study Screening and Selection

Detailed information about searching for qualitative evidence can be found in the chapter on qualitative evidence synthesis in the *Cochrane Handbook for Systematic Reviews of Interventions* (Noyes et al., 2022). Studies identified through electronic database searches and other searches (e.g., hand searches) are typically screened against inclusion and exclusion criteria by two members of the research team independently reading titles and abstracts. This is referred to as double screening and is more robust than screening by one researcher alone (Waffenschmidt et al., 2019). While a qualitative evidence synthesis could be conducted by one researcher, several authors have emphasized the value of conducting a qualitative evidence synthesis as part of a research team (Cahill et al., 2018; Campbell et al., 2011). Our experience of working on qualitative evidence syntheses as part of a wider team has been positive, not only in terms of improving process such as screening but also in enriching the complex analytic phases through critical discussions and by facilitating reflexivity throughout the analysis process.

Studies selected based on title/abstract screening are then reviewed by reading the full text of the paper; again, this is usually conducted by two members of the research team independently. Disagreements throughout the screening process are usually resolved through discussion or involvement of a third member of the research team. Rayyan and Covidence are online applications which ease sharing of review results across a research team and allow comparison of independent reviewer's decisions during the study screening and selection phase (Johnson & Phillips, 2018; Kellermeyer et al., 2018). Katie has used Rayyan across several reviews. It is completely free to use and has been hugely beneficial for record keeping in terms of decision-making to describe the flow of studies through a qualitative evidence synthesis. Rayyan includes free access to a series of training articles and short YouTube videos. Although it is only used at the screening and study selection phase of a qualitative evidence synthesis, our experience has been that the short few hours needed to learn how to use it has been worthwhile especially when screening larger number of database results. Covidence requires a subscription but is a well refined and intuitive tool to use. Covidence has been used by Carolyn and Mandy for duplicate screening, plus it can be used for data extraction.

The PRISMA flow diagram was recently updated and provides a template for researchers to illustrate the flow of studies through the review from identification to inclusion (Page et al., 2022). The PRISMA flow diagram maps out visually the number of records identified through database searching or other searches, the number of studies included and excluded, and the reasons for exclusion. Further details and templates are available at https://prisma-statement.org/prismastatement/flowdiagram.aspx. We have used a PRISMA flow diagram in every qualitative evidence synthesis we have conducted and although the record keeping needed to accurately populate the flow diagram is extensive, we appreciate that it increases the transparency of the screening and study selection phases.

In our example, Carolyn and Mandy searched ten electronic databases from 1980 to 2016 and re-ran the search from 2016 to 2018. Both the original search and the updated search from 2016 to 2018 are clearly presented in their PRISMA flow diagram along with full results of all database searches and screening decisions. For example, they excluded 28 studies from their review because they did not discuss choice and control related to everyday life. From 8508 originally received results from database searches they finally included 29 studies in their synthesis. (Murray et al., 2019)

Critical Appraisal

A key aspect of any systematic review (except for scoping reviews) is the requirement to undertake critical appraisal of the research with the intent of only including those papers of the highest quality. Therein lies another process mismatch between quantitative meta-analysis and qualitative meta-synthesis (Malterud, 2019b; Sattar et al., 2021; Williams et al., 2020) because, oftentimes, despite the quality of the study, the decision is made to include it because the paper is information rich with participant quotes and has the potential to be a highly valuable addition to the review despite methodological limitations. Appraisal of qualitative studies requires a sound understanding of qualitative research and sufficient information to be reported in the study (Carroll et al., 2012; Korhonen et al., 2013; Williams et al., 2020).

Some questions have been raised about the value of appraising included studies in qualitative evidence synthesis, but the meta-synthesis is only as sound as the included papers and appraisal provides an important reflection point within a structured process to consider whether to include papers and how to justify this (Hannes & Macaitis, 2012). A further challenging issue in appraisal of studies in a qualitative evidence synthesis is that appropriate criteria for the appraisal of qualitative research are contested. More than 100 tools for quality appraisal of qualitative studies exist (Majid & Vanstone, 2018). Many researchers opt for simple tools that provide a score and are, therefore, easier to report (Korhonen et al., 2013); while others use more comprehensive tools such as the McMaster Qualitative Review Form (Letts et al., 2007).

In several meta-ethnographic syntheses, Katie has used the Critical Skills Appraisal Program (CASP, n.d.) Qualitative Checklist (https://casp-uk.net/images/checklist/documents/CASP-Qualitative-Studies-Checklist/CASP-Qualitative-Checklist-2018_fillable_form.pdf). This tool has benefits in terms of being quick to administer; however, in Katie's experience, the tool may give a researcher team less nuanced information on study quality to inform subsequent phases of analysis in comparison with tools like the McMaster Qualitative Review Form (Letts et al., 2007). In Carolyn and Mandy's synthesis on choice and control, they used the McMaster criteria. There was a consistent methodological limitation across the studies with limited attention paid to the role of the researchers, their motivations for conducting the study, and whether or not there were pre-existing relationships between researchers and participants (Murray et al., 2019).

In relation to appraising studies in a meta-ethnography, Noblit (2018) suggested that appraisal tools need to be justified on the basis that they are not excluding on genre rather than quality and warned that the criteria used for appraisal of quality need to be interrogated. Ultimately, selection of an appraisal tool for a qualitative evidence synthesis depends on several factors including the objectives of the synthesis, the expertise of the synthesis authors, and the available time (Majid & Vanstone, 2018). For a comprehensive description of the structure, content, and objectives of available appraisal tools see Majid and Vanstone (2018).

Carroll et al. (2012) proposed a system of excluding papers based on adequacy of reporting as opposed to trying to evaluate the procedural rigor of the study. If there is a clear yes against two or more of their four criteria, then the paper can be included and further evaluated according to procedural rigor. This step has merit because it avoids the challenge of trying to assess quality of papers where the information is not adequately reported. As part of their work in this area, Carroll et al. (2012) conducted a sensitivity analysis to check if valuable and insightful data were lost due to study exclusion and found there was negligible impact on results. The reporting assessment checklist (Carroll et al., 2012) was used in the qualitative evidence synthesis led by Luker et al. (2017) and resulted in the exclusion of one paper. In Carolyn's meta-ethnography exploring challenges in occupational therapy practice (Murray et al., 2015), a bespoke appraisal tool was developed that was organized into the headings of dependability, credibility, transferability, and confirmability. This resulted in the exclusion of five papers with reasons related to study quality.

Given the explosion in numbers of publications in the last ten years and the possibility that qualitative evidence synthesis may increasingly become more about quality rather than quantity of papers, there may be some merit in being selective based on study rigor and quality, as well as considering whether inclusion of the paper will enrich the findings or simply further condense an already saturated data-set. Critical appraisal and further decisions about inclusion often occur alongside data extraction which is the precursor to data analysis.

Qualitative Evidence Synthesis Reporting and Study Rigor

Reporting guides and registering of protocols for research are becoming an increasing necessity for peer review and publication, and qualitative evidence synthesis is no exception. If planning to undertake a meta-synthesis, it is recommended that researchers familiarize themselves with these protocols and reporting guides, alongside learning about their chosen approach.

Tong et al. (2012) developed a reporting guideline for syntheses of qualitative research; the enhancing transparency in reporting the synthesis of qualitative research (ENTREQ) statement. This statement consists of 21 items grouped into 5 domains (introduction, methods and methodology, literature search and selection, appraisal, and synthesis of findings). They reviewed 40 published qualitative systematic reviews from health and social science fields to develop the ENTREQ statement which provides a useful foundation for any occupational scientists or occupational therapists conducting meta-synthesis research. The reporting criteria follows similar steps to the well-established PRISMA systematic reviews processes (Page et al., 2021), with the exception being differences in the process of data collection (extraction), the need to explain coding, study comparison, and inductive development of findings. There is an expectation that the final synthesis includes quotations and is "rich and compelling" (Tong et al., 2012, p. 4). In their synthesis of the views of people with spinal cord injury Carolyn, Mandy, and colleagues used the ENTREQ reporting guideline and cite this as an example of their rigorous approach to the conduct of their review (Murray et al., 2019).

A specific reporting guideline for meta-ethnography—the eMERGe reporting guideline—was developed by France et al. (2019b). Based on a robust mixed-methods study design and evidence-based methods the guidelines identified 19 reporting criteria across the 7 phases of meta-ethnography (France et al., 2019b). Reporting guidelines, while helpful in improving transparency and reporting standards, can also serve as a useful guide for those who are new to the approach. Having a chosen reporting guide adds rigor to the study at the same time as guiding the researcher as to what constitutes rigorous research in qualitative evidence synthesis. As with all qualitative research, there is a need for the processes followed to address transparency, dependability, confirmability, and transferability. Methods to ensure this include having multiple researchers involved (including public and participant involvement if possible) and for researchers to be reflexive about their own possible interpretation biases and motives for doing the research. For example, open acknowledgement about how a researcher's experiences as an occupational scientist and occupational therapist may influence how they will view and interpret the data. This sensitivity can be a strength but only if tempered with self-awareness. In our experience working as part of a team is useful for promoting reflexivity throughout the analysis phase, particularly when using approaches such as meta-ethnography with a high degree of interpretation.

In terms of analysis, keeping an audit trail of all analytic decisions made is essential, as is regular team discussions and regularly returning to the original papers for context. The inductive interpretative process of qualitative evidence synthesis cannot be rushed or forced as construction of the findings needs to be grounded in the data. Having said that, in our experience, most journals require searches to have been completed within 12 months prior to submission. If they are older, this may require researchers to re-run their search and include any newly published papers into the qualitative evidence synthesis. Carolyn, Mandy, and colleagues completed a re-run of their search and found an additional nine papers for integration into their synthesis. This was a useful step as they found the extracted data blended well with the themes and sub-themes they had developed, thus reaching data saturation and supporting confirmability of the findings.

The GRADE-CERQual (Confidence in the Evidence from Reviews of Qualitative Research) approach allows assessment of how much confidence should be placed in findings from qualitative evidence synthesis and was developed to be used across the various approaches (Lewin et al., 2018). This approach provides a systematic and transparent framework to assess the extent to which a review finding is a reasonable representation of the phenomenon of interest (Lewin et al., 2018) and involves considering four components after findings have been developed: (1) methodological limitations, (2) coherence, (3) adequacy of data, and (4) relevance (Lewin et al., 2018). GRADE-CERQual results are usually presented in tables.

In Textbox 15.1, we put forth a number of questions readers may want to consider when assessing the rigor of a qualitative evidence synthesis.

Data Extraction and Analysis

The data extraction step is common to all qualitative evidence synthesis approaches. It begins with extracting data on the characteristics of included studies; for example, characteristics of the recruited participants, sample size, the study setting, approaches to data collection and analysis. This information is usually presented in a table. Data extraction then involves identifying relevant findings in the included studies for synthesis. Noblit and Hare (1988) recommended repeated reading of the included studies and extraction of key

---

Textbox 15.1   Key Considerations When Reading a Qualitative Evidence Synthesis

- Was the review *registered in advance* and have the authors justified why a qualitative evidence synthesis was warranted?
- Has the *selected approach* to synthesizing the studies (e.g., meta-aggregation) been described and justified?
- Has the search strategy and flow of studies throughout the review been described in a *clear and transparent manner* such that you could replicate the search?
- Has the *approach to sampling* studies for inclusion been described and justified?
- Have the authors *included a flow chart* of their search and screening process and outcomes?
- Have the authors presented a *clear description of the analysis* process?
- Do the findings offer a *new interpretation* of the topic being explored?
- Have the authors *reflected on the synthesis* and presented strengths and limitations of their synthesis?

---

concepts or metaphors or "what others may call themes, perspectives and/or concepts revealed by qualitative studies" (p. 14). The term 'second order construct' is also used to describe these concepts. In meta-ethnography, 'first order constructs' refer to quotes from participants in the included studies, while 'second order constructs' refer to the researchers' interpretations of first order constructs, and 'third order constructs' refer to the concepts developed by those conducting the meta-ethnography (Toye et al., 2014).

In meta-ethnography this stage of data extraction involves reading the included studies in an intensive, repetitive, and a highly active manner (Lee et al., 2015). The extracted details and text from the included papers are essentially the data for the qualitative evidence synthesis and, as such, we engage with and immerse ourselves in reading the included papers during this analytic phase. This phase mirrors our previous experience of immersion in raw data, for example, through transcribing interviews or field notes. The complex analytic phases of meta-ethnography follow data extraction and reading in meta-ethnography. These complex analytic phases originally purported by Noblit and Hare have not been very clearly delineated in the past. An excellent source for guidance is a recent review of meta-ethnography by France et al. (2019a).

Following extraction, the researchers consider how second order constructs relate to each other within a study, juxtaposing second order constructs across studies. Researchers determine how studies relate to one another by grouping studies by their focus or grouping common concepts from studies (France et al., 2019a). This can be done using lists, tables, or qualitative software programs such as NVivo. NVivo requires a license and some practice, but once mastered can create efficiencies. Software programs help to manage and sort the data extracted from the included studies during these phases. Extracted data from each included paper are imported into NVivo and the 'nodes' function can be used to identify/code all second order constructs across the papers. The researcher still does the analysis, but software can help to make this process easier to manage. In our reviews, we have managed this stage of analysis using software packages and also other manual methods such as MS Word and Excel, and sometimes printing out the data to manually sort.

In the next phase of meta-ethnography, the researchers aim to translate concepts from one study into another to generate concepts which represent more than one study (Cahill et al., 2018). Noblit and Hare (1988) described two types of translation: reciprocal translation refers to where accounts are directly compared, and refutational translation is conducted when accounts are in relative opposition to one another (France et al., 2019a). Translation does not have to be either reciprocal or refutational but can involve both (France et al., 2019a). In the final phase of meta-ethnographic analysis, the researchers view the studies as a whole, rather than as parts in order to generate a fresh interpretation of phenomena through developing new findings or a new conceptualization (Cahill et al., 2018; Noblit & Hare, 1988). This process is described as 'line of argument synthesis' where translations are interpreted to generate "a textual synthesis or narrative/storyline which expresses a new conceptualisation" (France et al., 2019a, p. 11). Using our example of choice and control for people with spinal cord injury, Carolyn, Mandy, and colleagues developed 15 categories from extracting and analyzing the data from 29 papers. Through written descriptions of the categories and scrutinizing the data, two broad overarching themes were developed and reported, each with sub-themes (Murray et al., 2015).

Katie, Mandy, and colleagues undertook a meta-ethnography of the lived experiences, views, and preferences of children and young people with developmental coordination disorder (O'Dea et al., 2021). They found 15 papers that were reciprocally translatable and led to the development of three interpretative themes: (1) 'It's harder than it should be': Navigating daily activities; (2) Fitting in; and (3) 'So what? I drop things': Strategies and supports to mitigate challenges (O'Dea et al., 2021). In the final phase of analysis, higher order interpretation of the three identified themes found that the experiences of children and young people with developmental coordination disorder could be understood as psycho-emotional disablism. This concept described the experiences and responses of people with impairments when they were hurt by the reactions and behaviors of those around them and were "made to feel worthless, of lesser value, worthless, unattractive," hopeless, stressed, or insecure (Thomas, 2004, p. 31).

Ethics

Generally, researchers do not require ethical approval from a human ethics research committee before commencing a qualitative evidence synthesis; however, there are still ethical issues to consider. A key issue is the ethical dilemma of study participants consenting to be involved in the primary research but not in the secondary analysis. It is essential that the researcher check that the primary studies report they obtained ethical clearance; and, if they did not, or this cannot be found out from the authors, then these papers are excluded. In addition, it is essential that researchers be respectful of those who contributed to the primary data set and their understanding of what they consented to.

Application to Occupational Science

Given the predominance of qualitative studies within occupational science with sample sizes appropriate for the type of inquiry, the potential of different types of qualitative evidence synthesis studies to contribute knowledge to the discipline is evident. However, on searching the *Journal of Occupational Science*, there are few examples where scholars have applied the approach to concepts within occupational science. While it is recognized that the *Journal of Occupational* Science is not the only holder of occupational science knowledge, it is a key publication within the discipline. Upon searching, the journal appears to have only a few examples of qualitative evidence syntheses. A meta-study exploring perceptions of persons living with dementia as to what enables or hinders social citizenship provides information about the contextual factors relating to society, culture, justice, and occupational opportunities that promote and prevent a sense of social citizen ship (Peoples et al., 2022). Walder and Molineux (2017) reported a grounded theory synthesis of studies exploring adults' experiences of adjustment to chronic disease or injury, which is an excellent example of a methodologically robust grounded theory synthesis that adds to knowledge within the concept of occupational adaptation. Further, a thematic synthesis of motives of retirement-aged workers revealed the importance of being, becoming, and belonging for those who prolong their working life beyond the act of 'doing' or financial motives (Bratun et al., 2022). These examples highlight the potential that the approach has for occupational science in bringing together studies with small sample sizes to synthesize the findings into something that accelerates conceptual development, and it appears that it is beginning to gain traction.

Application to Occupational Therapy

Qualitative evidence synthesis has much to offer occupational therapy as this approach can draw together findings on the acceptability and feasibility of an intervention and the importance of outcomes to service users (Flemming et al., 2019). These are important topics to address, alongside questions about the effectiveness of an intervention which are best addressed through systematic review of quantitative studies. Recent qualitative evidence synthesis studies of relevance for occupational therapy practice include a synthesis on how stakeholders narrate possible outcomes of reablement services (Bergström et al., 2022), synthesis of service user experiences of occupational therapy in acute mental health settings (Steede & Gough, 2022), and synthesis of the experiences of rehabilitation for adults with traumatic brain injury (Larsson-Lund et al., 2022). Syntheses of the experiences of people with various injuries, illness, and impairments have proliferated in recent years and are hugely informative for clinicians; recent examples include synthesis of the experience of lower limb amputation (Schober & Abrahamsen, 2022), chronic pain (Toye et al., 2021), and aphasia after stroke (Manning et al., 2019).

Implications for health professionals arising from the synthesis completed by Carolyn, Mandy, and colleagues include the need for health professionals to be vigilant for the thresholds of readiness for choice and control, and need to promote readiness by being willing to listen and be guided by the person with spinal injury, fostering psychological coping strategies in rehabilitation and understanding the systemic processes influencing choice and control to ensure service provision is balanced with ensuring people's rights to self-determination (Murray et al., 2019).

Authors' Reflections

In an era of plentiful information, Carolyn finds that qualitative evidence synthesis provides an opportunity to consolidate the findings from qualitative studies with a similar aim, creating larger sample sizes. While qualitative research is not reliant on large samples, this consolidation can lead to theory development or knowledge translation opportunities and recommendations that smaller qualitative studies cannot. Also, if there is much similar research, it could signal the need to look at problems from new perspectives or with different methodologies to avoid repeating the same research with no ensuing change. For Mandy, the opportunity to learn about meta-ethnography came by chance when invited on to the supervision panel for a PhD student. The student was having difficulty recruiting participants for her study, so the decision was made to change to doing a review of the literature using meta-ethnography. Working closely with other health professional academics who were experts in systematic reviews she could see the value and potential of meta-ethnography to provide knowledge from synthesizing the smaller qualitative studies. Identifying as a methodologist, she was keen to explore the utility of this approach. Katie has been involved in several qualitative evidence synthesis studies over the past few years mostly using a meta-ethnographic approach. She appreciates the potential of this well-delineated approach to both comprehensively review existing knowledge on a phenomenon and generate novel interpretations and conceptual innovation. Like Carolyn, Katie has increasingly seen the benefits of robust qualitative evidence synthesis in mapping the research conducted on a phenomenon to date and identifying gaps in knowledge or under-researched populations.

Synthesis of qualitative studies by meta-ethnography requires a research team with a broad range of skills, prior experience of qualitative research, and capacity to move beyond description to engagement in interpretative analysis. The resultant synthesis needs to provide a more conceptual understanding of the topic that could not have been derived by any single study. Achieving a more conceptual understanding requires in-depth engagement with the original studies and is a time-intensive process. A further challenge with qualitative evidence synthesis is to develop a question and search terms that yields inclusion of a manageable number of studies in the context of the research teams' resources, so the review is neither too big nor too small.

Qualitative evidence synthesis is usually conducted in a team and the interpretative work during the analytic phase benefits from involvement of multiple researchers. This opportunity to work collaboratively and the inclusion of multiple perspectives can prompt deep reflexive consideration which ultimately enriches the analysis. Qualitative evidence synthesis is a significant body of publishable work, and it is rewarding to arrive at meaningful higher order findings that gives useful insights into the area being explored.

Conclusion

There are a wide range of approaches to qualitative evidence syntheses. In this chapter we have expanded on one of those approaches, meta-ethnography. Drawing on our various experiences with the approach we have highlighted the advantages of bringing the findings from qualitative studies in occupational science or occupational therapy together and synthesizing the findings to arrive at a higher level of conceptual understanding. We have also discussed the methodological decisions that need to be made along the way and drawn attention to taking a rigorous approach. In doing so we have highlighted how qualitative evidence syntheses can contribute knowledge to occupational science and occupational therapy practice.

References

Ames, H., Glenton, C., & Lewin, S. (2019). Purposive sampling in a qualitative evidence synthesis: A worked example from a synthesis on parental perceptions of vaccination communication. *BMC Medical Research Methodology, 19*(1), 26. https://doi.org/10.1186/s12874-019-0665-4

Barnett-Page, E., & Thomas, J. (2009). Methods for the synthesis of qualitative research: A critical review. *BMC Medical Research Methodology*, *9*(1), 59. https://doi.org/10.1186/1471-2288-9-59

Bergström, A., Vik, K., Haak, M., Metzelthin, S., Graff, L., & Hjelle, K. M. (2022). The jigsaw puzzle of activities for mastering daily life; service recipients and professionals' perceptions of gains and changes attributed to reablement: A qualitative meta-synthesis. *Scandinavian Journal of Occupational Therapy*, *30*(5), 604–615. https://doi.org/10.1080/11038128.2022.2081603

Booth, A. (2006). Clear and present questions: Formulating questions for evidence based practice. *Library Hi Tech*, *24*(3), 355–368. https://doi.org/10.1108/07378830610692127

Booth, A., Noyes, J., Flemming, K., Gerhardus, A., Wahlster, P., van der Wilt, G. J., Mozygemba, K., Refolo, P., Sacchini, D., Tummers, M., & Rehfuess, E. (2016). *Guidance on choosing qualitative evidence synthesis methods for use in health technology assessments of complex interventions.* Available from www.integrate-hta.eu/downloads/

Booth, A., Noyes, J., Flemming, K., Gerhardus, A., Wahlster, P., van der Wilt, G. J., Mozygemba, K., Refolo, P., Sacchini, D., Tummers, M., & Rehfuess, E. (2018). Structured methodology review identified seven (RETREAT) criteria for selecting qualitative evidence synthesis approaches. *Journal of Clinical Epidemiology*, *99*, 41–52. https://doi.org/10.1016/j.jclinepi.2018.03.003

Booth, A., Noyes, J., Flemming, K., Moore, G., Tuncalp, O., & Shakibazadeh, E. (2019). Formulating questions to address the acceptability and feasibility of complex interventions in qualitative evidence synthesis. *BMJ Global Health*, *4*, e001107. https://doi.org/10.1136/bmjgh-2018-001107

Bratun, U., Asaba, E., & Zurc, J. (2022). Motives of retirement-aged workers and the importance of doing, being, becoming, and belonging: A systematic review of qualitative studies. *Journal of Occupational Science*, *30*(3), 420–437. https://doi.org/10.1080/14427591.2022.2057574

Cahill, M., Robinson, K., Pettigrew, J., Galvin, R., & Stanley, M. (2018). Qualitative synthesis: A guide to conducting a meta-ethnography. *British Journal of Occupational Therapy*, *81*(3), 129–137. https://doi.org/10.1177/03080226177450

Campbell, R., Pound, P., Morgan, M., Daker-White, G., Britten, N., Pill, R., Yardley, L., Pope, C., & Donovan, J. (2011). Evaluating metaethnography: Systematic analysis and synthesis of qualitative research. *Health Technology Assessment*, *15*(43), 1–164. https://doi.org/10.3310/hta15430

Carroll, C., Booth, A., & Lloyd-Jones, M. (2012). Should we exclude inadequately reported studies from qualitative systematic reviews? An evaluation of sensitivity analyses in Two case study reviews. *Qualitative Health Research*, *22*(10), 1425–1434. https://doi.org/10.1177/1049732312452937

CASP. (n.d.). *Qualitative research checklist.* https://casp-uk.net/images/checklist/documents/CASP-Qualitative-Studies-Checklist/CASP-Qualitative-Checklist-2018_fillable_form.pdf

Cooke, A., Smith, D., & Booth, A. (2012). Beyond PICO: The SPIDER tool for qualitative evidence synthesis. *Qualitative Health Research*, *22*(10), 1435–1443. https://doi.org/10.1177/1049732312452938

Downe, S. (2008). Metasynthesis: A guide to knitting smoke. *Evidence-Based Midwifery*, *6*(1), 4–8.

Flemming, K., Booth, A., Garside, R., Tunçalp, Ö., & Noyes, J. (2019). Qualitative evidence synthesis for complex interventions and guideline development: Clarification of the purpose, designs and relevant methods. *BMJ Global Health*, *4*(Suppl. 1), e000882. https://doi.org/10.1136/bmjgh-2018-000882

Flemming, K., & Noyes, J. (2021). Qualitative evidence synthesis: Where are we at? *International Journal of Qualitative Methods*, *20*. https://doi.org/10.1177/1609406921993276

France, E. F., Ring, N., Noyes, J., Maxwell, M., Jepson, R., Duncan, E., Turley, R., Jones, D., & Uny, I. (2015). Protocol-developing meta-ethnography reporting guidelines (eMERGe). *BMC Medical Research Methodology*, *15*(1), 1–14. https://doi.org/10.1186/s12874-015-0068-0

France, E., Uny, I., Ring, N., Turley, R., Maxwell, M., Duncan, E. S., Jepson, R., Roberts, R., & Noyes, J. (2019a). A methodological systematic review of meta-ethnography conduct to articulate the complex analytical phases. *BMC Medical Research Methodology*, *19*(1), 35. https://doi.org/10.1186/s12874-019-0670-7

France, E. F., Cunningham, M., Ring, N., Uny, I., Duncan, E. A., Jepson, R. G., Maxwell, M., Roberts, R. J., Turley, R. L., Booth, A., & Britten, N. (2019b). Improving reporting of meta-ethnography: The eMERGe reporting guidance. BMC medical research methodology. *BMC Medical Research Methodology, 19*(1), 1–13. https://doi.org/10.1186/s12874-018-0600-0

Halls, D., Murray, C., & Sellar, B. (2021). Why allied health professionals use evidence-based clinical guidelines in stroke rehabilitation: A systematic review and meta-synthesis of qualitative studies. *Clinical Rehabilitation, 35*(11), 1611–1626. https://doi.org/10.1177/02692155211012324

Hannes, K., & Macaitis, K. (2012). A move to more systematic and transparent approaches in qualitative evidence synthesis: Update on a review of published papers. *Qualitative Research, 12*(4), 402–442. https://doi.org/10.1177/1468794111432992

Johnson, N., & Phillips, M. (2018). Rayyan for systematic reviews. *Journal of Electronic Resources Librarianship, 30*(1), 46–48. https://doi.org/10.1080/1941126X.2018.1444339

Kellermeyer, L., Harnke, B., & Knight, S. (2018). Covidence and Rayyan. *Journal of the Medical Library Association, 106*(4), 580–583. https://doi.org/10.5195/jmla.2018.513

Kelly, M., Ellaway, R. H., Reid, H., Ganshorn, H., Yardley, S., Bennett, D., & Dornan, T. (2018). Considering axiological integrity: A methodological analysis of qualitative evidence syntheses, and its implications for health professions education. *Advances in Health Sciences Education, 23*(4), 833–851. https://doi.org/10.1007/s10459-018-9829-y

Korhonen, A., Hakulinen-Viitanen, T., Jylhä, V., & Holopainen, A. (2013). Meta-synthesis and evidence-based health care: A method for systematic review. *Scandinavian Journal of Caring Sciences, 27*(4), 1027–1034. https://doi.org/10.1111/scs.12003

Larsson-Lund, M., Pettersson, A., & Strandberg, T. (2022). Team-based rehabilitation after traumatic brain injury: A qualitative synthesis of evidence of experiences of the rehabilitation process. *Journal of Rehabilitation Medicine, 54.* https://doi.org/10.2340/jrm.v53.1409

Lee, R. P., Hart, R. I., Watson, R. M., & Rapley, T. (2015). Qualitative synthesis in practice: Some pragmatics of meta-ethnography. *Qualitative Research, 15*(3), 334–350. https://doi.org/10.1177/1468794114524221

Letts, L., Wilkins, S., Law, M., Stewart, D., Bosch, J., & Westmorland, M. (2007). *Critical review form−Qualitative studies (Version 2.0).* https://srs-mcmaster.ca/research/evidence-based-practice-research-group/#yJWcLhEC

Lewin, S., Booth, A., Glenton, C., Munthe-Kaas, H., Rashidian, A., Wainwright, M., Bohren, M., Tunçalp, Ö., Colvin, C., Garside, R., Carlsen, B., Langlois E. V., & Noyes, J. (2018). Applying GRADE-CERQual to qualitative evidence synthesis findings: Introduction to the series. *Implementation Science, 13*(Suppl. 1), 2. https://doi.org/10.1186/s13012-017-0688-3

Liamputtong, P. (2013). *Research methods in health: Foundations for evidence based practice.* Oxford University Press.

Lockwood, C., Munn, Z., & Porritt, K. (2015). Qualitative research synthesis: Methodological guidance for systematic reviewers utilizing meta-aggregation. *JBI Evidence Implementation, 13*(3), 179–187. https://doi.org/10.1097/xeb.0000000000000062

Luker, J., Murray, C., Lynch, E., Bernhardsson, S., Shannon, M., & Bernhardt, J. (2017). Carers' experiences, needs, and preferences during inpatient stroke rehabilitation: A systematic review of qualitative studies. *Archives of Physical Medicine and Rehabilitation, 98*(9), 1852–1862. https://doi.org/10.1016/j.apmr.2017.02.024

Marshall, C. A., Boland, L., Westover, L. A., Wickett, S., Roy, L., Mace, J., Gewurtz, R., Barbic, S., & Kirsh, B. (2020). Occupational experiences of homelessness: A systematic review and meta-aggregation. *Scandinavian Journal of Occupational Therapy, 27*(6), 394–407. https://doi.org/10.1080/11038128.2019.1689292

Majid, U., & Vanstone, M. (2018). Appraising qualitative research for evidence syntheses: A compendium of quality appraisal tools. *Qualitative Health Research, 28*(13), 2115–2131. https://doi.org/10.1177/1049732318785358

Malterud, K. (2019a). *Qualitative metasynthesis: A research method for medicine and health sciences* (1st ed.). Roultedge. https://doi.org/10.4324/9780429026348

Malterud, K. (2019b). Theoretical and methodologial challenges. In K. Malterud (Ed.), *Qualitative metasynthesis: A research method for medicine and health sciences* (1st ed., pp. 75–100). Routledge.

Malterud, K. (2019c). The impact of evidence-based medicine on qualitative metasynthesis: Benefits to be harvested and warnings to be given. *Qualitative Health Research, 29*(1), 7–17. https://doi.org/10.1177/1049732318795864

Manning, M., MacFarlane, A., Hickey, A., & Franklin, S. (2019). Perspectives of people with aphasia post-stroke towards personal recovery and living successfully: A systematic review and thematic synthesis. *PloS One, 14*(3), e0214200. https://doi.org/10.1371/journal.pone.0214200

Murray, C., Turpin, M., Edwards, I., & Jones, M. (2015). A qualitative meta-synthesis about challenges experienced in occupational therapy practice. *British Journal of Occupational Therapy, 78*(9), 534–546. https://doi.org/10.1177/0308022615586786

Murray, C., Van Kessel, G., Guerin, M., Hillier, S., & Stanley, M. (2019). Exercising choice and control: A qualitative meta-synthesis of perspectives of people with a spinal cord injury. *Archives of Physical Medicine and Rehabilitation, 100*(9), 1752–1762. https://doi.org/10.1016/j.apmr.2019.01.011

Noblit, G. W. (2018). Meta-ethnography adaptation and return. In L. Urrieta & G. W. Noblit (Eds.), *Cultural constructions of identity meta-ethnography and theory* (pp. 34–50). Oxford University Press.

Noblit, G. W., & Hare, R. D. (1988). *Meta-ethnography: Synthesising qualitative studies.* SAGE.

Noyes, J., Booth, A., Cargo, M., Flemming, K., Harden, A., Harris, J., Garside, R., Hannes, K., Pantoja, T., & Thomas, J. (2022). Qualitative evidence. In J. P. T. Higgins, J. Thomas, J. Chandler, M. Cumpston, T. Li, M. J. Page, & V. A. Welch (Eds.), *Cochrane handbook for systematic reviews of interventions* (ver. 6.3, Chapt 21). Available from www.training.cochrane.org/handbook

O'Dea, Á., Stanley, M., Coote, S., & Robinson, K. (2021). Children and young people's experiences of living with developmental coordination disorder/dyspraxia: A systematic review and meta-ethnography of qualitative research. *PloS One, 16*(3), e0245738. https://doi.org/10.1371/journal.pone.0245738

Page, M. J., McKenzie, J. E., Bossuyt, P. M., Boutron, I., Hoffmann, T. C., Mulrow, C. D., Shamseer, L., Tetzlaff, J. M., Akl, E. A., Brennan, S. E., Chou, R., Glanville, J., Grimshaw, J. M., Hróbjartsson, A., Lalu, M. M., Li, T., Loder, E. W., Mayo-Wilson, E., McDonald, S., McGuinness, L. A., Stewart, L. A., Thomas, J., Tricco, A. C., Welch, V. A., Whiting, P., & Moher, D. (2021). The PRISMA 2020 statement: An updated guideline for reporting systematic reviews. *BMJ, 372*, n71. https://doi.org/10.1136/bmj.n71

Page, M. J., Moher, D., & McKenzie, J. E. (2022). Introduction to PRISMA 2020 and implications for research synthesis methodologists. *Research Synthesis Methods, 13*(2), 156–163. https://doi.org/10.1002/jrsm.1535

Patton, M. (2002). *Qualitative research and evaluation methods* (3rd ed.). SAGE.

Peoples, H., Varming, J., & Kristensen, H. K. (2022). Social citizenship when living with dementia: A qualitative meta-study. *Journal of Occupational Science, 30*(3), 453–471. https://doi.org/10.1080/14427591.2022.2061040

Sattar, R., Lawton, R., Panagioti, M., & Johnson, J. (2021). Meta-ethnography in healthcare research: A guide to using a meta-ethnographic approach for literature synthesis. *BMC Health Services Research, 21*(1), 50. https://doi.org/10.1186/s12913-020-06049-w

Schober, T. L., & Abrahamsen, C. (2022). Patient perspectives on major lower limb amputation–A qualitative systematic review. *International Journal of Orthopaedic and Trauma Nursing, 46*, 100958. https://doi.org/10.1016/j.ijotn.2022.100958

Steede, K., & Gough, R. (2022). Service user experiences of occupational therapy in acute mental health settings: A qualitative evidence synthesis. *Occupational Therapy in Mental Health, 38*(4), 364–382. https://doi.org/10.1080/0164212X.2022.2064031

Suri, H. (2011). Purposeful sampling in qualitative research synthesis. *Qualitative Research Journal, 11*(2), 63–75. https://doi.org/10.3316/QRJ1102063

Taylor, C. E. V., Murray, C. M., & Stanton, T. R. (2022). Patient perspectives of pain and function after knee replacement: A systematic review and meta-synthesis of qualitative studies. *PAIN Reports, 7*(3), e1006. https://doi.org/10.1097/pr9.0000000000001006

Thomas, C. (2004). Rescuing a social relational understanding of disability. *Scandinavian Journal of Disability Research*, 6(1), 22–36. http://doi.org/10.1080/15017410409512637

Thorne, S. (2022). Qualitative meta-synthesis. *Nurse Author & Editor*, 32(1), 15–18.

Tong, A., Flemming, K., McInnes, E., Oliver, S., & Craig, J. (2012). Enhancing transparency in reporting the synthesis of qualitative research: ENTREQ. *BMC Medical Research Methodology*, 12(1), 181. https://doi.org/10.1186/1471-2288-12-181

Toye, F., Belton, J., Hannink, E., Seers, K., & Barker, K. (2021). A healing journey with chronic pain: A meta-ethnography synthesizing 195 qualitative studies. *Pain Medicine*, 22(6), 1333–1344. https://doi.org/10.1093/pm/pnaa373

Toye, F., Seers, K., Allcock, N., Briggs, M., Carr, E., & Barker, K. (2014). Meta-ethnography 25 years on: Challenges and insights for synthesising a large number of qualitative studies. *BMC Medical Research Methodology*, 14, 80. https://doi.org/10.1186/1471-2288-14-80

Waffenschmidt, S., Knelangen, M., Sieben, W., Bühn, S., & Pieper, D., (2019). Single screening versus conventional double screening for study selection in systematic reviews: A methodological systematic review. *BMC Medical Research Methodology*, 19(1), 1–9. https://doi.org/10.1186/s12874-019-0782-0

Walder, K., & Molineux, M. (2017). Occupational adaptation and identity construction: A grounded theory synthesis of qualitative studies exploring adults experiences of adjustment to chronic disease, major illness or injury. *Journal of Occupational Science*, 24(2), 225–243. https://doi.org/10.1080/14427591.2016.1269240

Williams, V., Boylan, A.-M., & Nunan, D. (2020). Critical appraisal of qualitative research: Necessity, partialities and the issue of bias. *BMJ Evidence-Based Medicine*, 25(1), 9–11. https://doi.org/10.1136/bmjebm-2018-111132

Additional Resources

Cochrane training video: https://training.cochrane.org/resource/meta-ethnography

Dr Andrew Booth video on Qualitative Evidence Synthesis Protocol development: www.youtube.com/watch?v=YjkUX97z9KQ

Introduction to Meta-Ethnography Ruth Garside (You Tube Video) www.youtube.com/watch?v=vMcteRM4RGA

NVIVO™ training video (You Tube): www.youtube.com/watch?v=2mS4lWyHuWg

Rayyan support/training videos: https://help.rayyan.ai/hc/en-us/articles/4412340931345-Rayyan-Systematic-Review-Tutorial-

16 Netnography

Amy Wallis

Netnography is an adaptation of ethnography that has evolved due to advances in data communication technology (Kozinets, 2010). Therefore, to understand netnography, its genesis, in the roots of ethnography, must first be considered. Ethnography has its origins in what is known as sociological research and was first used in the early 1800s as a means of providing anthropologists insight into the lives of people of varying races and cultures living outside of Europe (Ryan, 2017). Historically, observation has been the main tool used to gather information; however, interviews and focus groups are now also used in ethnography, although less commonly. Originally, the focus of ethnography was to learn about non-industrialized people, communities, and culture using written records (Rees & Gatenby, 2014), taking particular interest in the influences of cultural and historical contexts. Researchers would immerse themselves in the communities of interest, often living within the community for long periods of time (Kaoukaou, 2021). It is this immersion of the researcher into the community or population that provides the in-depth information and adds strength to the findings, setting ethnography apart from other methodologies that may also use observation. For a more detailed history of ethnography see Chapter 9.

Ethnography is considered one of the early qualitative approaches, with its main purpose to assist researchers gain insight and learn *about people* rather than *study* people, as is done in other qualitative approaches. It is key to note that ethnography helps researchers to learn about what may be defined as 'traditional' populations and communities, such as when people live or gather together in groups in person, which have historically been the subject of sociology in scientific research. However, since the inception, development, and regular use of modern technology, and the start of the so-called digital revolution (Toledano, 2017), there has been a significant shift in how populations and communities are now defined. Digital communities are growing in numbers demonstrating how populations and communities have evolved over time (Dover & Kelman, 2018). The nature and structure of people's lives, how they interact with others, how they share views and find information are just a few examples of how the digital revolution has altered life.

In recent times, the internet has become an important place where people of all ages can learn new information, connect with others, and share experiences. Attending online forums; being part of social networking sites, podcasts, blogs, videocasting, and photo-sharing communities; as well as participating in online gaming/virtual worlds is ever increasing in popularity and common practice (Bowler, 2010). This shift in how people interact and seek information came to the attention of qualitative researchers in the early 1990s, and in 1996 the term 'virtual ethnography' was first used by researcher Bruce Mason (1996). Mason described ethnographic research of virtual interactions and used

DOI: 10.4324/9781003456216-16

offline ethnographic approaches to understand online communication and behaviors. The term netnography was then coined in 1998 by Robert Kozinets, an American marketing and journalism professor (Kozinets, 1998).

Broken down, netnography is comprised of two parts: (1) 'net' (internet) and (2) 'nography' (a version of ethnography); thus, this methodology is one that is conducted solely online. Netnography enables unobtrusive observation of an online forum or community, providing insight into personal experiences, opinions, thoughts, and online practices of virtual community members (Costello et al., 2017). Thus, given that netnography predominantly uses observational data without the need to immerse in the community or population it provides a less intrusive research experience than traditional ethnography (Heinonen & Medberg, 2018). Hence, this approach to research is considered more naturalistic than obtaining data through traditional methods of interviews, surveys, focus groups, and experiments, which can be influenced by the researcher's values and beliefs.

There are clearly similarities between ethnography and netnography; however, Kaoukaou (2021) has identified the following five distinctions:

1 *Intermittent engagement.* Researchers immerse themselves in the community in both ethnography and netnography. In traditional ethnography the researcher fully immerses themselves in the community for lengthy periods of time. In netnography, the immersion is unique whereby the researcher enters the virtual community for shorter periods of time and, while still immersing themselves, comes and goes from the community. This intermittent engagement is also a characteristic of participants in online communities.
2 *Digital transparency.* Data available online is considered transparent, meaning it is accessible instantly and can be considered an active form of archiving. Information is stored instantly, providing the netnographer with instant access to data. This is a unique point of difference of netnography. For our study's purpose, as there are no current guidelines for netnography, we decided to adhere to traditional research ethics requirements and securely store the data from the blogs for seven years. Netnographers need to be aware that bloggers may choose to remove their post/s from the online community during the time of the netnographer's study. Again, there are no current guidelines for this event; therefore, I suggest it would be up to the netnographer to choose whether or not to continue to use the previous posts in their study.
3 *Virtual interviewee paradox.* A major distinction lies in the provision of consent in netnography. Data are openly shared online by participants and, hence, researchers are not required to seek approval to use that information. The paradox lies in the fact that participants imply consent through the act of publishing their blogs; however, they have no control over how the information is used or presented in research by netnographers. Netnography does not allow for co-construction of information and dialogue.
4 *Interpretation applied in the digital space.* Researchers need to be aware in this methodology that different voices may be present in the data and can interfere with interpretation, something that is not common in ethnography and can cause confusion in clarity and interpretation for the netnographer.
5 *Information flows and the limitation of the research scope.* As data available on the internet are commonly available in large amounts, it is key for the netnographer to devote time prior to beginning a study to exploring the information availability, reliability, and the flow of information, while simultaneously defining the sample to be utilized in the study. Again, something that is particular to netnography.

Netnography is a unique, contemporary, and useful way to investigate and gain rich information about how people are living and communicating in the digital era where new ways to connect are continually being developed.

Netnography found its origins in the world of marketing and business research where it was used to identify consumer patterns and behaviors (Tavakoli & Wijesing, 2019). Over the last few decades, due to its broad study of social interaction, it has become popular in other fields of research including health, education, tourism, politics, and geography (Hetland & Morch, 2016; Kozinets, 2018)—all sites rich with potential for exploring occupation.

Online communities represent contemporary ways in which many people are now communicating and socializing, and one of the ways cybercultures are established. Cyberculture is the concept of the social environment and the result of online interactions that are created through computer-mediated communication (You, 2020). Globally, online communities have also increased interaction between people from differing levels of education, socioeconomic backgrounds, and geographical locations (Vohra & Bhardwaj, 2019). Digital platforms provide the virtual space for users to express themselves instantly, openly, and unreservedly. The naturalistic and uninfluenced (by researchers) data available online can provide the occupation-focused researcher with insight into daily experiences, meaning, and influences on meaningful engagement and participation that is raw and 'in the here and now.' Therefore, I argue that netnography is a very useful qualitative methodology for occupational scientists and occupational therapists seeking to gain insight into the behaviors and influences on communities and populations.

Epistemology, Ontology, Axiology

The underpinning of netnography lies in the epistemologies of participant observation of anthropology and the value of cultural or community understanding (Hetland & Morch, 2016). Further, netnography heavily relies on means of communication and information digitally presented and archived, setting netnography apart from the more traditional ethnography. Within epistemology, there are three main paradigms: realism, positivism, and interpretivism (Lincoln & Guba, 1985). The interpretivist paradigm, which sees reality to be complex and multi-layered (Kozinets, 2015), and has the potential to present multiple interpretations of one phenomenon, tends to best fit with netnography (Salmons, 2016).

Based on a participant-observational approach, both active or passive netnography (explained later in the chapter) enable researchers to delve into users' digital narratives to study online social and cultural trends and interactions (Darawsheh, 2014; Kozinets, 2010). This methodology is useful when studying sensitive topics, providing greater access to geographically dispersed groups, spontaneous self-expression, and trustworthy interpersonal communications within online communities (Dehkhoda et al., 2020).

Netnography's epistemology is positioned as the human input behind the technology through which it is presented. The ontology of netnography, however, is positioned as relativism which values the human interpretation that comes through in the data (Tamminen & Poucher, 2020). Ontology is the study of the construction of human and non-human realities (Berryman, 2019) and is defined as circumstances through which individuals view and comprehend the nature of reality. Relativism postulates that reality is dependent upon a person's lived experience, their interpretation of experiences, and the impact of social/environmental context; hence, people will have different interpretations depending on internal and external factors within their induvial contexts (Tamminen &

Poucher, 2020). Netnography research utilizes this form of ontology to understand a variety of interpretations, helping to gain insight into why people view experiences the way they do.

Herron and Reason (1997) add another paradigm of inquiry to participation known as axiology. Axiology considers both aesthetics and ethics and offers a practical understanding of the world. Axiology asks what the intent and purpose of research is, acknowledging that research always has motivations; that is, who does it aim to empower or what does it aim to justify. Axiological orientation in terms of netnography is considered critical, humanist, and moral (Herron & Reason, 1997).

A true axiological perspective proposes that researchers should not avoid sharing information about ethical challenges and questions with all involved in the research process. It suggests that researchers should be aware of honesty in the process, and the added value that sharing of process, information, challenges, and knowledge helps communities to foster relationships and collaboration within the research process (Kozinets & Nocker, 2018). Netnography's epistemology and axiology recognizes the human input behind the technology it is presented through and values the human interpretation that comes through in the data and research process.

Keeping all of this in mind, my research team utilized netnography to explore the experience of occupational participation for bloggers living with leukemia and to understand the possibility of multiple and potentially complex phenomena for this population. Our study relied on humanistic communications, interpretations, and digital interactions, which incorporated an interpretivist epistemology. I will refer to this study throughout the chapter.

Topics and Questions Best Suited for Netnographical Studies

Kozinets (2010) suggested netnography research questions should: (1) Seek to answer one or two central questions with no more than seven related sub-questions; (2) Utilize probing or exploratory verbs for example 'explore,' 'describe,' or 'understand'; and (3) Employ open-ended questions. In our study we took these points into consideration when exploring the experience of occupational participation for bloggers living with leukemia. Specifically, we addressed the following two research questions: (1) What do bloggers living with leukemia write about their experiences of living with cancer and how does it impact their participation in occupations? and (2) What factors influence participation in these occupations for people living with leukemia?

To date, occupation-focused studies utilizing netnography are not evident in the literature base. Netnography has the potential to provide a different and interesting way to understand how communities and populations interact, communicate, and function. Hence, I believe it would be fascinating and forward thinking if the occupational therapy profession and occupational science community seized this research opportunity. I suggest the extension of our research project, as reported here, would be of interest to the occupational therapy profession, using netnography. Exploring the impact of a child's cancer diagnosis on the parenting and sibling roles would lend itself well to netnography.

Recruitment and Sampling

In addition to formulating the research question, Kozinets (2010) has contended that the 'entrée' (or entering process) into a study utilizing netnography is important and must include identification of a suitable online community or population to study. Researchers need to decide exactly what they are interested in studying, how they will study it, how they will represent themselves in the online community, and, very importantly, how they will ethically conduct their project. Additionally, researchers are required to consider how much disruption they may potentially create in the online communities or population in which they conduct their studies. For our research, the decision about how to address immersion and disruption was made based on the premise communication with the bloggers would affect the nature of the data, shifting the focus to the blogger themselves rather than looking specifically at the blog content.

Kozinets (2010) suggested guidelines for netnographical recruitment. He proposed that the researcher should search for online communities that relate to the research focus, are active or have recent posts or communications, have a large data set to allow for in-depth analysis should the study be using a passive approach, and, where possible, several contributors. A significant feature of netnography is that researchers have the potential to *recruit* participants extensively and quickly due to the internet providing large amounts of available online interactions.

Recruitment in netnography most commonly utilizes purposive sampling as researchers aim to identify specific trends or experiences that occur online or in online forums. Maximum variability sampling, which identifies potential participants with the greatest differences in experience and characteristics between them (Ames et al., 2019), is also commonly used by the netnographer. Maximum variability sampling highlights unique and shared patterns across different people, populations, and communities (Ames et al., 2019). This type of sampling was especially relevant to our study population, as people living with leukemia are not a homogenous group, with varieties in diagnosis, treatment, age, culture, and gender differences amongst the population (Australian Institute of Health and Welfare, 2018). For our study, we employed a passive approach (to be discussed below in data collection methods in more detail), with blogs being freely accessible online; hence, there was no need to advertise when seeking participants. For netnographical studies that use active researcher participation, access to and permission to use the blogs, and participation in the community needs to be approved by the communities' 'gatekeepers'/website administrators.

Data Collection

There is a wealth of data online just waiting to be collected. Data collection is one of the most critical parts of netnography as methodical work is key to ensuring rigor and trustworthiness of studies. Data are commonly collected from well-known search engines such as Google, online blogging platforms, and more customized or specialized social network sites such as Facebook and Snapchat. Data sources from these collection points are commonly in the form of interviews, fieldnotes, blog posts, archives, images, or videos (Costello et al., 2017), and various data collection methods are available to the netnographer depending on the type of data they want to collect (Lugosi & Quinton, 2018).

For data to be collected, netnography primarily requires participation of some form in the desired online community (Kozinets, 2010; Kulavuz-Onal & Vásquez, 2013). Participation ranges from passive, observation only participation, through to active or complete participation where the researcher is a group member (Costello et al., 2017). Passive approaches to data collection utilize inert participation, with researchers acting as bystanders and observers within the community (DeWalt & DeWalt, 2011). A passive approach is suited to sensitive data as it provides a sense of anonymity, allowing free, non-biased, and naturalistic data collection (Langer & Beckman, 2005). It is often not suitable or possible, due to gatekeepers or the type of research question posed by the research team, to become an active part of online communities, which is why a passive approach was chosen for our study with online bloggers with leukemia.

While passive participation may be appropriate for some online environment studies, such as ours, the opportunity for co-creation in digital communities is missed. Therefore, active participation is often the preferred data collection method. Here, the netnographer has an opportunity to conduct their research in an immersive way that adds value, allows for clarification to be sought, and for continuity of narratives in virtual environments. Narrative influence by the researcher does need to be considered in terms of presenting certain bias when active participation is the main method of data collection as clarification can be sought from the participant by the researcher (Costello et al., 2017).

Finally, it needs to be highlighted that there are multiple ways to collect data from an online source. Sequential-top-down posting is when data are gathered from the most recent post down, working backwards chronologically. Alternatively, data collection can be performed in the reverse post order, or even random order (Weller et al., 2018). All ways of gathering posts are recognized to be effective and correct if they help to best answer the research question/s. In our study we chose to gather data sequentially top-down from the chosen blogs, which had been accessed from multiple sites, which provided recent data that met our search criteria date wise and provided contemporary data. All blogs accessed were freely accessible and found on sites that did not have administrators; hence, permission was not required to utilize the blogs in our study.

Data Analysis

The next step of conducting a study using netnography is the analysis and interpretation stage, where data are classified and coded. In this process, the netnographer attempts to understand and communicate the reality of the community studied by detailing nuanced interpretations, that are culturally based. In the analysis stage it is the job of the netnographer not to determine certain facts, but to provide insight into the lives of others (Kozinets, 2018). This is also the stage where the netnographer utilizes personal journals or memos to maintain a reflexive approach to analysis (Hammersley, 2006), which is a particular ethnographic tradition.

So how is analysis done in netnography? First, classification occurs. This step requires the researcher to organize all information that has been gathered to enable it to be analyzed easily—order is key in this process. Commonly, data are grouped by purpose (topic, content, media/photographic, or written). Researchers need to ask themselves whether their data are 'informative' or 'social' in nature and purpose (Bowler, 2010). Data with a social purpose are information from community members that primarily share stories, provide social connections, or simply comments on other online forum information. Informative data relies on pertinent information and informs community members of important information. This grouping was achieved manually in our study; for example, by grouping information about diagnosis or treatment and information which centered on personal experiences/stories about the cancer journey together. All data were placed into a Word document to be manually coded by the research team. Data in our study were all in written form, with no photographs or images utilized.

After categorizing the data, coding data into categories occurs. This is a process that can be performed manually (perhaps an 'old school' way but one that I personally prefer), or by using software packages. NVivo and Leximancer, are examples of software that can manage large data sets and assist in identifying prevalent and common information (Sotiriadou et al., 2014). Whether you prefer a hands on/old school approach or the digital form of analysis is totally up to you, as long as rigor processes are considered.

Generating codes and the development of themes followed Braun and Clarke's (2006) framework. Initial coding included the searching for codes in each line of text, which comprised 75,368 words and resulted in the creation of 95 unique codes. Once discussed as a team and clarity around meaning emerged, 59 relevant codes were identified and grouped to further identify 15 sub-themes. Sub-themes emerged from the similarities and differences noted across the data. Sub-themes were then discussed by the research team in more depth to ensure representation of the data was clear and accurate; eight sub-themes were then finalized. Three themes answering the research question were then created. These themes can be seen in Figure 16.1.

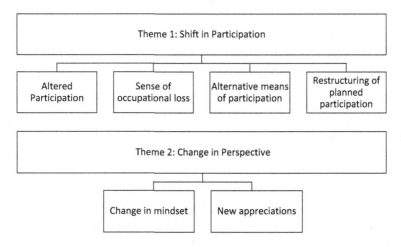

Figure 16.1 Visual presentation of themes and sub-themes. Author created

As highlighted in Figure 16.1, occupationally three things were identified. First, that there was a shift in participation. People needed to change how they participated in chosen and required occupational roles due to treatment side effects, often meaning a reduction in participation or changes in occupations. Alternative means of participation clearly occurred meaning people blogged rather than attended in person social activities, providing them with the ability to still engage in meaningful occupations. Second, changes in perspectives about doing and the need to participate in relationships was evident. People realized they could still be active in communities from a social standpoint through blogging, enabling meaningful participation. Third, people blogged about the need for normality versus acceptance of their new normal; re-defining how they engaged in meaningful ways.

Rigor and Ethics

Rigor and trustworthiness are important to any research, and with new and ever-changing data sources for the netnographer to access, they are key to address. Credibility, dependability, confirmability, and trustworthiness should be addressed when considering rigor (DePoy & Gitlin, 2016). Below I present the ways in which rigor was addressed and achieved in our study. I then discuss some unique ethical issues that may arise when using netnography.

Credibility:

- Regular peer debriefing sessions among the research team (Stanley, 2015).
- Analytical examination of transcripts and memos to question or validate findings between the codes, categories, and themes that the research team arrived at (Dehkhoda et al., 2020; Liamputtong, 2020; Thomas & Magilvy, 2011).
- Reviewing all transcripts, looking for similarities within the participants' experiences and checking for representativeness across the data (Thomas & Magilvy, 2011).
- Reflexivity: continual critical self-reflection (recording expectations, thoughts, emotions, and assumptions) and making these intellectual and personal biases explicit throughout the research process (Darawsheh, 2014; Liamputtong, 2020).

Dependability:

- Clear audit trail of the entire study process including memos detailing internal feelings, thematic logs, and minutes from all research team meetings (Darawsheh, 2014; Liamputtong, 2020).
- Recording and saving analysis as it progresses to document the analytical and methodological decisions made at each stage (Stanley, 2015).

Confirmability:

- Maintaining a sense of openness and awareness as the study unfolds and making certain that the findings are clearly linked to the data and not derived from the researcher's imagination or need to answer the research question a certain way (Liamputtong, 2020; Thomas & Magilvy, 2011).

Transferability:

- Research process was well documented, traceable, and logical, allowing an outsider to follow, critique, and audit the entire research process (Liamputtong, 2020).

Conducting ethical netnographical research presents a variety of unique challenges (Morais et al., 2020). While advantages of netnography include access to data and large amounts of data availability, Corrêa and Rozados (2017) identified the need for the netnographer to decide whether to conduct research within traditional ethical boundaries or adapt ethical standards and requirements to the characteristics of the digital and virtual environment. Should researchers opt to follow traditional ethical guidelines they are in jeopardy of not collecting enough data size wise and enough data in terms of richness to showcase new knowledge or expansion of existing knowledge. However, researchers also need to be careful not to deviate too far from traditional ethical standards. As Ackland (2013) contended, "Ethical guidelines for use of digital trace data are still a moving target" (p. 74). And no doubt a target that will need to develop as technology and use of digital data transforms. Some common current ethical considerations for the netnographer include the following:

1 *Public vs private content and consent.* Online interactions are either private or public. On the one hand, if communications are considered private, informed consent should be sought to allow data to be utilized in research. On the other hand, public online interactions suggest that consent exists already as data are freely available and made that way

by choice and a want to share information. For our study, consent was assumed as we targeted freely available blogs; and based on this understanding we received an exemption from the ethics department by the university through which our study was completed. As digital research increases over time and shifts in its digital footprint style, consent is an area requiring attention. Researchers are encouraged to check their national ethical standards guidelines to ensure up-to-date ethical processes are followed in regard to consent when researching within online communities.

2 *Data reliability.* Data reliability is a big challenge for the netnographer. How is it ascertained for certain that online data are trustworthy, authentic, and not posted by phony profiles? According to Borkar and Purohit (2019), the construction of false online profiles is often driven by the creator's desire to build a social network with a specific purpose—the want to defame a person or organization, to advertise or campaign with a motive, or to take personal or specific industry data for benefit. In our study, the likelihood of fake profiles we believed, armed with the previous reasoning, was minimal due to our sourcing of profiles not being from fundraising sites or sites seeking gains. Hence, we saw minimal opportunity of advantageous gains by bloggers to have fake profiles

In our study of blogging in the leukemia population, the ethical debate around the use of social media posts for research purposes inevitably arose. It was the unclear nature of the ownership of these posts that caused the debate. After much discussion and ethical consideration, the consensus within our research team was that the data could be used for our study without consent from the author. Blogs were evaluated based on how public they were intended to be, as it can be argued overtly public or relatively anonymous blogs can be used without permission (Barker, 2008; Burles & Bally, 2018; Lamprell & Braithwaite, 2018). All blog content we collected were through passive observation with no blogger interaction, on the premise communication with bloggers would affect the nature of the data, shifting the focus to the blogger themselves rather than looking specifically at the blog content. We identified the importance of anonymity; therefore, to meet this ethical requirement, the names of all bloggers and blogs were removed from the data, and any names mentioned in quotations were de-identified. Images were also excluded from analysis to preserve anonymity. Finally, we reported the data collection in such a way as to not identify individual blogs; rather, give an idea of the method used to locate the entire sample to ensure the recruitment was rigorous without sacrificing anonymity.

The netnographer needs to attempt to counteract these potential ethical issues—informed consent and reliability—by using a type of disclosure whereby they can identify such risks. To avoid potential ethical challenges faced by the netnographer, Kozinets (2002) suggested four guidelines to consider.

1 A researcher should alert the online community members of their presence.
2 Confidentiality and anonymity of the online participants should be guaranteed by the netnographer.
3 Feedback from the online community participants should be sought.
4 Permission should be sought to directly quote specific posts.

Now, these ethical principles are well suited for traditional research, and perhaps netnographical research when the researcher identifies themselves to the community of interest, but what happens when the researcher does not need to or is not able to identify themselves and/or be part of the online community? Langer and Beckman (2005) argued that netnography analysis is like content analysis of more traditional forms of media (e.g., television or newspapers) and, therefore, ethical principles need to be specific and unique to the type of netnography performed. It is also argued in the available literature that disturbing the community flow, data may become disjointed or biased. In more recent years, Kozinets (2010) acknowledged that it could be ethically sound to study certain digital communities without seeking permission. Thus, ethics is an ever-changing challenge for the netnographer that will no doubt continue to change over time.

Best Practice

Being conscious of best practice when using netnography is key, ensuring all methodological decisions are explicit and transparent contributes to best practice. Through the use of reflexive processes, the netnographer is able to identify their positionality to the data and the research process and provide the space for true and honest reflection. Reflexive processes such as journaling, note taking, and de-briefing with their research teams allow netnographers to consider ethical issues that arise when working with online communities and, in particular, when passively participating in the community.

Application to Occupational Therapy

For the occupational therapist, netnography is a way to gain insight into contemporary experiences, opinions, and interactions people have in a way that is socially and culturally relevant. Online engagement is growing as technology enhances and societies continue to demonstrate a need to connect with others differently, that being virtually in the digital world. Online forums provide people in our developing society a place to connect with likeminded and experienced people, as well as offering a place to be heard, often without being seen. These developing ways of involvement in the occupation of online interaction and socialization provide the opportunity of a strong evidence base to draw from for the occupational therapist who can gain value in understanding new ways of meaningful participation.

Our study showed the need for a sense of belonging/meaningful participation sought by bloggers living with leukemia while experiencing a sense of occupational deprivation due to times of isolation due to treatment requirements. The study identified how an online environment can provide people with a sense of community and feeling they are not alone in their experiences. Our study also showed that blogging gave people a sense of purpose and provided an occupation with meaning that they were able to participate in despite often feeling unwell. Netnographical studies are further relevant to the occupational therapist as they help develop an in-depth insight and understanding of healthcare experiences, cultures, and complex phenomenon in real-life contexts.

Application to Occupational Science

Occupational scientists are interested in how people participate in their chosen occupations, and the development of new and often innovative ways that enable people to participate meaningfully (Yerxa, 1990). Occupational scientists present an occupational perspective of identifying and gaining insight into the way that people 'do' (Kristensen & Petersen, 2015). This concept of observing people 'doing' and participating in their natural environments is congruent with netnography, as is the idea of, and interest in, new, developing, and innovative ways to participate; hence, the two go hand in hand. Additionally, Zemke and Clark (1996) identified the importance of studying human occupation and the importance of meaning, connection, and purpose for people. The netnographer is also very keen to identify how people and community members gain a sense of meaning from posting and connecting online and being part of digital communities. Netnography aims to increase the understanding of human online interactions, mirroring one of the aims of occupational science which is to build evidence of observable human interaction. It is exciting to think that this new way of observing how people interact and participate will enable occupational scientists to investigate new and emerging data sources that seem to be constantly changing. Imagine the wealth of data that may come from this data as occupation-focused online communities continue to develop and emerge as technology changes.

Our study contributes to the occupational science knowledge base as it identified what it is like to live with leukemia and how participation changes through the disease trajectory; it also highlighted the need for participation, connection to others, and establishing belonging. Whalley-Hammell (2014) identified that by establishing a sense of belonging and connectedness within communities and between people, a positive correlation to well-being is established. Through common or shared experiences and feelings of belonging to a group or community, meaningful occupation is experienced. Our study identified the challenges of connection for people living with leukemia as they are often required to isolate, avoiding human interaction during treatment to avoid additional illness and complications. Our study then identified how online interactions can assist people to connect, participate, and belong despite these medical limitations.

Critiquing Netnographical Studies

There is a paucity of netnography studies in occupational science and occupational therapy; therefore, occupational science and occupational therapy researchers wishing to use netnography will need to look to other disciplines. With this in mind, in Textbox 16.1 I suggest some questions to ask yourself as you read the literature and consider your netnographical process.

Textbox 16.1   Critiquing Netnographical Studies – Questions to Ask

1 Is the research *question and scope* clearly defined?
2 Are *recruitment strategies and sampling* processes clearly outlined and appropriate?
3 Is the *platform or forum* public/easily accessible or closed?
4 Do the researchers state if they were or were not actively involved in, or observers of the online community?
5 Is the *platform or forum* used to collect data most appropriate?
6 Is there *variation in the available data*?
7 Is there *enough content online* to answer the research problem?
8 Have *relevant digital ethical standards* met?
9 Have researchers used reflective pondering as part of rigor?
10 Has the *analysis process* been clearly articulated?
11 Are all themes identified *rich in description*?

Author Reflections

"Blogging is to writing, what extreme sports are to athletics: more free-form, more accident-prone, less formal, more alive. It is, in many ways, writing out loud" (Sullivan, 2022). The idea of gaining insight into how people experience living with leukemia and how they reflect on their experiences of the disease process and trajectory in raw form is what drew me to consider netnography in my research. There are not many opportunities in research when researchers are able to gather data that are unedited, unapproved, or uninfluenced by the research process. I was particularly intrigued by the fact that blogging is considered 'alive' or 'instant' in the way it is published. As a result of this interest, I began thinking of how I could best research blogging and bloggers and netnography was my answer.

Personally, I find using netnography interesting and contemporary. On reflection of the challenges netnography poses, I have found myself, at times, wondering, what happens next for participants? As our study did not use researcher interaction there were times that I wanted to know more about what participants wrote online and I was unable to ask. However, the beauty of netnography really does lie in the instantaneous thought processes and experiences presented in the data.

Summary

The online world has opened a whole new scale of data and wealth of information which directly offers researchers in all fields endless exciting study possibilities. Netnography provides those researchers with the means to deal with large digital data sets, identify current trends, opinions, and experiences, and navigate challenging ethical issues identified in the virtual research space as it develops (Kozinets, 2018). This chapter has presented one way of doing netnography through the example of one study which identified the experience of occupational participation for bloggers living with leukemia. This chapter reveals how this form of qualitative methodology can be useful for the occupational therapy profession as it provides the means to do research in a way that aligns with the values of occupational therapy: client centered, participatory centric with a focus on meaningful engagement. For the occupational scientist, netnography is a means to gain rich insight into contemporary issues experienced by communities and populations.

References

Ackland, R. (2013). *Web social science: Concepts, data and tools for social scientists in the digital age.* SAGE. https://dx.doi.org/10.4135/9781446270011

Ames, H., Glenton, C., & Lewin, S. (2019). Purposive sampling in a qualitative evidence synthesis: A worked example from a synthesis on parental perceptions of vaccination communication. *BioMed Central Medical Research Methodology, 19*(1), 1–9. https://doi.org/10.1186/s12874-019-0665-4

Australian Institute of Health and Welfare. (2018). *Cancer data in Australia; Australian cancer incidence and mortality (acim) books: Leukaemia (all types).* Australian Government. www.aihw.gov.au/reports/cancer/cancer-data-in-australia/

Barker, K. K. (2008). Electronic support groups, patient-consumers, and medicalization: The case of contested illness. *Journal of Health and Social Behavior, 49*(1), 20–36. https://doi.org/10.1177/002214650804900103

Berryman, D. R. (2019). Epistemology, ontology, methodology, and methods: Information for librarian researchers. *Medical References Services Quarterly, 38*(3), 271–279 https://doi.org/10.1080/02763869.2019.1623614

Borkar, B. S., & Purohit, R. (2019). Recognition of fake profiles in social media: A literature review. *Journal of Engineering and Technology, 5*(2), 1119–1121.

Bowler, G. M. (2010). Netnography: A method specifically designed to study cultures and communities online. *Qualitative Report, 15*(5), 1270–1275. http://doi.org/10.46743/2160-3715/2010.1341

Braun, V., & Clarke, V. (2006). Using thematic analysis in psychology. *Qualitative Research in Psychology, 3*(2), 77–101. http://eprints.uwe.ac.uk/11735

Burles, M. C., & Bally, J. M. G. (2018). Ethical, practical, and methodological considerations for unobtrusive qualitative research about personal narratives shared on the internet. *International Journal of Qualitative Methods, 17*(1), 1–9. https://doi.org/10.1177/1609 406918788203

Corrêa, M. V., & Rozados, H. B. F. (2017). Netnography as a research method. *Information Science, 22*(49), 1–18; 441–455. https://doi.org/10.46743/2160-3715/2020.4227

Costello, L., McDermott, M. L., & Wallace, R. (2017). Netnography: Range of practices, misperceptions, and missed opportunities. *International Journal of Qualitative Methods, 16*, 1–12. https://doi.org/10.1177/1609406917700647

Darawsheh, W. B. (2014). Reflexivity in research: Promoting rigor, reliability and validity in qualitative research. *International Journal of Therapy and Rehabilitation, 21*(12), 560–568. https://doi.org/10.12968/ijtr.2014.21.12.560

Dehkhoda, A., Owens, R. G., & Malpas, P. J. (2020). A netnographic approach: Views on assisted dying for individuals with dementia. *Qualitative Health Research, 30*(13), 2077–2091. http://doi.org/10.1177/1049732320925795

DePoy, E., & Gitlin, L. N. (2016). *Introduction to research: Understanding and applying multiple strategies* (5th ed.). Elsevier/Mosby. https://doi.org/10.1016/B978-0-323-26171-5.00030-6

DeWalt, K. M., & DeWalt, B. R. (2011). *Participant observation: A guide for fieldworkers* (2nd ed.). Altamira Press.

Dover, Y., & Kelman, G. (2018). Emergence of online communities: Empirical evidence and theory. *PLOS One, 13*(11), 1–17. https://doi.org/10.1371/journal.pone.0205167

Hammersley, M. (2006). Ethnography: Problems and prospects. *Ethnography and Education, 1*, 3–14. https://doi.org/10.1080/17457820500512697

Heinonen, K., & Medberg, G. (2018). Netnography as a tool for understanding customers: Implications for service research and practice. *Journal of Services Marketing, 32*(6), 657–679. https://doi.org/10.1108/JSM-08-2017-0294

Herron, J., & Reason, P. (1997). A participatory inquiry paradigm. *Qualitative Inquiry, 3*, 274–294. https://doi.org/10.1177/107780049700300302

Hetland, P., & Morch, A. I. (2016). Ethnography for investigating the internet. *Seminar.Net, 12*(1), 11–17. https://doi.org/10.7577/seminar.2335

Kaoakaou, M. (2021). Netnography: Towards a new sociological approach of qualitative research in the digital age. *SHS Web Conferences, 119*, 1–7. http://doi.org/10.105/shsconf/202111901006

Kozinets, R. V. (2015). *Netnography: Redefined.* SAGE. https://doi.org/10.1002/9781118767771.wbiedcs067

Kozinets, R. V. (1998). On netnography: Initial reflections on consumer research investigations of cyberculture. *Advances in Consumer Research, 1*(25), 366–371.

Kozinets, R. V. (2002). The field behind the screen: Using netnography for marketing research in online communities. *Journal of Marketing Research, 39*, 61–72. https://doi.org/10.1509/jmkr.39.1.61.18935

Kozinets, R. V. (2010). *Netnography: Doing ethnographic research online.* SAGE. https://doi.org/10.4324/9781003001430

Kozinets, R. V. (2018). Netnography for management and business research. In C. Cassell, A. Cunliffe, & G. Grandy (Eds.), *The SAGE handbook of qualitative business and management research methods* (pp. 384–397). SAGE. https://methods.sagepub.com/book/the-sage-handbook-of-qualitative-business-and-management-research-methods-v2/i2745.xml

Kozinets, R. V., & Nocker, M. (2018). Netnography: Engaging with the challenges. In A. Bryman & D. A. Buchanan (Eds.), *Unconventional methodology in organization and management research* (pp. 127–146). Oxford University Press.

Kristensen, H. K., & Petersen, K. S. (2015). Occupational science: An important contributor to occupational therapists' clinical reasoning. *Scandinavian Journal of Occupational Therapy*, *23*(3), 240–243. https://doi.org/10.3109/11038128.2015.1083054

Kulavuz-Onal, D., & Vásquez, C. (2013). Reconceptualising fieldwork in a netnography of an online community of English language teachers. *Ethnography and Education*, *8*(2), 224. https://doi.org/10.1080/17457823.2013.792511

Lamprell, K., & Braithwaite, J. (2018). When patients tell their own stories: A meta-narrative study of web-based personalized texts of 214 melanoma patients' journeys in four countries. *Qualitative Health Research*, *28*(10), 1564–1583. https://doi.org/10.1177/1049732317742623

Langer, R., & Beckman, S. C. (2005). Sensitive research topics: Netnography revisited. *Qualitative Market Research: An International Journal*, *8*(2), 189–203. https://doi.org/10.1108/wellb13522750510592454

Liamputtong, P. (2020). *Qualitative research methods* (5th ed.). Oxford University Press.

Lincoln, Y., & Guba, E. G. (1985). *Naturalistic inquiry*. SAGE.

Lugosi, P., & Quinton, S. (2018). More-than-human netnography. *Journal of Marketing and Management*, *34*(3), 287–313. https://doi.org/10.1080/0267257X.2018.1431303

Mason, B. (1996). Moving toward virtual ethnography. *American Folklore Society News*, *25*(2), 4–5. http://doi.org/10.7577/seminar.2335

Morais, G. M., Santos, V. F., & Gonçalves, C. A. (2020). Netnography: Origins, foundations, evolution and axiological and methodological developments and trends. *The Qualitative Report*, *25*(2), 441–445. https://doi.org/10.46743/2160-3715/2020.4227

Rees, C., & Gatenby, M. (2014). Critical realism and ethnography. In P. K. Edwards, J. O'Mahoney & S. Vincent (Eds.), *Studying organizations using critical realism: A practical guide* (pp. 1–17). Oxford University Press.

Ryan, G. S. (2017). An introduction to the origins, history and principles of ethnography. *Nurse Researcher*, *24*(4), 397–402. http://doi.org/10/7748.nr2017.e1470

Salmons, J. (2016). *Choosing methodologies and methods for online studies*. SAGE. https://dx.doi.org/10.4135/9781473921955

Sotiriadou, P., Brouwers, D., & Le, T.A. (2014). Choosing a qualitative data analysis tool: A comparison of NVivo and Leximancer. *Annals of Leisure Research*, *17*(2), 218–234. http://doi.org/10.1080/11745398.2014.902292

Stanley, M. (2015). Qualitative descriptive. In S. Nayar & M. Stanley (Eds.), *Qualitative research methodologies for occupational science and therapy* (pp. 21–37). Routledge.

Sullivan, A. (2022, June 19). *Why I blog*. www.theatlantic.com/magazine/archive/2008/11/why-i-blog/307060/

Tamminen, K. A., & Poucher, Z. A. (2020). Research philosophies. In D. Hackfort & R. J. Schinke (Eds.), *The Routledge international encyclopedia of sport and exercise psychology* (pp. 535–549). Routledge.

Tavakoli, R., & Wijesing, R. S. (2019). The evolution of the web and netnography in tourism: A systematic review. *Tourism Management Perspectives*, *29*, 48–55. https://doi.org/10.1016/j.tmp.2018.10.008

Thomas, E., & Magilvy, J. K. (2011). Qualitative rigor or research validity in qualitative research. *Journal for Specialists in Pediatric Nursing*, *16*(2), 151–155. https://doi.org/10.1111/j.1744-6155.2011.00283.x

Toledano, M. C. M. (2017). Emergent methods: Using netnography in public relations research. *Public Relations Review*, *43*, 597–604. http://doi.org/10.1016/J.PUBREV.2017.03.007

Vohra, A., & Bhardwaj, N. (2019). Exploring active participation in virtual communities and the role of community benefits: An empirical study of university students in India. *Global Business Review*, *20*(2), 515–528. http://doi.org/10.1177/0972150918825211

Weller, W., Bassalo, L., & Pfaff, N. (2018). Collecting data for analyzing blogs. In U. Flick (Ed.), *The SAGE handbook of qualitative data collection* (pp. 482–495). SAGE. https://dx.doi.org/10.4135/9781526416070.n31

Whalley-Hammell, K. R. (2014). Belonging, occupation, and human well-being: An exploration. *Canadian Journal of Occupational Therapy*, *81*(1), 39–50. http://doi.org/10.1177/0008417413520489

Yerxa, E. J. (1990). An introduction to occupational science, A foundation for occupational therapy in the 21st century. *Occupational Therapy Health Care*, *6*(4), 1–17. http://doi.org/10.1080/J003v06n04_04

You, W. (2020). The influence of cyberculture on lifestyle under the background of new media. *Frontiers in Educational Research*, *3*(5), 90–93. http://doi.org/10.25236/FER.2020.030518

Zemke, R., & Clark, F. (Eds.). (1996). *Occupational science: The evolving discipline*. F. A. Davis.

Additional Resources

Robert Kozinets on netnography. YouTube. www.youtube.com/watch?v=IBBQixBe3i8

Robert Kozinets: Netnography: The essential guide to qualitative social media research. YouTube. www.youtube.com/watch?v=CUnLAvyuQB8

An example of an organizational blog: www.cancer.org.au/about-us/news-and-media/blog?query=&hitsPerPage=9&page=1

An example of a consumer blog: www.thepatientstory.com/cancers/faq/cancer-blogs/

17 Big Qualitative Data

Mandy Stanley

One of the oft-heard critiques of qualitative research is that sample sizes are small. Generally, I am one of the first to defend a small sample and tell students to never apologize for the size of their sample as the depth and richness far outweighs the breadth of data. However, there is a relatively untapped opportunity to contribute to occupational science knowledge and occupational therapy practice through the use of qualitative Big data. In the context of this book, Big qualitative data is defined as data from 100 or more participants (Brower et al., 2019). In this chapter, I begin by further explicating what Big qualitative data is, before describing what it has to offer to researchers engaging in the study of occupation. To inform this chapter, I draw on work I have been undertaking with colleagues from the Centre for Research in Aged Care at Edith Cowan University, Australia, using publicly available data from an Australian Royal Commission into Quality and Safety in Aged Care (2021). As part of this work, I will refer to my study of risk and how risk was talked about (herein referred to as the 'dignity of risk study') within the Royal Commission data to illuminate points related to theoretical orientation, sampling, data collection and analysis, and ethical issues. I will also draw on two other studies conducted by my Research Center colleagues—the chemical restraint study, and the transfer to emergency departments study (Cain et al., 2022).

Before I go any further, it is important to clarify here that I am not arguing in favor of a well-known English saying, 'The bigger the better.' Rather, I contend that there is a research opportunity for occupational scientists and occupational therapists that has potential to be explored. Currently, it appears that very little academic attention has been paid to data repositories and to the use of Big qualitative data. I make no claims to being an expert with Big qualitative data; however, in an emerging field, I write this chapter as a researcher who can share their experience and that of their colleagues and open up possibilities for other researchers. It is a new and rapidly developing area of research which is generating debate within the methodological literature. Indeed, Brower et al. (2019) argued that Big qualitative data is lacking roots in deep qualitative philosophical thinking as that is yet to come. I find it mildly amusing that the convention used within the literature is the term Big Qual, making it a proper noun, but I will stay with that convention.

While Big Qual has been used in a variety of disciplines, the majority of work being undertaken is secondary analyses; thus, occupational science and occupational therapy researchers need to be aware of the developments, the methodological debates, and to consider the possibilities for contribution to knowledge and practice. With rapidly developing changes in artificial intelligence and machine learning, and the proliferation of data

DOI: 10.4324/9781003456216-17

that are collected about everyday occupations, it seems prudent to consider the possibilities for occupation focused research.

There appear to be three broad approaches to Big Qual within the literature. These are as follows:

1   *As Part of Large Mixed Method Studies*

Many large mixed method studies comprise sizable data sets for quantitative studies, often longitudinal, which have a qualitative component. There is increasing recognition that quantitative studies and the subsequent data and results cannot provide the whole story, or the full answer to a research problem, and that data from a qualitative component enriches the understanding of the quantitative results. The development of Big qualitative data in this space is, perhaps, a natural development of the increasing growth in mixed method studies. Some of the very large longitudinal population studies are likely to have either subsets of data that are qualitative—perhaps semi-structured in-depth interview data or responses to open ended questions within questionnaires that are analyzed qualitatively. Readers will either be aware of these large population studies in their own region or, once aware of their existence, be able to explore the possibilities for being involved in data analysis. For example, there is the Raine study (Straker et al., 2015) which is the oldest pre-birth longitudinal study in the world and extensively studies pregnancy, childhood, and adulthood (https://rainestudy.org.au/). The data are available to researchers once they meet certain requirements, particularly around data management and safety. On looking through the available data as listed on the study website, there are not large amounts of qualitative data available; however, I could identify open-ended questions about the food children eat or concerns a parent might have, which would still yield large amounts of data for analysis. Alternatively, there are the data from the Australian Longitudinal Survey of Women's Health (https://alswh.org.au/), which has qualitative data available from an open-ended question at the end of the surveys. Given these examples, it is likely that readers will be able to locate further studies relevant to their own context, and it is highly likely that there are data sets with much richer qualitative data of interest to occupational scientists or occupational therapists than the examples provided here.

2   *Curation of Large Data sets*

Another type of qualitative data set can be found within government documents, library archives, archived data sets, or, indeed, online. Winskell et al. (2018) described the process of data management and analysis that they used to analyze what they labelled "big, thick, long and wide" (p. 1629) data. The data were drawn from an archive of more than 75,000 narratives submitted to contests by young people who pitched film ideas related to HIV between 1997 and 2014. The study aimed to identify how cultural meanings and context informed sexual behaviors and social practices of young people across sub-Saharan Africa. While this study was within public health it is not too difficult to see how occupational scientists or occupational therapists could engage with similar data sets, given all the right permissions and approvals, to explore topics from an occupational perspective.

Another example of a publicly available data set is the Timescapes data (Neale et al., 2012). This data set was established by a network of researchers from five universities in the United Kingdom, from a variety of disciplines. The data set includes seven studies that spanned the life course with a different focus at each life stage; for example, work-life balance in families with young children. Drawn into a collective that includes data from over

300 individuals, the data were collated into an archive which began operating in 2010 with the intention to have the data available for secondary analysis (Neale & Bishop, 2012). Further exploration of some of the other topics include motherhood across the generations, men as fathers, and grandparents and social exclusion. It does not take much imagination to see how such a data archive would be of interest to occupational scientists or occupational therapists. The Timescapes data is also a great example of the research collaboration that could be replicated within occupational science and occupational therapy to expand the possibility of studies across time, lifespan, and geographies. The World Federation of Occupational Therapists' occupational narratives database project (https://occupational-narratives.wfot.org/) has the potential to be such a data archive if attention was given to wider sampling (beyond occupational therapists and occupational therapy students) and a longitudinal approach was adopted. Further sources of data are government websites and documents, and data repositories.

3 *Data Mining of Social Media*

The proliferation of social media in an increasingly digital world presents multiple opportunities for data mining and exploration of everyday occupational engagement. Various forms of social media provide big databases that are searchable and offer social and occupational data on an unprecedented scale. For example, a study of disruption to the organization and delivery of healthcare in the United Kingdom during the COVID-19 pandemic combined data from telephone interviews with health care workers and accounts of health care workers' experiences published on YouTube and Twitter (Dowrick et al., 2021). They found 16,600 posts in English language (after retweets) and eight YouTube videos. Sentiment analysis was used to assess the range of feelings expressed together with software for discourse analysis to examine the expression of emotion within the social media impressions.

Another example of use of social media as naturally occurring data that might be of interest to occupational therapists is a study of the use of Twitter by those who self-harm (Hilton et al., 2017). They employed thematic analysis (Braun & Clarke, 2013) to analyze posts from 317 Twitter users. The findings provide a rich understanding of how social media is used as a source of support and of the attitudes and beliefs of the general public about self-harm.

I will focus in this chapter on the second approach to Big qualitative data—curation of large data sets—as that is where the dignity of risk study and the other studies we have conducted from the Royal Commission data fit. To give some context, a Royal Commission in Australia (Parliament of Australia, n.d.) is a public inquiry which investigates matters of public importance. They are commissioned by the government with terms of reference and a timeline; and are generally granted broad powers to investigate, including the ability to summons witnesses or to request documents as evidence. It is the highest level of inquiry within the country.

Positioning the Researcher

Having positioned myself as a learner and not an expert in this approach, I need to further position myself as a researcher. I am a grounded theorist at heart with a natural tendency to focus on process, and I often find that when I am bothered by things in life it is because there is no clear process or the process has not been followed appropriately. I realized sometime after completing my PhD, back in 2006, that it was not at all surprising that I had chosen grounded theory for that work and, indeed, it was a good fit for me at a much more personal level, not just a good fit for the research question that I was asking. Since then, much of my qualitative research work, including a funded program of research, has been utilizing a qualitative descriptive study design (see Chapter 4). Over the years working with students, I have enjoyed learning and 'playing' with other research designs such as narrative (Maywald & Stanley, 2015) and focused ethnography. More recently, I have developed an interest in critical discourse analysis. Interestingly, when I approached the dignity of risk study, that I draw on for this chapter, my plan was to take a descriptive qualitative approach and use thematic analysis. Once I began to look at the data, and having recently completed a critical discourse analysis of portrayals of older people, risk, and COVID-19 in the media (Skoss et al., 2022), I could not help but use a critical lens for this study. As a researcher, once you take a critical view of data that examines power and the societal structures that perpetuate power differentials it is very hard to not take that view.

I am not usually an early adopter of technology, although I enjoy using technology when it is fit for purpose, and I understand it! To be honest, I find the notion of artificial intelligence quite scary and, in some respects, threatening, bringing further signs of a dystopian world. Having said that, I am open to new challenges within qualitative research methodology and approach Big Qual in that vein.

Epistemology, Ontology, and Axiology

The epistemological and ontological positioning of Big Qual studies will depend on the approach chosen to collate and analyze the data. Given the origins and nature of Big Qual, it could easily be positioned within a post positivist paradigm. That is a position that recognizes that ideas and the identity of the researcher influence the outcome of the research but still aim towards a fairly objective outcome (Guba & Lincoln, 2005). While there might be a temptation to stay within a post positivist paradigm given the quantity of data, a pragmatic paradigmatic positioning is more appropriate for qualitative researchers working with Big data. An astute reader will identify that my positioning as a researcher appears to conflict with the statements I have just made about paradigms. Indeed, all three studies that have been conducted with the same data set have all taken different epistemological and ontological positions but, I argue, still fit within pragmatism in taking the approach that best fits with the logistics of working with Big data and the research question being asked. It would be nice to write that our journey into Big data was a well-planned one; however, although it was well considered with reference to appropriate methodological literature, it was a journey of significant learning and discovery along the way.

Research is often not a smooth linear process as reported in journal articles, rather a 'one step forward, two steps backwards' experience. In this case, we began with exploring data with searches using key words for each topic (explicated in more detail below). Once we had a better idea of what the data looked like, we chose the approach to the analysis and retrospectively fitted the epistemology and ontology. While not ideal or perfect, I share this experience as the reality of doing research and to demonstrate the need for researchers to be keen to explore, experiment, have fun, push the boundaries, and learn. The chemical restraint study adopted a constructivist approach, and the emergency departments transfer study a critical realist epistemology. In the dignity of risk study, as researchers we took a critical stance with a subjectivist epistemology where the research adopts a position of political advocate to address situations of inequity in power (Guba & Lincoln, 2005). The ontology is historical realism recognizing that situations exist as a result of social, political, cultural, and economic realities which shape identities and human doing. In terms of axiology, the research team valued the position of humans as occupational beings with the right to engage in occupations of choice that bring meaning and fulfillment. Further, my colleagues and I placed value on older people having a right to receive care that respects their dignity as a person with an occupational history.

Topics and Questions Best Suited for Big Qual Data

The research questions pursued within Big qualitative data will depend on the data source and, conversely, the research questions will point to a Big data source. Researchers may start with a research question and turn to thinking about where would be best or how would be the best way to go about answering that question. In the use of Big data, it is probably more likely to be "here is my data set, what questions can I ask within it?" That was certainly the case for the studies my colleagues and I have conducted within the Royal Commission data. The interim report (Royal Commission into Aged Care Quality and Safety, 2019) gave some cues as to the questions or topics that could be explored in more depth and that prompted the first study that members of the research center conducted with the Royal Commission data exploring the use of chemical restraint. Further research questions for that data set were driven from our own interests and in noting that the 148 recommendations in the final report (Royal Commission into Aged Care Quality and Safety, 2021) did not comment specifically on these topics which piqued our curiosity. For some time, I have been interested in how risk is accounted for within practice with older people and the how the principles of occupational rights and the dignity of risk are applied. Given the focus of the Royal Commission on safety and quality in residential aged care, this provided an ideal site for progressing that research interest. Other questions that have been formed in relation to the same data set are presented in Textbox 17.1.

The question for the third study arose from knowledge that transitions in care are sources of tension and the potential for communication breakdown, Thus, the question arose, "What does the Royal Commission data set have to say about transfers to and from the emergency department?" Indeed, one of the recommendations in the final report from the Royal Commission related to improving communication between facilities and exploring systems changes such as multi-disciplinary outreach services. Care provision in residential aged care is becoming increasingly complex and needing to be managed with a workforce that has a low level of training and supervision by limited numbers of

---

Textbox 17.1 Further Sample Questions for the Royal Commission Data Set

1 How is care understood within the context of the Royal Commission into Safety and Quality in residential aged care?
2 What does the Royal Commission data reveal about how diversity is accounted for in residential aged care (e.g., culture, GLBTIQ+)?
3 What is said about the provision of allied health services, specifically occupational therapy within the Royal Commission data?

qualified and experienced nurses. There are frequent occasions where a decision about the need for transfer to acute care needs to be made with international reviews finding that the outcomes did not always justify the transfer and in some cases were detrimental (Cain et al., 2022).

Sampling and Data Management

The sampling of Big qualitative data can make use of data mining tools. This is a rapidly developing space especially with the development and spread of artificial intelligence into everyday occupations such as using a mobile phone or writing an email. However, the challenge is to resist more positivist approaches to sampling and to still take a qualitative approach. It is not necessary to collect every single piece of data but to think through the logic of the approach to sampling as it applies to the project. For my exploration of the Royal Commission data, the research team had curated a data set from the Royal Commission by downloading all of the documents from the website and exporting them into NVivo. This is publicly available data which amounted to 11 GB of data comprising over 10,000 submissions from the public, special interest groups, aged care providers, and health professionals. There were general submission (1183 items), transcripts of hearings and post hearing submissions (227 items), exhibits (5712 items), and Commissioner reports (17 items). During the process of curating the data set there were some important learnings about the size of data set that NVivo can accommodate; thus, the data set was curated within 4 NVivo files for ease of use.

Data Collection Methods

The approach the research team took to data collection has been informed by Seale and Charteris-Black's (2010) key word analysis. Key words are selected for searching the data set for data of interest in order to extract it for data analysis. The team brainstormed the key words that were relevant for each topic, searched the data set for those words, and reviewed the associated excerpts in order to retrieve relevant data to form a new data set. Records were kept of the results of the searches and the volume of data extracted so that the team could reflect on the "keyness" (Seale & Charteris-Black, 2010, p. 539) of the different words. As a starting point, the team chose to begin the searches in the general submissions before moving to hearing transcripts and exhibits. Given the very large amount of data within the exhibits (9 GB) we had to make judicious decisions about the return on investment of time and effort in doing the searches; hence, for the dignity of risk study the exhibits were only searched when it was indicated by content from the hearing transcripts that had already been extracted. We did random checks of a few exhibits and found that it did not yield any additional data.

We learnt a great deal from the chemical restraint study which was the first foray into the data set. An extensive list of 230 key words was generated including terms: chemical and restraint; drug names; and actions and behaviors known to be associated with restraint. The data extracted contained a lot of repetition and certain stories appeared repeatedly. For the emergency department transfer study, a list of 102 key words were generated and used for searching the submissions and transcripts; however, 29 of those words provided the most relevant content. These words were more likely to be exclusive to the emergency department transfer scenario than to other scenarios within the data and thus were used in the remaining searches.

Based on the learnings from the first two studies, a much smaller list of 15 key words was generated for the dignity of risk study. The list included terms such as risk, dignity, safety, and autonomy. Data were extracted from submissions, hearings, exhibits, and Commissioner reports into a new NVivo data set.

Data Analysis

The research team drew on Davidson et al.'s (2019) 'breadth and depth method' to inform the approaches to analysis. For the dignity of risk study, we chose a critical discourse analytic approach (van Dijk, 2009) informed by the Foucauldian concept of governmentality (Foucault & Gordon, 1980; Wodak & Myer, 2016). The first reading of the data was undertaken to identify the key discourses within the segments of text. In the second reading, we followed a similar approach to that of Rudman and Molke (2009). This approach had been previously used (Skoss et al., 2022) in making note of how risk was constructed and problematized within the text, how the subjects (older residents) were positioned in relation to risk, and how risk was constructed discursively within the public documents. In reviewing the documents, attention was paid to the silences, or what was not talked about. Through an iterative process of examining the segments of text, the team were able to identify the dominant subject positions and the use of power and surveillance, and the key discursive features which perpetuated the subject positions.

In the chemical restraint study the same 'stories' kept appearing in the data, so the decision was made to approach analysis using a case study methodology (Yin, 2014). There were four dramatic cases where chemical restraint led to abuse and neglect, and four less dramatic cases that were complex distressing situations but did not appear to involve abuse. For the emergency department transfer study, the team used reflexive thematic analysis (Braun & Clarke, 2022) to identify the key themes.

What can be seen here is that different approaches to analysis were adopted based on the team's sense of the best approach to each research question and topic, and the researcher's interest and skill set. The team were flexible in their approach and prepared to change their thinking based on what was revealed within each data set. Once a decision had been made about the approach to be taken, it was then important to ensure that the approach was applied consistently and that rigor strategies congruent with the approach were utilized.

Rigor and Trustworthiness

The researcher has a range of strategies for rigor available to them which need to be selected to ensure credibility, transferability, dependability, and confirmability following Guba's model (as cited by Krefting, 1991). In the dignity of risk of risk study the research team chose to use 'thick' description of methods and findings to ensure dependability and transferability. Reflexivity and peer debriefing were used for credibility and confirmability. We also kept an audit trail of analytical decisions. Our reflexive discussions centered around the subject positions and power, and the discursive elements used in invoking the 'safety clause' to justify the removal of choice from the resident and family members. During those discussions we came to see the binary between quality and safety and that these two ideas were always seen as options and mutually exclusive. In the other two studies there was also triangulation of researchers where the data were analyzed by different members of the team and compared which brought different perspectives to the analysis.

A limitation of using Big data and conducting secondary analysis is the inability to use probing questions to further explore meaning with individuals or groups, or to clarify meaning and interpretation. That limitation needs to be acknowledged and rigor strategies such as reflexivity employed to further examine the research assumptions in interpreting the data and questioning of each other in peer examination.

Ethical Issues

At first glance, researchers may think that ethical approval is not required for using Big data as no human participants are directly involved. However, researchers will potentially need permission from the 'owners' of the data. For the studies presented in this chapter, the research team sought permission from the Commission to access the data even though it was publicly available. Seeking permission will not be applicable in all cases, for example using data from social media. In the National Health and Medical Research Council and Universities Australia (2007, updated 2018) Statement on Ethical Conduct in Human Research, which provides guidance for all research with humans in Australia, the definition of human research includes "access to this information (in individually identifiable, re-identifiable or non-identifiable form) as part of an existing published or unpublished source or database" (p. 7). Therefore, we submitted an ethics protocol to the University Human Research Ethics Committee where it was assessed as low risk and approved. While the Australian Royal Commission data are publicly accessible and identifiable, the research team chose to remove all identifying information out of respect to individuals and organizations. The decision to do so was that although individuals made submissions to the Commission or appeared at hearings and gave consent for their information to be published, at the time they did not give explicit consent for their information to be used in other ways that they probably could never have imagined it would be used. Researchers will need to consider their own data sources, consult the ethical guidelines and requirements for the jurisdiction that they work within, and make their own decisions. It is possible to seek guidance from local ethics committees if unsure, but overall the research needs to meet the guiding principles of merit, integrity, justice, beneficence, and respect.

One aspect of ethics that I had not appreciated was the risk to the researchers in reading and re-reading stories of neglect, abuse, and suffering of older people living in residential aged care, which began to cause some distress for one of the team. Fortunately, it was identified by a team member early in the analysis and support was provided through the Employee Assistance Program. The issue of vicarious distress and trauma for researchers is not a new one; however, it may not be anticipated in what is often seen as a (re)-analysis of data or at least removed from the human experience of the telling and less likely to raise concerns to have preventative measures in place. My experience reveals that reading texts without having any contact with the narrator of the story can potentially be disturbing and, if the risk is not anticipated and mitigated, has the potential to harm the researcher.

Dekas and McCune (2015) posed five ethical questions for large companies in their use of social media data, which were further modified by Mills (2018) for a more wider research audience. These questions (see Textbox 17.2) provide prompts for researchers to consider the ethical questions raised with Big Qual data throughout the study.

Textbox 17.2   Core Ethical Questions (Mills, 2018, p. 597)

1 How comfortable would the original contributors be with the use of data analytics?
2 Would the original contributors consider that the research presents no unmanaged risk to them?
3 Can the original contributors trust that the researcher and any collaborating organization have their best interests at heart?
4 Would the original contributors experience any sense violation if they learned about the study findings and conclusions?
5 Can the original contributors trust the analytic processes to be unbiased?

Best Practice

At present there is little guidance in the literature on what constitutes best practice in Big Qual. There are a number of worked examples of data sampling and analysis which provide some guidance. One such example of interest to occupational scientists and occupational therapists is the analysis of a large longitudinal and cross-national narrative data set—The Global Dialogues (Winskell et al., 2018). The data arose from a contest which invited young people to submit ideas for short films about HIV and related topics with more than 200,000 young people in sub-Saharan Africa taking part between 1997 and 2014. The authors provide an excellent account of their theoretical framework, the sampling strategy, data management, and narrative analysis.

Best practice will require researchers to understand and recognize the limitations of the data set in use. A limitation of the Royal Commission data set and analyses was the selection bias of the material for the hearings which was within a legalistic frame, with the material being chosen as the best evidence to support their legal argument. The lawyers were not restricted by attention to rigor to present evidence that was emblematic or even representative. Any secondary analysis needs to keep the limitations in mind and acknowledge the implications.

Application to Occupational Science

Analysis of the dignity of risk study revealed a binary of quality OR safety, which is an interesting paradox within a commission specifically addressing quality AND safety. Older people were positioned as vulnerable and unable to exercise choice and control so that when situations of risk brought safety concerns into focus, the power rested with the nursing staff to overrule the older person and their family. Safety was always chosen as the proxy for quality care, so that safe care was always the higher priority. Decisions in the name of safety legitimized and sanctioned certain occupations and out ruled others. Older people did not have the choice and control to engage in occupations that they valued, such as going for a walk as it was considered to be unsafe.

Big qualitative data provides many opportunities for occupational scientists to study humans as occupational beings to add to knowledge within occupational science. I can even see the possibility of using citizen science within occupational science where citizen sciences is defined as "the collection and analysis of data relating to the natural world by members of the general public, typically as part of a collaborative project with professional scientists" (Oxford Languages, 2023). Big data could be generated by members of the general public being meaningfully engaged to collect and contribute data about occupational engagement to then be analyzed from a variety of perspectives such as the influences of culture, geography, climate, stage of lifespan, gender, and so on.

Application to Occupational Therapy

The analysis of the emergency department transfer study revealed themes of shortfalls and failings in care; hesitancy and misunderstanding; and discovery and exposure (Cain et al., 2022). All three themes related to workforce and access to healthcare issues that have been well documented and require significant structural reform in the industry to address them. In addition, the analysis revealed significant breakdowns in communication between the residential aged care facility and the emergency department at the acute hospital, and that little attention was paid to advance care directives. The situation for residents from diverse cultural backgrounds was amplified and highlights the need for urgent attention to how culture is accounted for in residential aged care.

Identifying these issues provide avenues for change that do not require such major structural reform. While not directly related to occupational therapy, it can be seen from this example that similar analyses could provide knowledge that could lead to improvements in occupational therapy service provision and, thus, the health and well-being of service recipients.

There may be other opportunities within the mixed method approach to identify data which would give consumer feedback on what is important to consumers or the ways in which consumers would like to receive information. What is perhaps more obvious at present is how the occupational therapy profession could be informed about its status and optic through mining of social media data. Researchers could search Twitter or other social media accounts using the key words occupational therapy and occupational therapists to explore the questions: How is the occupational therapy profession portrayed? or What is the profession portraying about itself? There is the example from Walsh (2018) who conducted an environmental scan of three media outlets to explore the public perception of occupational therapy. They included Google images and Twitter feeds. The author did not situate their study within Big data but did use data analytical tools to suggest it could be. Another avenue for exploration could be, what is being said about racism and decolonizing of occupational therapy?

Critiquing Literature

There is very little guidance available in the literature on how to appraise Big Qual studies. The lack of guidance would be due to the rapid emergence of this methodology and lack of consensus about best practice. Therefore, I have devised a set of questions that I believe are useful to use in critiquing Big Qual studies (see Textbox 17.3). This set of questions has been compiled based on my reading of the literature, my discussions about rigor with my research center colleagues, and my background and experience as a qualitative researcher.

Textbox 17.3   Critiquing Big Qual Studies

1   Has it been made clear *which type of Big Qual* study they are reporting on?
2   Is the *epistemological, ontological and axiological positioning* of the study made explicit?
3   Have the *researchers explicitly positioned themselves* in relation to the research topic?
4   Has the *choice of data set* been made explicit and justified?
5   Have *data sampling choices* been made explicit and a rationale provided?
6   What *data management considerations* have been described?
7   Does the analysis account for both *depth and breadth*?
8   Are the *data sampling and analysis procedures* consistent with the epistemological, ontological and axiological positioning of the study?
9   Are the steps in *analysis described in detail*?
10 Do the findings *add to knowledge*?

Author Reflection

As someone who likes to identify as a qualitative methodologist, I am always keen to learn and to try different methodologies. When I was first made aware of the opportunity to use the data from the Royal Commission that I have described above, I was excited about trying something new. To be honest, it was also a golden opportunity presented to me given the occurrence of the global pandemic, which was making research in aged care difficult, if not impossible, and where there was a data set that did not require any involvement with the residential aged care facilities that were struggling to manage staffing and providing care and were significant sites of COVID-19 infections. As the research team progressed working on the different projects and altered the approach to suit each focus topic, we could see the merit in writing a methodological paper. Concurrently the research team were exploring the literature on Big qualitative data and adding depth and breadth to our knowledge. I was excited by the possibilities that I could see for occupational science and occupational therapy research. In many ways, the notion of Big data goes against my natural tendencies for qualitative analysis, which have always been very a 'hands on' manual approach and I have had to adjust and learn how to use NVivo, which is perhaps not a bad thing!

I have often reflected on the phrase that 'just because the data is there, it doesn't mean you have to do it.' Am I just being lured to the 'bright lights' of Big Qual data sets and trying to overcome the concern (shame, disappointment, jealousy …?) of small sample sizes within qualitative work? Maybe. However, the richness of the data set that my colleagues and I were working with overcame my hesitations. While I can see the opportunities that exist within social media as Big data, the appeal in the approach for me is in the documents produced within government repositories as it speaks to my interests in the use of critical discourse analysis to reveal the structures that govern the occupations that are or are not sanctioned. My interest is in taking the knowledge gained and examining that through the lens of occupational science theory and to then translate that knowledge into changing practice to transform the lives of older people or those with a disability.

Conclusion

In this chapter I have defined Big Qual as a methodology and drawn on my own work in relation to dignity of risk, and that of my colleagues' work in a Centre for Research in Aged Care. I have shared the learnings that we have had as the research team have ventured into Big Qual in analyzing the content from a Royal Commission in Australia which is publicly available data. In drawing on the three studies, I have been able to show that there is not one way to go about analyzing Big data and that researchers can explore methodological approaches to harness developments in technology and access to information. Having said that, we are a group of experienced qualitative researchers and were able to apply our knowledge and skill to ensure that the approaches taken were theoretically sound and rigorous.

My study of the dignity of risk within the Royal Commission data set using critical discourse analysis contributes to knowledge about how occupational engagement is talked about, what is privileged, and what is marginalized. I have also identified possibilities for research of relevance to occupational therapy practice. I encourage occupational scientists and occupational therapy researchers to explore their own contexts for Big Qual data sets, not just because Big might be better but for the opportunity to maximize the use of data that already exists to reveal the potential for occupational science and occupational therapy.

References

Braun, V., & Clarke, V. (2013). *Successful qualitative research: A practical guide for beginners*. SAGE.

Braun, V., & Clarke, V. (2022). *Thematic analysis: A practical guide*. SAGE.

Brower, R. L., Jones, T. B., Osborne-Lampkin, L. T., Hu, S., & Park-Gaghan, T. J. (2019). Big Qual: Defining and debating qualitative inquiry for large data sets. *International Journal of Qualitative Methods, 18*. https://doi.org/10.1177/1609406919880692

Cain, P., Alan, J., & Porock, D. (2022). Emergency department transfers from residential aged care: What can we learn from secondary qualitative analysis of Australian Royal Commission data? *BMJ Open, 12*(9), e063790. https://doi.org/10.1136/bmjopen-2022-063790

Davidson, E., Edwards, R., Jamieson, L., & Weller, S. (2019). Big data, qualitative style: A breadth-and-depth method for working with large amounts of secondary qualitative data. *Quality & Quantity, 53*(1), 363–376. https://doi.org/10.1007/s11135-018-0757-y

Dekas, K., & McCune, E. A. (2015). Conducting ethical research with big and small data: Key questions for practitioners. *Industrial and Organizational Psychology, 8*(4), 563–567. https://doi.org/10.1017/iop.2015.84

Dowrick, A., Mitchinson, L., Hoernke, K., Mulcahy Simmons, S., Cooper, S., Martin, S., Vanderslott, S., San Juan, S. V., & Vindrola-Padros, C. (2021). Re-ordering connections: UK healthcare workers' experiences of emotion management during the COVID-19 pandemic. *Sociology of Health and Illness, 43*, 2156–2177. https://doi.org/10.1111/1467-9566.13390

Foucault, M., & Gordon, C. (1980). *Power/knowledge: Selected interviews and other writings, 1972–1977*. Harvester Press.

Guba, E. G., & Lincoln, Y. S. (2005). Paradigmatic controversies, contradictions, and emerging confluences. In N. K. Denzin & Y. S. Lincoln (Eds.), *The SAGE handbook of qualitative research* (3rd ed., pp. 191–215). SAGE.

Hilton, C. E. (2017). Unveiling self-harm behaviour: What can social media site Twitter tell us about self-harm? A qualitative exploration. *Journal of Clinical Nursing, 26*, 1690–1704. https://doi.org/10.1111/jocn.13575

Krefting, L. (1991). Rigor in qualitative research: The assessment of trustworthiness. American *Journal of Occupational Therapy, 45*(3), 214–222. https://doi.org/10.5014/ajot.45.3.214

Maywald, A., & Stanley, M. (2015). Prescribing mobility scooters in Australia: Occupational therapists' narratives. *Australian Occupational Therapy Journal, 62*(2), 86–92. https://doi.org/10.1111/1440-1630.12131

Mills, K. A. (2018). What are the threats and potentials of big data for qualitative research? *Qualitative Research, 18*(6), 591–603. https://doi.org/10.1177/1468794117743465

National Health and Medical Research Council, Australian Research Council, & Universities Australia. (2007, updated 2018). *National Statement on Ethical Conduct in Human Research.* National Health and Medical Research Council. www.nhmrc.gov.au/about-us/publications/national-statement-ethical-conduct-human-research-2007-updated-2018#block-views-block-file-attachments-content-block-1

Neale, B., & Bishop, L. (2012). The Timescapes archive: A stakeholder approach to archiving qualitative longitudinal data. *Qualitative Research, 12*(1), 53–65. https://doi.org/10.1177/1468794111426233

Neale, B., Henwood, K., & Holland, J. (2012). Researching lives through time: An introduction to the Timescapes approach. *Qualitative Research, 12*(1), 4–15. https://doi.org/10.1177/1468794111426229

Oxford Languages. (2023). Oxford University Press. Retrieved from https://languages.oup.com/google-dictionary-en/

Parliament of Australia. (n.d.). *About Royal Commissions. Parliament of Australia.* Retrieved from www.royalcommission.gov.au/about-royal-commissions

Royal Commission into Aged Care Quality and Safety. (2019). *Interim report: Neglect.* Author. Retrieved from www.royalcommission.gov.au/aged-care/interim-report

Royal Commission into Aged Care Quality and Safety. (2021). *Final report: Care, dignity and respect.* Retrieved from www.royalcommission.gov.au/aged-care/final-report

Rudman, D., & Molke, D. (2009). Forever productive: The discursive shaping of later life workers in contemporary Canadian newspapers. *Work, 32*(4), 377–389. https://doi.org/10.3233/WOR-2009-0850

Seale, C., & Charteris-Black, J. (2010). Keyword analysis: A new tool for qualitative research. In I. Bourgeault, R. Dingwall, & R. De Vries (Eds.), *The SAGE handbook of qualitative methods in health* (pp. 536–558). SAGE. https://doi.org/10.4135/9781446268247

Skoss, M., Batten, R., Cain, P., & Stanley, M. (2022). Vulnerable, recalcitrant and resilient: A Foucauldian discourse analysis of risk and older people within the context of COVID-19 news media. *Ageing & Society,* 1–18. https://doi.org/10.1017/S0144686X22000897

Straker, L. M., Hall, G. L., Mountain, J., Howie, E. K., White, E., McArdle, N., Eastwood, P. R., & The Raine Study 22 Year Follow-up Investigator, G. (2015). Rationale, design and methods for the 22 year follow-up of the Western Australian Pregnancy Cohort (Raine) study. *BMC Public Health, 15*(1), 663. https://doi.org/10.1186/s12889-015-1944-6

van Dijk, T. A. (2009). Critical discourse studies: A sociolinguistic approach. In R. Wodak & M. Myer (Eds.), *Methods of critical discourse analysis* (2nd ed., pp. 62–86). SAGE.

Walsh, W. E. (2018). Investigating public perception of occupational therapy: An environmental scan of three media outlets. *American Journal of Occupational Therapy, 72*(3), 1–10. https://doi.org/10.5014/ajot.2018.024513

Winskell, K., Singleton, R., & Sabben, G. (2018). Enabling analysis of big, thick, long, and wide data: Data management for the analysis of a large longitudinal and cross-national narrative data set. *Qualitative Health Research, 28*(10), 1629–1639. https://doi.org/10.1177/1049732318759658

Wodak, R., & Myer, M. (2016). *Methods of critical discourse studies* (3rd ed.). SAGE.

Yin, R. K. (2014). *Case study research: Design and methods* (5th ed.). SAGE.

Additional Resources

Timescapes Archive: https://timescapes-archive.leeds.ac.uk/
Qualitative data archives: https://ukdataservice.ac.uk/help/other-data-providers/other-data-
   providers-qualitative-data/european-archives/
https://qualpage.com/2019/05/09/archiving-qualitative-data/

18 Best (or Better?) Practices

Shoba Nayar

Throughout this book the importance of language has been emphasized, and readers have been encouraged to become familiar with and mindful of the language they are using when designing and implementing their research programs. Indeed, in Chapter 3, Isla, Chontel, and Lana underscored the importance of an agreed vocabulary between researchers and participants or co-researchers as central to decolonial research. As the editors, Mandy and I, started the book with a discussion on what we mean when we talk about methodology and methods, and defining words such as paradigm, epistemology, ontology, and axiology. So, as I come to this closing chapter, it seems appropriate that I begin with returning to where we started—thinking about language. In this book, we have set out to make visible and accessible the application of a range of qualitative methodologies and their associated methods for undertaking research in the fields of occupational science and occupational therapy. But is it that simple? Unfortunately, no.

What are 'best practices'? What exactly does this phrase mean or call us to consider? According to the Oxford English Dictionary (2023), the adjective 'best' can be defined as "of the most excellent or desirable type or quality"; while 'practices' is defined as "the actual application or use of an idea, belief, or method." The definition of 'best' sits uncomfortably in a book on qualitative research given the inherent positivist overtones to posit that there is one way, the 'best way,' to do things—a singular path that ignores reasonable options (Davis Jr., 1997). Further, among qualitative researchers there is no consensus as to what exactly is 'best practice.' Indeed, Dixon-Woods et al. (2004) contended that there is "disagreement not only about the characteristics that define good quality qualitative research, but also on whether criteria for quality in qualitative research should exist at all" (p. 223).

In Chapter 3, Isla and colleagues wrote about decolonizing research in occupational science and occupational therapy and drew attention to the phrase 'wise practice,' a term being used counter to 'best practice' in Indigenous research. They note that wise practice encompasses good relations and where power and control lie within such relations. In this spirit, and in keeping with the intention of this book to show the variety and complexity of what are qualitative methodologies, I argue for the consideration of 'better practices' when thinking about the foundations to engaging in rigorous and robust qualitative research.

A Case for Better Practices

This book has served, in part, to showcase the diversity and complexity of qualitative research methodologies; yet it is certainly not exhaustive. There are other methodologies that have not been covered such as oral history (Charlton et al., 2007), heuristic

DOI: 10.4324/9781003456216-18

methodology (Moustakas, 1990), or appreciative inquiry (Cooperrider & Whitney, 2005). Given the extensive array, it is not surprising that there really is no consensus as to what constitutes best practice. In this book, Mandy and I sought out researchers with in-depth knowledge from around the globe to guide researchers in thinking about what is rigorous for each of the methodologies that have been included. Our rationale for seeking inclusion of more diverse perspectives and geographies was, in part, an attempt to push back on and bring some balance to the dominant ways of knowing which, historically, have been grounded in Western, philosophical thought and academic paradigms.

Throughout each of the chapters, the authors have offered insights and interpretations of best practice in relation to their chosen methodology. Some of these 'better practices' span methodologies such as researcher reflexivity (which I will discuss further below). Other forms of better practice, however, are more tailored to the specific methodology; for instance, Debbie and Silke in Chapter 10 on critical discourse analysis draw upon Ballinger's (2006) four considerations, Kirk (Chapter 6) followed the criterion outlined by Annells (1999) for phenomenology while Kate and I (Chapter 5) use Charmaz's (2006) four criterion as appropriate for a study employing a constructivist grounded theory methodology.

As such, I consider better practices to be a set of guiding principles. Indeed, to talk about a definitive set of 'best practices' would feel uncomfortable given that Mandy and I do not consider ourselves 'experts' but people who have a level of 'expertise' in qualitative research. Thus, from that stance, in this chapter, I draw together some of the ideas presented throughout this book, that I believe can be grouped into four principles to guide researchers in attending to better practice (see Textbox 18.1). The first two are practices that relate to the overall conceptualization and enactment of the research; while the second two practices deal more directly with the researcher's experience and story.

Needless to say, these principles might not represent or fit every scenario—including researcher, participants, and topic—and sometimes it may not be possible to address all of them to the standard that you or others might initially expect. However, I believe it is important that all occupational scientists and occupational therapists who are considering undertaking qualitative research bear these principles in mind and actively strive towards meeting them, as a way of knowing what the limitations might be. In doing so, there is increased likelihood of ensuring the research is grounded in lived reality which has meaning and benefit for the participants. Additionally, as qualitative research is increasingly used to inform policy and practice decisions (Anderson, 2010), applying these principles adds to the rigor of the research which is necessary for engaging with key stakeholders beyond that of the immediate study to move forward action for change in wider contexts. Let us consider each of the principles as outlined in Textbox 18.1.

Textbox 18.1 Guiding Principles for Better Practice in Qualitative Research

- Having a sound knowledge of the methodology that extends beyond using it solely as a method
- Demonstrating congruence throughout the study
- Use of reflexivity and disclosure of author positionality throughout the research process
- Being open to others' perspectives and critique

Sound Knowledge of Methodology Beyond Method

The varied epistemological and ontological perspectives underpinning the different methodologies may feel daunting if you are just embarking on your journey with qualitative research. These theoretical and philosophical standpoints often take time to understand and describe how they align and support the topic to be studied; and while one might have the luxury of doing this when writing a doctoral thesis, for instance, most journal articles and reports for funding bodies do not allow the time and space to detail these discussions. Thus, it is not surprising that greater emphasis tends to be placed on describing the methods used in the study. In doing so, it can often seem as though the methodology is merely a mixture of different methods that are best suited for collecting and analyzing data. For example, it is common to see researchers write of using 'grounded theory methods' such as theoretical sampling or axial coding without a discussion of the broader methodology— whether it be grounded theory or not—within which the study is being framed and conducted. Or perhaps in writing up their studies, authors claim they used phenomenology and in-depth interviews but do not take the time to describe which branch of phenomenology and how their choice influenced the way they analyzed the data. In this sense, there is the risk that methodology and methods become separated, viewed as two standalone entities that contribute to the research in different ways. I would argue, however, that methods cannot exist without methodology and having a sound knowledge of which methodology is being used for the study will subsequently inform the choice of methods.

While methods and methodology go hand in hand, the authors of each of the chapters in this book have shown that there is no one set path or 'shoulds' when it comes to employing methodology and methods. This can be unnerving for new researchers who, understandably, would appreciate clearer guidance on how to 'do' the analysis or how to determine when 'enough' data have been gathered. Indeed, the concept of saturation, while having "attained widespread acceptance as a methodological principle in qualitative research" (Saunders et al., 2018, p. 1893), continues to be the focus of debate regarding its conceptualization and consistency of use. In Chapter 4 on qualitative descriptive, Mandy reflected on how her recommendation of three to five themes in the first edition of this book has been interpreted by some as a 'definitive instruction' where she had intended and offered it more as a guide. This is one example of better practice where having a sound knowledge of methodology as extending beyond mere method can guide both the process and rigor of the research.

As researchers, we may be drawn to certain methodologies because they have resonance with who we are as individuals—our values, the way we like to work, what we hold to be important in the world. For instance, when it comes to qualitative research I have a leaning towards grounded theory methodology, which aligns with and reflects my interest in 'process.' In my everyday life, when faced with a problem, more often than not, it is not the end point that matters to me; rather, what I deem important is the process of coming to that position. I may not agree with the outcome; however, if I can see that a transparent, robust process has been followed, I am more likely to understand the situation and accept the conclusion. Knowing this about myself helps me be aware of my bias towards shaping a study or forming the research question to suit the methodology, and recognizing when a particular topic may call for another methodology more appropriate to bringing forth the understandings being sought. As Anderson (2010) rightly stated, "Qualitative research is not appropriate to answer every research question and researchers need to think carefully about their objectives" (p. 1). Extending this better practice principle of having a sound knowledge of methodology leads into a second area of better practice in which I encourage the researcher to think about how they implement methodological congruence throughout the different aspects of the study.

Demonstrating Congruence Throughout the Study

Occupational therapists are interested in seeing the establishment of policies and interventions that can be implemented to bring about positive change in the settings within which therapists work and interact with clients. Qualitative studies can offer rich understandings of those settings and thus provide essential information to inform the development of needed policy and action. However, the strength of the findings as a platform for change is dependent on the robustness of the study and the application and congruence of chosen methodology, methods, and positionality.

Methodological congruence can be described as the "fit between the research problem and the question, fit between research question and the method, and, of course, fit among the method, the data, and the way of handling data" (Morse & Richards, 2002, p. 32). To achieve this congruence requires the researcher to critically assess each step of the research design as it unfolds. Continually assessing to determine the suitability of a chosen method and the fit between method and research question necessitates a degree of flexibility within the research design and by the researcher to make changes when needed. For instance, you may have originally designed the study with the intention of doing in-person observations with participants only to find that a global pandemic required people to isolate and made this form of data collection no longer possible! Waiting out the pandemic and hoping that one day in the not too distant future the research will be able to continue as planned may be an option, but not if there is a schedule which means that, pandemic or not, the research must be completed within a certain timeframe.

Qualitative research involves working with humans and interacting with the environment; neither of which are fixed entities. Therefore, while I believe in the importance of taking the time to design a study and not simply entering the field without a clear intention of what you want to do and why you want to do it (though it is unlikely that such a study would get the necessary ethical approval to proceed), qualitative researchers must be prepared to adapt to the research context. This may mean seeking an amendment to ethics to include more participants or employ another means of collecting data. Such adaptations, however, need to be made keeping in mind the broad umbrella of the methodology and determining whether the chosen methods align with the methodology and will best serve to answer the research question. Within this book Mandy and I have worked with chapter authors to showcase how methodological congruence can be achieved for each of their chosen methodologies. In and of themselves, I consider each chapter to be an example of better practice for that particular research study.

It is often recommended that qualitative researchers keep a journal documenting their research process, the decisions they make, any changes that occur to the original plan; as well as more general ongoing insights and reflections (as Kirk discussed in Chapter 6). A journal may be an informal way of demonstrating congruence in a study. However, there are also more formal means which, increasingly, many journal editors and reviewers are looking for when it comes to publishing studies. For instance, when thinking about best practice in relation to qualitative research, researchers might immediately call to mind the CASP Qualitative Studies Checklist (CASP UK, 2022) or the JBI Checklist for Qualitative Research (Joanna Briggs Institute, 2022) or the Standards for Reporting Qualitative Research (O'Brien et al., 2014). However, Busetto et al. (2020) noted that "none of these have been elevated to the 'gold standard' in the field" (p. 6). A possible reason for this situation is that, as this book has demonstrated, qualitative research is diverse and as a broad umbrella encompasses a variety of epistemological, ontological, and axiological standpoints. A point previously noted by Meyrick (2006) who commented that often "within qualitative research, the means of establishing quality have been representative of single epistemological standpoints (p. 803).

Reporting guidelines and critical appraisal tools offer a way to be more critical of what is being read, but they can perpetuate certain ways of knowing and doing. Thus, while journal editors may require authors to follow the standards set out in reporting guidelines, I would urge researchers not to blindly adopt this process simply for the sake of getting one's study published. Better practice would suggest that researchers need to use reporting guidelines judiciously and weigh up whether they are indeed congruent with the study's methodology. For example, it is common to hear researchers talking about member checking as an essential process necessary for ensuring credible qualitative research when it is just one among many techniques for promoting a study's rigor; and, indeed, may not always be appropriate for the study being reported (Motulsky, 2021). Upholding methodological congruence requires researchers to be continually engaging in a process of critical reflection.

Reflexivity and Author Positionality Throughout the Research Process

Since the first edition of this book, the notion of reflexivity has become a much-discussed topic in the field of qualitative research and is increasingly recognized as one way of demonstrating rigor in a study alongside other well-known criteria such as use of a conceptual framework or theory, prolonged engagement in the field, and triangulation, to name a few. However, it remains poorly understood by many, which can often be seen by the limited ways in which it is addressed in qualitative research publications (Olmos-Vega et al., 2022). So, what is meant by researcher reflexivity? Palaganas et al. (2017) offered the following:

> The journey of discovering how researchers shaped and how they were shaped by the research process and output is an iterative and empowering process. More so when their positionality/ies is/are challenged and the researchers acknowledge that reflexivity should be recognized as a significant part of the research findings.
>
> (p. 426)

In this 'journey of discovery,' I contend that one part of critical reflexivity as a means of better practice is to attend to being aware of, and taking actions to address, one's preconceptions (see Textbox 18.2). This process involves taking time to reflect on all dimensions of one's being – what is it that makes you who you are and how do these aspects potentially shape what you see or expect to find entering the field of study?

While examining one's own motivations and competencies for engaging in research is important, reflexivity must go further. Thus, beyond the individual, a second aspect of critical researcher reflexivity is the need to be inclusive of, and accountable, to the 'teams, groups, and communities' (see Emery-Whittington et al., Chapter 3) in order to produce actions and results that have a meaningful outcome. Walsh (2003) and Olmos-Vega et al. (2022) have categorized reflexivity in four ways (see Textbox 18.3)—personal, interpersonal, methodological, contextual. Each of the items in Textbox 18.2 (and the many more not listed) are an example of what could be

---

Textbox 18.2   Influences on One's Preconceptions

Consider which of the following factors may have a bearing on the research you are conducting:

1 Age
2 Gender
3 Socio-economic status
4 Ethnicity
5 Family structure
6 Religion
7 Political views
8 Level of education
9 Profession and level of experience
10 Area of residence

There are many more that could be added to this list.

Exercise: Think of another five to ten factors that may influence the way you interact with your study participants and topics. When you have your list, consider ranking the items, starting with those you think might have the biggest impact. Take the time to write down your thoughts or discuss your list with a peer, reflecting on why you have chosen the top three and how you might take these into consideration when planning your research.

Textbox 18.3   Four Dimensions of Reflexivity

1 *Personal*: How are your unique perspectives influencing the research?
2 *Interpersonal*: What relationships exist and how are they influencing the research and the people involved? What power dynamics are at play?
3 *Methodological*: How are you making methodological decisions and what are their implications?
4 *Contextual*: How are aspects of context influencing the research and people involved?

(Adapted from Olmos-Vega et al., 2022, pp. 4–5)

---

considered under 'personal reflexivity.' However, these factors also have the potential to influence the course of the research process at any point—from the design of the study and the topics chosen, to the recruitment of participants, the collection and analysis of data, through to the writing up of the study (Shaw et al., 2020). Using the four dimensions of reflexivity as outlined in Textbox 18.3 is a helpful framework to think about engaging in critical reflexivity beyond that of an individual researcher's lens throughout your study.

As part of the chapters, Mandy and I asked the authors to offer a personal reflection. Author positionality is also part of implementing and demonstrating congruence throughout a study (see the preceding principle), and a reminder that these principles for better practice do not stand in isolation of each other. Being deeply aware of one's positionality is necessary whether or not the researcher may be part of the community included in the study. For instance, in Chapter 9 on ethnography, Suzanne positioned herself as a "Canadian-born Francophone of European settler ancestry" who "has never lived abroad and has no personal experience of international migration". Thus, while she had some knowledge about the topic she was studying, it was only one perspective; hence the need to recruit participants. With the understanding that "qualitative researchers and the participants of their studies interact in a social process" and hence "researchers influence the research process" (Korstjens & Moser, 2017, p. 274), having knowledge of the researcher's position, can help readers determine how effectively methods for data collection were employed and the quality of analysis. For instance, an interview where the researcher offers more of their experience rather than allowing the participant's voice to be heard, may result in limited data which may then affect the quality and depth of analysis. Thus, in the words of Wijekoon and Peter (2022):

> Disclosure of positionality also allows readers to know the researchers' views, perspectives, and biases, and how they come to know what they know, and make a better-informed judgment as to the researcher's influence on the research process and their belief in the 'truthfulness' of the research data.
>
> (p. 12)

Palaganas et al. (2017) have argued, "it is impossible to remain 'outside of' one's study topic while conducting research" (p. 426). Equally, however, it is impossible for the actual research to remain outside of the researcher. Reflexivity captures the understanding that the qualitative research process and the researcher's subjectivity are inherently intertwined. They each exert an influence upon the other that shapes the ultimate outcome of the study. Therefore, it is also necessary that the act of reflexivity involves the researcher taking time to recognize how they have been impacted by the research (Finefter-Rosenbluh, 2017; Olmos-Vega et al., 2022); how the research process has changed their understandings both as a researcher and as a person more broadly.

Thus, I do not consider that engaging in reflexivity is a check box exercise, done once and never to be revisited. Like others (Barrett et al., 2020; Olmos-Vega et al., 2022; Palaganas et al., 2017), I am a firm believer that reflexivity is an ongoing process and, thus, should not be confined to a few sentences buried somewhere in the depths of the presentation and write up of the study. Rather, when considering reporting the study, reflexivity can be fore fronted in the introduction (what is the researcher's positionality), the methods (what decisions were made and why), and the discussion (how has the researcher been influenced by the study).

There are many different ways to engage in reflexivity, as has been discussed throughout the various chapters in this book; for example, undertaking a pre-suppositions interview prior to starting the research, member checking, or utilizing supervision with peers or mentors, and memo-ing. Barrett et al. (2020) noted that "reflexivity is not only an individual process but one that needs to be considered a collective process within a research team" (p. 9). Therefore, having an openness to others' perspectives and being willing to receive and provide critique can further support a process of better practice.

Being Open to Others' Perspectives and Critique

Going hand in hand with reflexivity is the practice of being open to others' perspectives and critiques. Now this does not mean just any person's point of view—although sometimes a conversation with a stranger who does not know your research may introduce a new idea of which you had not previously thought! Rather, as part of the research process, I suggest that better practice includes a mindful and considered gathering of individuals or communities who have some connection with the research and are willing to offer you frank and honest feedback regarding all aspects of the research, from the study design to the implementation, analysis, and writing up of findings. Three groups in particular come to mind: (1) participants, (2) co-researchers, peer researchers, or supervisors, and (3) an advisory group.

A theme that has arisen many times throughout different chapters in this book is the idea of doing research with participants which goes beyond simply working with participants to collect the data; whether that be in the form of interviews, observations, mapping, or visual/tactile creations. Busetto et al. (2020) have talked about participants as active contributors to the broader research process, arguing that their unique perspectives and experiences "add value beyond their own single story" (p. 7). Thus, participant feedback on analysis of the data can offer a greater richness to the findings then if viewed through the researcher's eyes alone. To this end, checking interpretations of the data with participants not only at the end of analysis but during the analytic process can heighten the study rigor. However, researchers need to be mindful that participants are made aware of the possibility of their involvement at the start of the study as it does present an additional time requirement that some participants may not be able to undertake.

As well as the contribution of participants, having other voices—be these of people within the study team, peer researchers or industry stakeholders, or supervisors—can be helpful for discussing interpretation of the data. At times these may be people who have some insight into the phenomena being studied, or perhaps have experience in the use of the chosen methodology. I remember when I was doing my PhD I was fortunate to belong to a 'grounded theory group.' This group comprised fellow students and staff from across the university. Thus, while our professional backgrounds differed—occupational therapists, psychologists, nurses, physiotherapists—we had the common experience of using grounded theory. In this space we would bring data to analyze and explore together. We would talk about the challenges of writing up a grounded theory study, and we used the forum to learn about emerging concepts within grounded theory. It was a wonderful experience of group learning and a safe space in which to have ideas gently challenged and new perspectives offered.

Another function of consulting with fellow researchers or stakeholders may be to check whether the resultant findings 'ring true.' The 'phenomenological nod' was a phrase coined by Munhall (1994) and is described as occurring "when people reading or hearing the phenomenological description nod in agreement" (Nelms, 2015, p. 17). While it is considered one way of determining the rigor and merit of phenomenological studies, I have seen the phenomenological nod happen in participants, conference audiences, and stakeholders in response to qualitative studies that have employed various different methodologies. Thus, I am of the opinion that any qualitative study in which the researchers have taken the time to be open to considering others' perspectives and critiques and integrating these into analysis of data is capable of eliciting the phenomenological nod.

Third, at the start of the study, you may want to consider establishing an advisory group. Increasingly, advisory groups are being used "to organize community–researcher partnerships and to improve relevance of research questions and findings, ethical procedures and access to participants" (Pinto et al., 2015, p. 329). Whether you are a member of the community amongst whom you are conducting the study, which has often been my research experience (Nayar, 2009; Nayar & Wright St. Clair, 2018), establishing a new relationship with a community (Thomas et al., 2017), or an experienced researcher with a longstanding community relationship, having an advisory group offers the opportunity to receive feedback on all stages of the study from conceptualization through to implementation and dissemination of findings. Indeed, many ethics committees and research funders often require evidence that consultation has been undertaken with key stakeholders in health and social research (Boivin et al., 2018).

Advisory groups are also one way of building reciprocal relationships in working towards patient and public involvement (Backman et al., 2022) and holding the researcher accountable to doing research 'with' rather than 'on' study participants. Engaging with an advisory group is not a one-off event and requires multiple, sustained conversations; therefore, as a researcher it is important to factor this into timelines and flexibility of the study. It may be that more time and space is required at the start to allow for meaningful engagement and robust discussion to occur and adjustments made to the design of the study to ensure the safety of all involved which needs to be factored into research proposals and planning.

Advisory groups can be both formal and informal. For instance, I conducted an occupational study with my colleague Valerie Wright St. Clair exploring the ways in which older Chinese, Korean, and Indian immigrants contribute to Aotearoa New Zealand society (Wright St. Clair & Nayar, 2018, 2019). While I had knowledge of, and connections to, the Indian community, both of us were 'outsiders' to the Chinese and Korean communities. Initially we spoke to postgraduate students from each of the communities with whom we were acquainted. They, in turn, gave us the names of senior representatives from each of the three communities. We sent letters to the representatives explaining the intention of the study and inviting them to be part of an advisory group. What made this group 'formal' was that we scheduled regular meetings and, as the researchers, were responsible for consulting with this group regarding our decisions throughout the process. Alternatively, an advisory group may be more 'informal,' and consist of those with knowledge in the area who can be called upon as and when needed for mentorship.

Being willing to consult with and consider other people's views and being adaptable to change course during the study in response (e.g., going back to data analysis or adopting a new recruitment method) are key dimensions of better practice when it comes to undertaking qualitative research. However, they are not the only ones. As discussed in this section, employing a combination of having a sound knowledge of the methodology that extends beyond using it solely as a method, implementing and demonstrating congruence throughout the study, and use of reflexivity and disclosure of author positionality throughout the process, along with being open to others' perspectives and critique will ultimately add to the robustness of the study.

Better Practices in Relation to Ethics

When the term best practice is talked about, what commonly comes to mind are approaches to rigor and, indeed, that is what has been largely discussed above with respect to the four principles for better practice. However, equally important when engaging in qualitative research is the need to consider better practices in relation to ethics; a view supported by Camfield (2019) who proposed a close relationship exists between rigor and research ethics.

Within each of the chapters presented in this book, the authors have included a section on ethics to highlight different tensions that are particular to the methodology discussed. Some of the ethical conflicts may be familiar to researchers such as who owns the data and gets to determine how it is used, as discussed in the chapters on visual methodologies by Laura and Katie (Chapter 12), and Eric and colleagues (Chapter 13); or the understanding of informed consent and voluntary participation as highlighted by Jens and colleagues in Chapter 8 on narrative methodology. However, as research evolves so too do ethical issues; for example, Debbie and Silke, in their exploration of critical discourse analysis (Chapter 10), and Amy, in Chapter 16 on netnography, all discuss the ethics of using data that are available in the public domain—whether this be printed material or social media groups online. Recognizing the diversity of ethical issues calls upon the researcher to be constantly reflecting on and acting with ethical integrity throughout the process (ethics in practice; see Guillemin & Gillam, 2004), not just for the sake of gaining study approval from an institutional review board (procedural ethics; see Guillemin & Gillam, 2004). In this sense, I contend that it can only ever be a case of 'better' practice in relation to ethics and research.

Recently, Patterson et al. (2023) undertook a systematic review "to identify factors which contribute to the enhancement of rigor for the practical implementation of qualitative research" (p. 1). They developed three analytical themes, the first of which was 'ethical co-construction,' which addresses issues of communicating truth and gaining the participants' trust. This theme relates to the third principle above—use of reflexivity and disclosure of author positionality throughout the process. The subjective nature of qualitative research means that aside from the standard ethical procedures (e.g., obtaining consent, ensuring anonymity or confidentiality etc.), qualitative researchers have an ethical obligation to engage with participants and readers of the study in a manner which upholds the trust that researchers are offered when participants agree to take part in the study and explicitly reflects the realities of both participants and researchers.

Acknowledging the 'realities' of research participants connects to the practice of compensation—a practice that is not without its debates and ethical tensions (Head, 2009; Saleh et al., 2020). It is common in research to offer participants some token of compensation as recognition of the time and knowledge that they have contributed to the study. Such compensation may be monetary such as cash or a voucher (e.g., for Amazon or a grocery store) or perhaps food; for instance, during my postgraduate research I took my participants a box of Indian sweets and a selection of herbal teas. There are no set guidelines as to what constitutes an 'appropriate' level of compensation and the tension lies in what is considered 'fair' recompense. Thus, it is incumbent on the researcher to ensure participants are fully aware of what their involvement in the study entails. For instance, does participation involve just the 60-minute interview or does it also include reviewing the transcript, a follow-up meeting to discuss emerging analysis, a request for participants to spread the word about the research and thus potentially send prospective participants to the researcher? Being explicit about the participants' level of involvement in the research and how they are being compensated is another layer of better practice that supports the rigor and ethics of the study.

In furthering the discussion of research that reflects the realities of both participants and researchers, Wijekoon and Peter (2022) examined racial, ethnic, and cultural diversity in occupational science research. From their work, they offer two recommendations to researchers to support better practice: (1) "engage in racial and cultural introspection in their research" and (2) "exercise transparency of their critical racial and cultural consciousness within their publications" (pp. 12–13). These recommendations echo Isla, Chontel, and Lana's (Chapter 3) call for researchers to question their motivations, skills, and expertise when engaging in decolonizing research and working with Indigenous communities. Increasingly, qualitative research within occupational science and occupational therapy is being conducted in complex and diverse cultural spaces. Given this trajectory, I support Wijekoon and Peter's recommendations and would claim that should occupational science and occupational therapy researchers choose not to do so, they risk breaching the ethical integrity of their work.

Summary

In writing this chapter, a tension I have grappled with throughout is the rub between offering a set of principles to promote better practice and positivist notions of 'the right way to do things.' It is not my intention to say all qualitative researchers 'must' adhere to these principles; I recognize that there are many elements that contribute to better practice in qualitative research. Rather, in considering the ways in which authors have talked about best practice in relation to their chosen methodology throughout this book, I have highlighted what I see as recurring themes. How researchers choose to engage with and demonstrate better practice principles will depend on the researcher and the type of study being undertaken. That said, Meyrick (2006) contended that there are "two key common principles of good qualitative research, transparency and systematicity" (p. 803). As the editors of this book, Mandy and I would agree that these principles underly the practices that, when woven throughout the research process, form a solid foundation for better practice in qualitative research.

To recap, the principles underpinning better practices that I see as important for occupational therapy and occupational science researchers to demonstrate are:

1 Having a sound knowledge of methodology beyond method
2 Demonstrating congruence throughout the study
3 Reflexivity and author positionality throughout the research process
4 Being open to others' perspectives and critique

When it comes to qualitative research, however, there are bound to be mistakes made in the process—after all, we are but human! Thus, I support Oakley's (2000) proposition that "the distinguishing mark of all good research is the awareness and acknowledgement of error" (p. 72). In that sense, better practice would see qualitative researchers striving towards ethical integrity through the entire research trajectory—from the research aim, defining theoretical positioning, methodology and methods (Taquette & Borges da Matta Souza, 2022).

Meyrick (2006) claimed that the "policy making and practice worlds will not wait for methodological perfection but are happy to accept 'good enough' research evidence of what works" (p. 807). I would argue that in undertaking research with our fellow humans, occupational scientists and occupational therapists have a duty to be, to do, more than 'good enough.' However, there is no 'one way' or even a 'right way' to fulfil this duty. Thus, in this chapter I have offered suggestions for means by which qualitative researchers can engage in better practice principles to ensure that the research being undertaken is robust, serves the people and communities with whom they work, and has the means to bring about change on societal and global levels. Ultimately, qualitative research is contextual. It requires an openness to sit in spaces of discomfort, to ask the hard questions of both participants and ourselves. In doing so, we recognize that, as qualitative researchers, our work is never complete—there is always room for better, wiser practices and ways of knowing.

References

Annells, M. (1999). Evaluating phenomenology: Usefulness, quality, and philosophical foundations. *Nurse Researcher, 6*(3), 5–19.

Anderson, C. (2010). Presenting and evaluating qualitative research. *American Journal of Pharmaceutical Education, 74*(8), Art. 141. https://doi.org/10.5688/aj7408141

Backman, C. L., Davidson, E., & Martini, R. (2022). Advancing patient and community engagement in occupational therapy research. *Canadian Journal of Occupational Therapy, 89*(1). https://doi.org/10.1177/000841742110726

Ballinger, C. (2006). Demonstrating rigour and quality? In L. Finlay & C. Ballinger (Eds.), *Qualitative research for allied health professionals: Challenging choices* (pp. 235–246). John Wiley & Sons.

Barrett, A., Kajamaa, A., & Johnston, J. (2020). How to … be reflexive when conducting qualitative research. *The Clinical Teacher, 17*, 9–12. https://doi.org/10.1111/tct.13133

Boivin, A., Richards, T., Forsythe, L., Grégoire, A., L'Espérance, A., Abelson, J., & Carman, K. L. (2018). Evaluating patient and public involvement in research. *BMJ, 363*. https://doi.org/10.1136/bmj.k5147

Busetto, L., Wick, W., & Gumbinger, C. (2020). How to use and assess qualitative research methods. *Neurological Research and Practice, 2*(14), 1–10. https://doi.org/10.1186/s42466-020-00059-z

Camfield, L. (2019). Rigour and ethics in the world of big-team qualitative data: Experiences from research in international development. *American Behavioural Scientist, 63*(5), 604–621. https://doi.org/10.1177/0002764218784636

CASP UK. (2022). *CASP checklists.* https://casp-uk.net/casp-tools-checklists/

Charlton, T. L., Myers, L. E., & Sharpless, R. (2007). *History of oral history. Foundations and methodology.* Altamira Press.

Charmaz, K. (2006). *Constructing grounded theory: A practical guide through qualitative analysis.* SAGE.

Cooperrider, D. L., & Whitney, D. (2005). *Appreciative inquiry: A positive revolution in change.* Berrett-Koehler Publishers.

Davis Jr., O. L. (1997). Editorial: Beyond "best practices" toward wise practices. *Journal of Curriculum and Supervision, 13*(1), 92–113.

Dixon-Woods, M., Shaw, R. L., Agarwal, S., & Smith, J. A. (2004). The problem of appraising qualitative research. *Quality and Safety in Health Care, 13*(3), 223–225. https://doi.org/10.1136/qhc.13.3.223

Finefter-Rosenbluh, I. (2017). Incorporating perspective taking in reflexivity. *International Journal of Qualitative Methods, 16*(1). https://doi.org/10.1177/1609406917703539

Guillemin, M., & Gillam, L. (2004). Ethics, reflexivity, and 'ethically important moments' in research. *Qualitative Inquiry, 10*(2), 261–280. https://doi.org/10.1177/1077800403262360

Head, E. (2009). The ethics and implications of paying participants in qualitative research. *International Journal of Social Research Methodology, 12*(4), 335–344. https://doi.org/10.1080/13645570802246724

Joanna Briggs Institute. (2022). *Critical appraisal tools.* https://jbi.global/critical-appraisal-tools

Korstjens, I., & Moser, A. (2017). Series: Practical guidance to qualitative research. Part 2: Context, research questions and designs. *European Journal of General Practice, 23*(1), 274–279. https://doi.org/10.1080/13814788.2017.1375090

Meyrick, J. (2006). What is good qualitative research? A first step towards a comprehensive approach to judging rigour/quality. *Journal of Health Psychology*, *11*(5), 799–808. https://doi.org/10.1177/1359105306066643

Morse, J. M., & Richards, L. (2002). *Readme first for a user's guide to qualitative methods*. SAGE.

Motulsky, S. L. (2021). Is member checking the gold standard of quality in qualitative research? *Qualitative Psychology*, *8*(3), 389–406. https://doi.org/10.1037/qup0000215

Moustakas, C. (1990). *Heuristic research: Design, methodology and applications*. SAGE.

Munhall, P. (1994). *Revisioning phenomenology*. National League for Nursing Press.

Nayar, S. (2009). *The theory of 'Navigating Cultural Spaces'* [Unpublished doctoral thesis, AUT University]. Auckland, New Zealand.

Nayar, S., & Wright St. Clair, V. (2018). Strengthening community: Senior Asian immigrants contributing to New Zealand society. *Journal of Cross-Cultural Gerontology*, *33*(4), 355–368. https://doi.org/10.1007/s10823-018-9357-5

Nelms, T. (2015). Phenomenological philosophy and research. In M. de Chesnay (Ed.), *Nursing research using phenomenology* (Chapt. 1). Springer. https://doi.org/10.1891/9780826126870

Oakley, A. (2000). *Experiments in knowing: Gender and method in the social sciences*. Polity Press.

O'Brien, B. C., Harris, I. B., Beckman, T. J., Reed, D. A., & Cook, D. A. (2014). Standards for reporting qualitative research: A synthesis of recommendations. *Academic Medicine: Journal of the Association of American Medical Colleges*, *89*(9), 1245–1251. https://doi.org/10.1097/ACM.0000000000000388

Olmos-Vega, F. M., Stalmeijer, R. E., Varpio, L., & Kahlke, R. (2022). A practical guide to reflexivity in qualitative research: AMEE Guide No. 149. *Medical Teacher*, *45*(3), 241–251. https://doi.org/10.1080/0142159X.2022.2057287

Oxford English Dictionary. (2023). *OED online*. Oxford University Press. www.oed.com/

Palaganas, E. C., Caricativo, R. D., Sanchez, M. C., & Molintas, M. V. P. (2017). Reflexivity in qualitative research: A journey of learning. *The Qualitative Report*, *22*(2), 426–438. https://doi.org/10.46743/2160-3715/2017.2552

Patterson, E. W., Ball, K., Corkish, J., & Whittick, I. M. (2023). Do you see what I see? Enhancement of rigour in qualitative approaches to inquiry: A systematic review of evidence. *Qualitative Research Journal*, *23*(2), 164–180. https://doi.org/10.1108/QRJ-06-2022-0086

Pinto, R. M., Spector, A. Y., Rahman, R., & Gastolomendo, J. D. (2015). Research advisory board members' contributions and expectations in the USA. *Health Promotion International*, *30*(2), 328–338. https://doi.org/10.1093/heapro/dat042

Saleh, S., Sambakunsi, H., Nyirenda, D., Kumwenda, M., Mortimer, K., & Chinouya, M. (2020). Participant compensation in global health research: A case study. *International Health*, *12*(6), 524–532. https://doi.org/10.1093/inthealth/ihaa064

Saunders, B., Sim, J., Kingstone, T., Baker, S., Waterfield, J., Bartlam, B., Burroughs, H., & Jinks, C. (2018). Saturation in qualitative research: Exploring its conceptualization and operationalization. *Quality & Quantity*, *52*(4), 1893–1907. https://doi.org/10.1007/s11135-017-0574-8

Shaw, R. M., Howe, J., Beazer, J., & Carr, T. (2020). Ethics and positionality in qualitative research with vulnerable and marginal groups. *Qualitative Research*, *20*(3), 277–293. https://doi.org/10.1177/1468794119841839

Taquette, S. R., & Borges da Matta Souza, L. M. (2022). Ethical dilemmas in qualitative research: A critical literature review. *International Journal of Qualitative Methods*, *21*. https://doi.org/10.1177/16094069221078731

Thomas, Y., Gray, M. A., & McGinty, S. (2017). The occupational wellbeing of people experiencing homelessness. *Journal of Occupational Science*, *24*(2), 181–192. https://doi.org/10.1080/14427591.2017.1301828

Wijekoon, S., & Peter, N. (2022). Examining racial, ethnic, and cultural diversity in occupational science research: Perspectives of persons of color. *Journal of Occupational Science*, *30*(3), 322–341. https://doi.org/10.1080/14427591.2022.2119269

Wright St. Clair, V., & Nayar, S. (2018). Late-life Asian immigrants managing wellness through contributing to socially embedded networks. *Journal of Occupational Science, 25*(1), 51–64. https://doi.org/10.1080/14427591.2017.1370607

Wright St. Clair, V., & Nayar, S. (2019). Resettling amidst a mood of loneliness: Later-life Chinese, Indian and Korean immigrants in New Zealand. *Ageing and Society, 40*(11), 2393–2409. https://doi.org/10.1017/S0144686X19000655

Additional Resources

CASP Qualitative Checklist. (2018). https://casp-uk.net/wp-content/uploads/2018/01/CASP-Qualitative-Checklist-2018.pdf

JBI Checklist for Qualitative Research. (2019). https://jbi.global/sites/default/files/2019-05/JBI_Critical_Appraisal-Checklist_for_Qualitative_Research2017_0.pdf

Miller, T., Birch, M., Mauthner, M., & Jessop, J. (Eds.). (2012). *Ethics in qualitative research* (2nd ed.). SAGE.

Index

Pages in *italics* refer to figures and pages in **bold** refer to tables.

appraisal standards for 44, 120, 179, 273, 278, 322
audit trail 58, 62, 280, 296, 310
axiology 14, 16–17, 35, 53, 70, 90, 108, 128, 150, 189, 209, 231, 255, 273, 292, 308

best practice 41–43, 71, 119, 129, 132, 134, 136, 139–141, 162, 169, 174, 177–179, 182, 189, 198–200, 262, 298, 312–313, 318–329
Big data 8, 304–315

case study 7, 105–122, 310
categories 61, 73–74, 77–79, 99, 115, 160, 282; and categorizing 59–60, 176, 294; core category 79–80
Charmaz 18, 68–73, 77–81, 196, 319
coding 58–61, 77–78, 102, 114, 160, 195, 222, 262, 294–295, 320; and theoretical 79, 158, 160
colonization 12, 15, 21, 30, 33, 119; and colonial 30–46, 150; post-colonial 15
community based research 8, 163, 198, 235, 252–269
co-researchers 187, 189–197, 201–202, 232, 235, 244, 259, 318, 325
critical appraisal 120, 273, 278–279, 322
critical discourse analysis 8, 155–156, 158, 169–183, 315
critical theory 15, 150, 155
cultural context 72, 119–120
cultural group 25, 106, 153, 161
culture 9, 15, 18, 23–25, 34, 38, 72, 84, 91, 93, 131, 149–150, 152–153, 163, 246, 283, 289, 313

data analysis 14, 19–20, 24, 38–39, 56, 58–62, 78–79, 96–99, 114–116, 134–135, 158–161, 174–178, 194–196, 219–223, 241, 262–263, 280–282, 294–295, 310;

and constant comparative 79–81; content 58–59, 298; thematic 39, 58–64, 96, 195, 262, 267, 310
data collection 18, 22, 24, 37–39, 55–58, 69, 74–78, 94–96, 112–114, 119, 131–134, 154–157, 174, 193–194, 260–261, 264, 267, 293–294, 309–310, 324
decolonial 4, 8, 30–46, **47**, 151, 254–255, 318
decolonizing 7, 23, 30–46, **47**, 162, 328
Dewey 8, 106, 108, 110, 128–130, 134–135, 142, 144
discourse analysis 13, 152, 169–170, 183, 306

epistemology 12, 14–18, 34, 53, 70, 90–91, 107–108, 128, 150–151, 189–190, 209–210, 231–232, 255–257, 273–274, 291–292, 307–308
ethics 17, 20, 22–23, 35, 39–41, 62–63, 81, 99–100, 118–119, 141–142, 161–162, 180, 194, 196–197, 200, 203, 223–224, 242–245, 264–265, 282, 295–298, 311, 326–328
ethnography 8, 149–165, **233–234**, 289–290; and meta-ethnography 272–273, 278, 280–281
evidence-based practice 2, 4, 169

field notes 76, 131, 135, 158, **159**, 281–282
fieldwork 25, 149–150, 153, 156
First Nations 38, **234**, 237, 239; *see also* Indigenous
Foucault 171, 221, 310
Freire 187, 190, 231–232, 235, 240, 252, 256

Gadamer 17, 89, 91–92, 94, 97
gatekeeper 153–154, 293–294
Glaser 17, 68, 71, 76, 79–81
grounded theory 4, 7, 16–18, 64, 68–84, 283, 319–320, 325

Heidegger 17, 88–91, 97, 100

Indigenous 4, 7, 15, 23–24, 30–46, **47**, 100,
119, 171, 237, 246, 254, 256, 265, 328;
see also First Nations
interpretivism 15, 291; and interpretivist 14,
16, **89**, 150, 256, 291–292
interviews 18, 56–58, 63, 73–75, 81, 91–92,
94, 106, 112, 131–132, 141, 144,
156–158, 193, 244, 289, 324; and focus
groups 56, 58, 74, 243, 289; pre-understandings 20, 91–92; semi-structured 209,
213, 218, 261; translation 137–138, 189,
282; yarning 37–38

journaling 62, 77, 217, 267, 298
Journal of Occupational Science 2, 4–5, 13, 25

literature, use of 54, 57, 59, 71, 79, 92–93,
108, 114, 128, 155
lived experience 13, 17, 24, 53, 63, 65, 71–72,
81, 83, 88, 93, 100, 102, 108, 149, 156,
212, 282, 291

mapping 97, 113, 115, 157, 217–218, 230,
325
member checking 62–63, 81, 118, 137, 322;
see also peer debriefing
memos 74, 76–78, 115, 160, 217, 221, 294,
296, 324
meta-synthesis 276, 278–279; *see also* qualitative evidence synthesis
methodology 2, 4, 6–7, 9–10, 12, 15, 17–18,
22, 24, 36, 38, 43, 52–53, 65, 68–71, 73,
80, 88–89, 95, 99, 105, *106*, 107, 116, 150,
163, 170, 173, 180, 187–188, 194, 208,
213, 225, 232, 243, 266, 269, 276,
290–291, 298, 313, 318–321, 325–326,
328
methods 4, 6–7, 9–10, 12, 15, 17–18,
21–25, 34, 36–39, 42, 56, 58–59, 69–70,
72, 74, 76, 78–79, 81, 91, 94, 100, 108,
113, 119, 132–133, 144, 150, 154–158,
162, 170, 174–175, 189, 193, 195,
208–210, **212**, 214–216, 223–224,
230–231, 236, 238, 240, 243, 260, 267,
273, 280–281, 293–294, 309–310, 318,
320–321, 324
mixed method 1, 260, **275**, 305, 313

narrative 8, 18, 53, 68, 73, 101, 127–145, 172,
194, 219, 235, 241, 272, 291, 307
netnography 8, 289–300, 327
NVivo 62, 80, 158, 160, 281, 295, 309;
see also software

observation 56, 74–76, 106, 113, 119, 150,
156, 158–160, 267, 290
occupational justice 14, 150, 188, 196, **211**,
224, 256, 260
occupational science, application to 43, 64, 82,
100–101, 120, 142, 163, 180–181, 197,
224, 267–268, 282–283, 298–299,
312–313
occupational therapy, application to 44, 64,
82–83, 101, 120, 142, 163–164, 181, 198,
225–226, 268, 283, 298, 313
online 3, 12, 21–23, 26, 74–75, 94, 216, 242,
277, 289–294, 296–300, 305, 327
ontology 14–16, 34, 53, 70, 90, 94, 107, 128,
150, 162, 189, 209–210, 231, 255–256,
273, 277, 292, 308

paradigm 6–7, 14–16, **45**, 53, **89**, 108, 110,
150, 181, 189, 196, **199**, 203, 209–210,
224, 231, 255, 291, 307
participant(s) 4, 16–23, 25, *42*, **45**, 53, 55–58,
60–61, 63, 69–81, 83, 90–91, 93–102,
111–113, 115, 118–119, 121, 128–145,
149–165, 180, 187–189, 193–194, 197,
199, 200, 208–219, 221–224, 226,
232–245, 247, 254, 257–260, 265–267,
273–274, 278, 280–282, 284, 290–291,
293–294, 296–297, 300, 304, 311,
318–321, 323–327, 329
participatory action research 8–9, 187–203;
and action research 4, 252, 255
partnership 20, 69–70, 100, 119–120, 153,
244–245, 252, 255, 258, 261, 265, 267;
and industry partner 54–55; partnering 72,
83, 154, 156, 236–237, 256, 259, 266;
see also co-researchers
peer debriefing 25, 62–63, 261, 296, 310
phenomenology 7, 17, 53, 88–103, 319–320
philosophy 9, 53, 72, 88–89, 92, 100, 110,
127–128, 226, 267
photo elicitation 132, 193, 230
photovoice 8, 193, 230–247, 260
positionality 19, 21, 26, 32, 41, 81, 151,
161–162, 194, 219, 230, 257, 261, 298,
322–324, 327
positivism 15, 291; and positivist 14, 68, 80,
88, **89**, 150, 169, 183, 209–210, 217, 256,
276, 309, 318, 328; post-positivist **89**,
107–108, 224, 307
power 8–9, 14, 20–21, 33, 35, 38–39, 42–44,
46, 119, 150, 155, 157, 163, 170–172,
175, 180, 182, 188–189, 194, 196, 200,
209, 226, 230, 232, 236, 244, 247, 254,
257, 261, 307, 310
pragmatism 8, 108, 128, 144

qualitative descriptive 4, 7, 52–66, 69, 81, 307, 320
qualitative evidence synthesis 272–284

recruitment 36, 55–56, 72–73, 93–94, 100, 112, 130, 153–155, 190–193, 214–216, 236–238, 258–260, 292–293
reflective thematic analysis 58, 262, 310
reflexivity 9, 18–21, 23, 35, 40–41, 44, 77, 84, 151, 161–162, 179–180, 182–183, 187, 190–191, 194, 197, **200**, 209, 231–232, 259, 261, 264, 277, 280, 296, 310, 319, 322–324, 327
research question(s) 1, 15, 21, 23, 34–36, 54, 65, 71–72, 91, 99–100, 109–110, 112, 114, 118–119, 130, 152, 173–174, 190, 213, 216, 221, 236, 244, 258, 292, 294, 308, 320; and review question 274
rigor 9, 13, 18, 21, 37, 39, 41, 55, 62–63, 80–82, 99–100, 107, 118–119, 139–141, 161–162, 164, 178–179, 196–197, 223–224, 242–245, 264, 276, 279–280, 293, 296–198, 310–311, 319, 322, 326–327

sampling 36, 55–56, 72–73, 93–94, 130, 153–155, 190–193, 214–216, 292–293; and maximum variation 55, 73, 130, 276; purposive 55, 72–73, 93, 112, 259, 273, 276, 293; representative 55, 236, 266; snowball 36, 94, 259; theoretical 73–75, 81, 276, 320
saturation 56, 74, 276, 280, 320
social constructivism 17; and social constructivist 65
social media 8, 21–22, 75, 94, 173, 180, 223, 239, 297, 306, 311, 313, 327
software 62, 80–81, 158, 239, 281, 295, 306
Strauss 17, 68, 73, 79–80
symbolic interactionism 17–18, 70

thematic analysis 39, 59, 62, 64, 195, 267, 306–307; *see also* reflective thematic analysis
triangulation 76, 81, 118, 272, 310, 322
transcription 58, 63, 94, 143, 243; and transcript 60–61, 63, 74, 76, 78–79, 96, 115, 133–134, 136–137, 139, 157–158, 160, 195, 222, 296, 309

visual arts 8, 131, 208–226, 230

Printed in the United States
by Baker & Taylor Publisher Services